Perioperative Care in Cardiac Anesthesia and Surgery

Perioperative Care in Cardiac Anesthesia and Surgery

EDITED BY

DAVY C. H. CHENG, MD, MSc, FRCPC

Professor and Chair
Department of Anesthesia & Perioperative Medicine
University of Western Ontario

Chief
Department of Anesthesia & Perioperative Medicine
London Health Sciences Centre and
St. Joseph's Health Care

Medical Director
Cardiac Surgery Recovery Unit
London Health Sciences Centre
London, Ontario, Canada

TIRONE E. DAVID, MD, FRCSC

Professor
Department of Surgery
University of Toronto

Head
Division of Cardiovascular Surgery
The Peter Munk Cardiac Centre
Toronto General Hospital
Toronto, Ontario, Canada

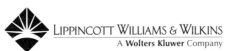

LIPPINCOTT WILLIAMS & WILKINS
A **Wolters Kluwer** Company
Philadelphia • Baltimore • New York • London
Buenos Aires • Hong Kong • Sydney • Tokyo

Acquisitions Editor: Brian Brown
Developmental Editor: Louise Bierig
Project Manager: Dave Murphy
Managing Editor: Franny Murphy
Senior Manufacturing Manager: Ben Rivera
Marketing Manager: Angela Panetta
Design Coordinator: Terry Mallon
Production Services: Laserwords Private Limited
Printer: Edwards Brothers

© 2006 by Lippincott Williams & Wilkins
530 Walnut Street
Philadelphia, PA 19106

Cover: Courtesy of the University of Pennsylvania Art Collection, Philadelphia, Pennsylvania

Printed in the United States

Library of Congress Cataloging-in-Publication Data
Perioperative care in cardiac anesthesia and surgery / edited by Davy C. H. Cheng, Tirone E. David.— 1st ed.
   p. ; cm.
   Includes bibliographical references and index.
   ISBN 0-7817-5774-6
   1. Heart—Surgery—Patients—Medical care—Handbooks, manuals, etc. 2. Therapeutics, Surgical—Handbooks, manuals, etc. 3. Operating room nursing—Handbooks, manuals, etc. 4. Postoperative care—Handbooks, manuals, etc. I. Cheng, Davy C. H. II. David, Tirone E. III. Title.
   [DNLM: 1. Coronary Disease—surgery—Handbooks. 2. Perioperative Care—methods—Handbooks. 3. Anesthesia—methods—Handbooks. 4. Cardiac Surgical Procedures—methods—Handbooks. WG 39 P445 2005]
   RD598.P45 2005
   617.4'12—dc22

                                    2005023363

To our Residents, Fellows, and Students

CONTENTS

SECTION III: SURGICAL TECHNIQUE AND POSTOPERATIVE CONSIDERATION *193*

SECTION IV: CARDIAC SURGICAL RECOVERY UNIT *339*

CONTRIBUTORS

Peter Allen, CPC, CCP
Clinical Partner
Cardiovascular Perfusion Program
Michener Institute for Applied
    Health Science

Chief Perfusionist
Perioperative Services
St. Michaels Hospital
Toronto, Ontario, Canada

Neal H. Badner, MD, FRCPC
Associate Professor
Department of Anesthesia & Perioperative
    Medicine
University of Western Ontario

Site Chief
Department of Anesthesia & Perioperative
    Medicine, Victoria Hospital
London Health Sciences Centre
London, Ontario, Canada

Daniel Bainbridge, MD, FRCPC
Assistant Professor
Department of Anesthesia & Perioperative
    Medicine
University of Western Ontario

Director
Perioperative Transesophageal
    Echocardiography
Department of Anesthesia & Perioperative
    Medicine
London Health Sciences Centre
London, Ontario, Canada

Atilio Barbeito, MD
Cardiothoracic Anesthesiology and Critical
    Care Fellow
Department of Anesthesiology
Duke University Medical Center
Durham, North Carolina

Michael A. Borger, MD, PhD
Assistant Professor
Department of Surgery
University of Toronto

Staff Surgeon
Division of Cardiovascular Surgery
The Peter Munk Cardiac Centre
Toronto General Hospital
Toronto, Ontario, Canada

W. Douglas Boyd, MD
Associate Professor
Department of Surgery
University of South Florida College
    of Medicine
Tampa, Florida

Chief
Division of Cardiothoracic Sugery
Director, Minimally Invasive and Robotic
    Surgery
Cleveland Clinic Florida
Weston, Florida

Stephanie J. Brister, MD
Associate Professor
Department of Surgery
University of Toronto

Staff Surgeon
Division of Cardiovascular Surgery
The Peter Munk Cardiac Centre
Toronto General Hospital
Toronto, Ontario, Canada

Ronald J. Butler, MD, MSc, FRCPC
Associate Professor
Department of Anesthesia & Perioperative
    Medicine
University of Western Ontario

Site Chief
Intensive Care Unit-University Hospital
London Health Sciences Centre
London, Ontario, Canada

Douglas A. Cameron, MD, FRCPC
Assistant Professor
Department of Medicine
University of Toronto

Cardiologist/Electrophysiologist
Department of Medicine
Toronto General Hospital
Toronto, Ontario, Canada

Lois K. Champion, MD, FRCPC
Associate Professor
Department of Anesthesia & Perioperative
  Medicine
University of Western Ontario
Consultant Intensivist
London Health Sciences Centre
London, Ontario, Canada

Davy C. H. Cheng, MD, MSc, FRCPC
Professor and Chair
Department of Anesthesia & Perioperative
  Medicine
University of Western Ontario

Chief
Department of Anesthesia & Perioperative
  Medicine
London Health Sciences Centre and
  St. Joseph's Health Care

Medical Director
Cardiac Surgery Recovery Unit
London Health Sciences Centre
London, Ontario, Canada

Tirone E. David, MD, FRCSC
Professor
Department of Surgery
University of Toronto

Head
Division of Cardiovascular Surgery
The Peter Munk Cardiac Centre
Toronto General Hospital
Toronto, Ontario, Canada

Achal K. Dhir, MBBS, DA, FRCA
Assistant Professor
Department of Anesthesia & Perioperative
  Medicine
University of Western Ontario

Consultant Anesthesiologist
Department of Anesthesia & Perioperative
  Medicine
London Health Sciences Centre
London, Ontario, Canada

George N. Djaiani, MD, FRCA
Assistant Professor
Department of Anesthesia
University of Toronto

Staff Anesthesiologist
Cardiac Anesthesia and Intensive Care
Department of Anesthesia
Toronto General Hospital
Toronto, Ontario, Canada

Wojciech Dobkowski, MD, FRCPC
Associate Professor
Department of Anesthesia & Perioperative
  Medicine
University of Western Ontario

Site Chief
Department of Anesthesia & Perioperative
  Medicine, University Hospital
London Health Sciences Centre
London, Ontario, Canada

Shafie Fazel, MD, MSc
Research Fellow
Department of Surgery
University of Toronto

Resident Physician
Division of Cardiac Surgery
Toronto General Hospital
Toronto, Ontario, Canada

Christopher M. Feindel, MD, MHCM, FRCSC
Professor
Department of Surgery
University of Toronto

Medical Director
The Peter Munk Cardiac Centre
Toronto General Hospital
Toronto, Ontario, Canada

Stefan Fischer, MD, MSc
Fellow
Division of Thoracic Surgery
Toronto General Hospital
Toronto, Ontario, Canada

Thomas L. Higgins, MD, MBA
Associate Professor
Departments of Medicine and Anesthesiology
Baystate Medical Center/Tufts University
    School of Medicine

Director
Adult Intensive Care Service
Departments of Medicine, Surgery, and
    Anesthesiology
Baystate Medical Center
Springfield, Massachusetts

Charles W. Hogue, Jr., MD
Associate Professor
Department of Anesthesiology
Washington University School of Medicine
St. Louis, Missouri

Helen M. K. Holtby, MBBS, FRCPC
Assistant Professor
Department of Anesthesia
University of Toronto

Director
Cardiac Anesthesia
Hospital for Sick Children
Toronto, Ontario, Canada

Ivan Iglesias, MD
Assistant Professor
Department of Anesthesia & Perioperative
    Medicine
University of Western Ontario

Consultant Anesthesiologist
Department of Anesthesia & Perioperative
    Medicine
London Health Sciences Centre
London, Ontario, Canada

Keyvan Karkouti, MD, MSc, FRCPC
Assistant Professor
Departments of Anesthesia
    & Health Policy, Management,
    and Evaluation
University of Toronto

Staff Anesthesiologist
Department of Anesthesia
Toronto General Hospital
Toronto, Ontario, Canada,

Jacek M. Karski, MD
Associate Professor
Department of Anesthesia
University of Toronto

Director
Cardiac Anesthesia and Intensive Care
Department of Anesthesia
Toronto General Hospital
Toronto, Ontario, Canada

Rita Katznelson, MD
Assistant Professor
Department of Anesthesia
University of Toronto

Staff Anesthesiologist
Department of Anesthesia
Toronto General Hospital
Toronto, Ontario, Canada

Shaf Keshavjee, MD, MSc, FRCSC, FACS
Professor and Chair
Division of Thoracic Surgery
Department of Surgery
University of Toronto

Director
Toronto Lung Transplant Program
Head
Division of Thoracic Surgery
Toronto General Hospital
Toronto, Ontario, Canada

Bob Kiaii, MD, FRCSC
Assistant Professor
Department of Surgery
University of Western Ontario

Director
Minimally Invasive and Robotic Cardiac
    Surgery
Department of Surgery
London Health Sciences Centre
London, Ontario, Canada

Igor E. Konstantinov, MD, PhD
Research Fellow
Department of Surgery
University of Toronto

Clinical Fellow
Division of Cardiovascular Surgery
Hospital for Sick Children
Toronto, Ontario, Canada

Patrick C. Lee, MD, FACS
Associate Professor
Department of Surgery
Tufts University School of Medicine

Chief
Trauma & Emergency Surgical Services
Department of Surgery
Baystate Health System
Springfield, Massachusetts

Susan C. M. Lenkei-Kerwin, MD, FRCPC,
    FACP, FACC, FCCP
Professor
Department of Medicine
University of Toronto

Senior Cardiology Consultant
Division of Cardiology
Department of Medicine
Toronto General Hospital
Toronto, Ontario, Canada

Janet Martin, BScPhm, RPh, PharmD
Lecturer
Department of Physiology
    & Pharmacology
University of Western Ontario

Coordinator
Pharmacy Services
London Health Sciences Centre
London, Ontario, Canada

R. Scott McClure, MD
Resident Physician
Department of Surgery
University of Western Ontario
London, Ontario, Canada

Karen McRae, MDCM, FRCP
Assistant Professor
Department of Anesthesia
University of Toronto

Co-Director
Anesthesia for Thoracic Surgery and Lung
    Transplantation
Department of Anesthesia
Toronto General Hospital
Toronto, Ontario, Canada

Alan H. Menkis, MD, FRCSC
Professor & Chair
Department of Cardiac Surgery
University of Manitoba

Medical Director
Department of Cardiac Sciences Program
St. Boniface General Hospital
Winnipeg, Manitoba, Canada

Lynda L. Mickleborough, MD, FRCSC
Professor Emeritus
Department of Surgery
University of Toronto
Toronto, Ontario, Canada

John M. Murkin, MD, FRCPC
Professor
Department of Anesthesia & Perioperative
    Medicine
University of Western Ontario

Director
Cardiac Anesthesiology
Department of Anesthesia & Perioperative
    Medicine
London Health Sciences Centre
London, Ontario, Canada

Patricia Murphy, BSc, MD, FRCPC
Associate Professor
Department of Anesthesia
University of Toronto

Clinical Director
Cardiac Anesthesia
Department of Anesthesia
Toronto General Hospital
Toronto, Ontario, Canada

Richard J. Novick, MD, MSc, FRCSC, FACS
Professor
Department of Surgery
University of Western Ontario

Chief/Chair
Division of Cardiac Surgery
London Health Sciences Centre
London, Ontario, Canada

Christopher A. Palin, MA, MBBS, FRCA
Specialist Registrar
Department of Anesthesia
Royal Brompton Hospital
London, United Kingdom

Jonathan Prychitko, MD
Anesthesia Resident
Department of Anesthesia &
    Perioperative Medicine
University of Western Ontario
London, Ontario, Canada

Fiona E. Ralley, BSc, MBChB, FFA
Professor
Department of Anesthesia & Perioperative
    Medicine
University of Western Ontario

Director
Perioperative Blood Conservation Program
Consultant Anesthesiologist
Department of Anesthesia & Perioperative
    Medicine
London Health Science Centre
London, Ontario, Canada

Vivek Rao, MD, PhD
Associate Professor
Alfredo and Teresa DeGasperis Chair in Heart
    Failure Surgery
Department of Surgery
University of Toronto.

Director
Cardiac Transplantation
Division of Carcliovascular Surgery
The Peter Munk Cardiac Centre
Toronto General Hospital
Toronto, Ontario, Canada

Steve K. Singh, MD
Resident
Department of Surgery
University of Toronto
Toronto, Ontario, Canada

Peter Slinger, MD, FRCPC
Professor
Department of Anesthesia
University of Toronto

Staff Anesthesiologist
Department of Anesthesia
Toronto General Hospital
Toronto, Ontario, Canada

Bruce D. Spiess, MD, FAHA
Vice Chair of Anesthesiology
Director of VCURES
Director of Research
Department of Anesthesiology
Virginia Commonwealth University
    Medical Center
Richmond, Virginia

**Mark Stafford-Smith, MD,
  CM, FRCPC**
Associate Professor
Department of Anesthesiology
Duke University and Duke University
    Medical Center
Durham, North Carolina

Ravi Taneja, MBBS, MD, FFARCSI, FRCA
Assistant Professor
Departments of Anesthesia & Perioperative
    Medicine
University of Western Ontario

Consultant Anesthesiologist
    and Intensivist
Department of Anesthesia & Perioperative
    Medicine
Cardiac Surgery Recovery Unit
London Health Sciences Centre
London, Ontario, Canada

Glen S. Van Arsdell, MD
Associate Professor
Department of Surgery
University of Toronto

Head
Division of Cardiovascular Surgery
Hospital for Sick Children
Toronto, Ontario, Canada

Annette Vegas, MD, FRCPC
Assistant Professor
Department of Anesthesia
University of Toronto

Staff Anesthesiologist
Department of Anesthesia
Toronto General Hospital
Toronto, Ontario, Canada

Richard D. Weisel, MD, FRCSC
Professor and Chairman
Division of Cardiac Surgery
Department of Surgery
University of Toronto

Staff Surgeon and Director
Toronto General Research Institute
Division of Cardiovascular Surgery
The Peter Munk Cardiac Centre
Toronto General Hospital
Toronto, Ontario, Canada

William G. Williams, MD
Professor
Department of Surgery
University of Toronto

Staff Surgeon
Division of Cardiac Surgery
Department of Surgery
Hospital for Sick Children
Toronto, Ontario, Canada

Terrence M. Yau, MD, MSc
Associate Professor
Department of Surgery
University of Toronto

Director of Research
Division of Cardiovascular Surgery
Toronto General Hospital
Toronto, Ontario, Canada

Raymond Yee, BMDSc, MD
Professor
Department of Medicine
University of Western Ontario

Director
Arrhythmia Service
Department of Cardiology
London Health Sciences Centre
London, Ontario, Canada

PREFACE

Cardiac anesthesia and surgery have evolved over the last five decades since the successful use of cardiopulmonary bypass circuit in 1953. There has been tremendous advancement in the practice of cardiac surgery from deep hypothermia to normothermic or tepid cardiopulmonary bypass regulation, cardioplegia solution, and oxygenators, and so on. Advancement in surgical technique and technology allows progress and ensures success in minimally invasive cardiac surgeries such as off-pump coronary artery bypass, robotic-assisted cardiac surgery, valvular surgery, congenital heart disease, and transplantation. Coupled with the advancement of cardiac surgery, cardiac anesthesia has progressed from a high-dose narcotic to a balanced narcotic–inhalational anesthesia using safer and effective anesthetic agents, regional anesthesia, and standard practice of fast-track recovery. There are continuing advancements in perioperative monitoring of myocardial (e.g., transesophageal echocardiography, epiaortic scan) and cerebral (e.g., electroencephalogram, oxygen saturation) conditions, and coagulation.

The modern practice of cardiac anesthesia and surgery has been characterized by cost containment, accountability, and evidence-based medical care. We have responded to these obligations by surgery with the same-day admission program, early tracheal extubation, improved operative techniques, and facilitated rehabilitation, all of which have reduced the intensive care stay and hospital stay.

This practical handbook describes the perioperative management of adult patients who undergo cardiac surgery. Although numerous authors have contributed to the current evidence of perioperative care, each chapter has been carefully edited to reflect the collective view of our cardiac care teams. The purpose of this handbook is to provide a succinct, problem-oriented source of practical information, on the basis of latest clinical and research experience, about patients undergoing cardiac surgery. The appendices section outlines the medical orders, protocols, and guidelines in the management of these patients. These appendices that serve as template examples are currently used in the cardiac surgical programs at Toronto General Hospital and London Health Sciences Centre. This handbook was designed for consultants and trainees in cardiac anesthesia and cardiac surgery, critical care nurses, perfusionist, and other allied health care personnel who are involved in the management of patients undergoing heart surgery.

Davy C. H. Cheng, MD
Tirone E. David, MD

ACKNOWLEDGMENTS

The editors wish to express their gratitude to the individual authors, who have contributed to the education of the trainees and the perioperative care of the cardiac surgical patients. They would also like to thank the cardiac program teams at Toronto General Hospital (TGH) and London Health Sciences Centre (LHSC), who are devoted to the continuous advancement of the clinical and research knowledge in cardiac anesthesia, surgery, and recovery care. They are grateful to numerous people who have helped in the development and publication of this handbook: Michelle LaPlante and Fran Murphy for their editorial assistance at Lippincott Williams & Wilkins; Linda Jussaume, CVICU Manager TGH; Pat Merrifield, critical care manager and Mary Kroh, Cardiac Surgery Recovery Unit coordinator at LHSC, for their input of the postoperative guidelines and protocols; and Dr. Janet Martin from LHSC, for her contribution to the cardiac pharmacology guidelines. Finally, Dr. Cheng would like to thank his administrative assistant, Jeanette Mikulic, who worked diligently to coordinate amongst Dr. Tirone David's office, the authors, and the publisher to ensure that the multitude of chapters were complete for publication.

Davy C. H. Cheng, MD
Tirone E. David, MD

Abbreviations

2,3-DPG	2,3-Diphosphoglyceraldehyde
AAA	Abdominal aortic aneurysm
ABG	Arterial blood gases
ACAS	Asymptomatic Carotid Atherosclerosis Study
ACB	Aortocoronary bypass
ACC	American College of Cardiology
ACE	Angiotensin-converting enzyme
ACEI	Angiotensin-converting enzyme inhibitors
ACLS	Advanced cardiac life support
ACST	Asymptomatic Carotid Surgery Trial
ACT	Activated clotting time
ACTH	Adrenocorticotropic hormone
ADH	Antidiuretic hormone
ADP	Adenosine diphosphate
AF	Atrial fibrillation
AHA	American Heart Association
AI	Aortic insufficiency
AMVL	Anterior mitral valve leaflet
ANP	Atrial natriuretic peptide
AoEDP	Aortic end diastolic pressure
APS	Acute physiology score
AR	Aortic regurgitation
ARDS	Acute respiratory distress syndrome
ARF	Acute renal failure
AS	Aortic stenosis
ASA	Acetylsalicylic acid
ASD	Atrial septal defect
ASE	American Society of Echocardiography
AT	Antithrombin
AT III	Antithrombin III
ATN	Acute tubular necrosis
ATP	Adenosine triphosphate
AV	Atrioventricular
AVR	Aortic valve replacement
BAV	Bicuspid aortic valve
BCPS	Bidirectional cavopulmonary shunt
BHACAS	Beating Heart Against Cardioplegic Arrest Studies
BIS	Bispectral Index
b.i.d.	Twice a day
BiVAD	Biventricular assist device
BLT	Bilateral lung transplant
BNP	B-type natriuretic peptide
BP	Blood pressure

BSA	Body surface area
BT	Blalock-Taussig
BUN	Blood urea nitrogen
BVS	Biventricular support
CABG	Coronary artery bypass grafting
CAD	Coronary artery disease
cAMP	Cyclic adenosine monophosphate
CAPD	Continuous abdominal peritoneal dialysis
CASH	Cardiac Arrest Study Hamburg
CAVHD	Continuous arterial-venous hemodialysis
CBC	Complete blood count
CBF	Cerebral blood flow
CCU	Coronary care unit
CEA	Carotid endarterectomy
cGMP	Cyclic guanine monophosphate
CHD	Congenital heart disease
CHF	Congestive heart failure
CI	Cardiac index
CIDS	Canadian Implantable Defibrillator Study
CK	Creatine kinase
CK-MB	Creatine kinase isoenzyme fraction
CMV	Cytomegalovirus
CNS	Central nervous system
CO	Cardiac output
COPD	Chronic obstructive pulmonary disease
COX	Cyclooxygenase
CPAP	Continuous positive airway pressure
CPB	Cardiopulmonary bypass
CPR	Cardiopulmonary resuscitation
CRT	Cardiac resynchronization therapy
CSF	Cerebral spinal fluid
CSRU	Cardiac surgery recovery unit
CT	Computed tomography
CTOPP	Canadian Trial of Physiologic Pacing
CUSUM	Cumulative sum
CVA	Cerebral vascular accident
CVICU	Cardiovascular intensive care unit
CVP	Central venous pressure
CVVHD	Continuous venous–venous hemodialysis
CXR	Chest x-ray
DC	Direct current
DDAVP	Desamino-D-arginine-vasopressin
DFT	Defibrillator thresholds
DHCA	Deep hypothermia and circulatory arrest
DIC	Disseminated intravascular coagulation

DKA	Diabetic ketoacidosis
DLCO	Diffusing capacity of lung for carbon monoxide coefficient
DLT	Double lumen tube
DNA	Deoxyribonucleic acid
DPG	Diphosphoglycerate
DVT	Deep vein thrombosis
ECASA	Enteric-coated aspirin
ECG	Electrocardiogram
ECMO	Extracorporeal membrane oxygenation
EDA	End-diastolic cross-sectional area
EDP	End diastolic pressure
EEA	Early extubation anesthesia
EEG	Electroencephalograph
EF	Ejection fraction
ELISA	Enzyme-linked immunosorbent assay
EMI	Electromagnetic interference
ESHF	End-stage heart failure
ETT	Endotracheal tube
ETVC	Endotracheal ventilation catheter
FAC	Fractional area change
FDA	Food and Drug Administration
FDG	Fluoro-deoxy-glucose
FEV	Forced expiratory volume
FEVI	Forced expiratory volume in one second
FFP	Fresh frozen plasma
FTCA	Fast-track cardiac anesthesia
FTT	Failure to thrive
GFR	Glomerular filtration rate
GI	Gastrointestinal
HATT	Heparin-associated thrombocytopenia and thrombosis
Hb	Hemoglobin
HCA	Hypothermic circulatory arrest
HCT	Hematocrit
HDR	Heparin dose response
HIPA	Heparin-induced platelet activation
HIT	Heparin-induced thrombocytopenia
HIV	Human immunodeficiency virus
HLA	Human leukocyte antigen
HLHS	Hypoplastic left heart syndrome
HOCM	Hypertrophic obstructive cardiomyopathy
HPT	Heparin protamine titration
HR	Heart rate
HTN	Hypertension
IABP	Intraaortic balloon pump
ICD	Implantable cardioversion defibrillators

ICU	Intensive care unit
ID	Infectious disease
IDDM	Insulin-dependent diabetes mellitus
IHD	Ischemic heart disease
IHSS	Idiopathic hypertrophic subaortic stenosis
IMA	Internal mammary artery
INR	International normalized ratio
IPF	Idiopathic pulmonary fibrosis
IPPV	Intermittent positive pressure ventilation
ISHLT	International Society of Heart and Lung Transplantation
IT	Intrathecal
ITA	Internal thoracic artery
IVC	Inferior vena cava
IVS	Interventricular septum
KIU	Kallikrein inhibitor units
LAD	Left anterior descending
LAP	Left arterial pressure
LBBB	Left bundle branch block
LED	Light-emitting diode
LITA	Left internal thoracic artery
LM	Left main
LMWH	Low-molecular-weight heparin
LOS	Length of stay
LPD	Low potassium dextran
LSVC	Left superior vena cava
LVAD	Left ventricular assistive device
LVEDP	Left ventricle end diastolic pressure
LVEDV	Left ventricle end diastolic volume
LVEF	Left ventricular ejection fraction
LVF	Left ventricular function
LVH	Left ventricle hypertrophy
LVOT	Left ventricular outflow track
LVR	Lung volume reduction
MADIT	Multicenter Automatic Defibrillator Implantation Trial
MAO	Monamine oxidase
MAP	Mean arterial pressure
MH	Malignant hyperthermia
MI	Myocardial infarction
MIDCAB	Minimally invasive direct coronary artery bypass
MIRAMVR	Minimally invasive robotically assisted mitral valve repair
MMS	Mini-Mental State
MOST	Mode Selection Trial
MPS	Myocardial protection system
MR	Mitral regurgitation
MRA	Magnetic resonance angiography

MRI	Magnetic resonance imaging
MRSA	Methicillin-resistant Staphylococcus aureus
MS	Mitral stenosis
MVP	Mitral valve prolapse
MVR	Mitral valve replacement
MVV	Maximal voluntary ventilation
NAPA	n-acetyl procainamide
NAT	Nucleic acid testing
NG	Nasogastric
NIDDM	Non–insulin-dependent diabetes mellitus
NIF	Negative inspiratory force
NIRS	Near infrared spectroscopy
NO	Nitric oxide
NSAID	Nonsteroidal anti-inflammatory drug
NTG	Nitroglycerin
NYHA	New York Heart Association
OLV	One lung ventilation
OPCAB	Off-pump coronary arterial bypass
OR	Operating room
PA	Pulmonary artery
PAC	Pulmonary artery catheter
Pap	Papanicolaou
PAP	Pulmonary artery pressure
PCA	Patient controlled analgesia
PCI	Percutaneous coronary intervention
PCWP	Pulmonary capillary wedge pressure
PD	Peritoneal dialysis
PDA	Patent ductus arteriosis
PDE	Phosphodiesterase
PE	Pulmonary embolism
PEEP	Positive end-expiratory pressure
PET	Positron emission tomography
PFO	Patent foramen ovale
PI	Pulmonary insufficiency
PIV	Posterior interventricular
PLV	Partial left ventriculectomy
POD	Postoperative day
PPM	Permanent pacemaker
PRBC	Packed red blood cell
PS	Pulmonary stenosis
PSV	Pressure support ventilation
PT	Prothrombin time
PTCA	Percutaneous transluminal coronary angioplasty
PTT	Partial thromboplastin time
PVB	Paravertebral block

PVC	Premature ventricular contraction
PVR	Pulmonary vascular resistance
RA	Right atrium
RAP	Right arterial pressure
RAVECAB	Robotically assisted video-enhanced coronary artery bypass
RBBB	Right bundle branch block
RBC	Red blood cells
RCA	Right coronary artery
RCP	Retrograde cerebral perfusion
RGEA	Right gastroepiploic artery
RITA	Right internal thoracic artery
RPA	Right pulmonary artery
RPM	Revolutions per minute
RRT	Renal replacement therapy
RT	Respiratory therapist
RV	Residual ventricle
RVAD	Right ventricle assist device
RVF	Right ventricular failure
RVH	Right ventricular hypertrophy
RVOT	Right ventricular outflow tract
SACP	Selective antegrade cerebral perfusion
SAM	Systolic anterior motion
SARS	Severe acute respiratory syndrome
SBP	Systolic blood pressure
SCA	Society of Cardiovascular Anesthesiology
SDA	Same day admission
SIADH	Syndrome of inappropriate antidiuretic hormone secretion
SIRS	Systemic inflammatory responses syndrome
SLT	Single lung transplant?
SNP	Sodium nitroprusside
STICH	Surgical Therapy for Ischemic Congestive Heart
STS	Society of Thoracic Surgeons
SVC	Superior vena cava
SVGs	Saphenous vein grafts
SVR	Systemic vascular resistance
SVT	Supraventricular tachycardia
SWMA	Segmental wall motion abnormalities
TA	Tranexamic acid
TAA	Thoracic aortic aneurysm
TBW	Total body water
TCCCA	Toronto Congenital Cardiac Center for Adults
TCD	Transcranial Doppler
TECAB	Totally endoscopic coronary artery bypass
TEE	Transesophageal echocardiography
TEF	Transesophageal fistula

TEG	Thromboelastography
TG	Transgastric
TGA	Transposition of the great arteries
TGH	Toronto General Hospital
TIA	Transient ischemic attack
TIF	Tracheo-innominate fistula
TIVA	Total intravenous anesthesia
TLC	Total lung capacity
TMR	Transmyocardial revascularization
TNF	Tumor necrosis factor
TOF	Tetralogy of Fallot
TPN	Total parenteral nutrition
TR	Tricuspid regurgitation
TRALI	Transfusion-related acute lung injury
TTE	Transthoracic echocardiography
TV	Tidal volume
UKPACE	United Kingdom Pacing and Cardiovascular Events
PTT	Partial Thromboplastin time
VAS	Visual analog score
VC	Vital capacity
VF	Ventricular fibrillation
VSD	Ventricular septal defect
VT	Ventricular tachycardia
vWF	von Willebrand factor
WBC	White blood cell

Introduction

Chapter 1

Prognostic Risks and Preoperative Assessment

Davy C. H. Cheng and Tirone E. David

Cardiac surgery is one of the most expensive surgical procedures. In this era of cost containment and physician report cards, we are increasingly held accountable for patients' outcomes in terms of mortality, morbidity, quality of life, length of stay (LOS), and costs of care.

According to the national database (2003) of the Society of Thoracic Surgeons (STS), the risk-adjusted mortality is 2% in isolated coronary artery bypass graft (CABG), 3% in aortic valve replacement (AVR), 5.4% in AVR + CABG, 5% in mitral valve replacement (MVR), and 12% in MVR + CABG. The mean post-procedure LOS is 7 days (the median is 5.2 days) for isolated CABG, 8.2 days for AVR, 9.8 days for AVR + CABG, 10.2 days for MVR, and 13 days for MVR + CABG.

Results during the decade from 1990 through 1999 demonstrate a progressive increase in preoperative risk and a decline in both observed mortality and the observed to expected mortality ratio. These results are likely a reflection of the ongoing advances in perioperative cardiac surgical care in spite of an increasing proportion of high-risk patients, particularly patients >75 years.

PROGNOSTIC RISKS AND COMPLICATIONS

Perioperative morbidity and mortality of patients who have undergone cardiac surgery are strongly influenced by their preoperative severity of illness and postoperative complications. These risk factors include age, sex, left ventricular function, type of surgery, urgency of surgery, repeat surgery, aortic stenosis, unstable angina, congestive heart failure (CHF), peripheral vascular disease, cerebral vascular disease, left ventricular aneurysm, left main coronary artery disease, renal insufficiency/failure, and diabetes (see Tables 1-1 and 1-2).

▶ **TABLE 1-1** **Summary of Isolated Coronary Artery Bypass Grating Outcomes by Risk Category for Fiscal Year 2001**

Risk Category	In-hospital Mortality (n = 7,840)		Mean Postoperative LOS (n = 7,620)		30-day Mortality (n = 7,595)	
	%	Rate	%	Days	%	Rate
Low	32.7	0.4	33.5	6.1	30.0	0.6
Medium	33.8	0.6	34.3	6.9	34.5	0.9
High	33.5	4.5	32.2	8.4	35.5	4.0

LOS, length of stay.
Reprinted with permission from Guru V, Gong Y, Rothwell D, et al. Report on cardiac surgery in Ontario: fiscal years 2000 & 2001. *Cardiac Surgery Report Card (July 2004).* Available at: http://www.ccn.on.ca/.

It has been shown that resource use, which is measured as LOS and cost of care, is strongly influenced by severity of illness, postoperative complications, and efficiency of nursing unit, and that there are large variations in resource use among different institutions.

The strongest predictors of cost are hospital LOS, intensive care unit (ICU) LOS, operating room time, and patient age. The most important predictors of high charges

▶ **TABLE 1-2** **Common Complications Following Heart Surgery**

Complication	Incidence	Risk Factors
Stroke	2%–4%	Age Previous stroke/TIA PVD Diabetes Unstable angina
Delirium	8%–15%	Age Previous stroke Duration of surgery Duration of aortic cross clamp Atrial fibrillation Blood transfusion
Atrial fibrillation	Up to 35%	Age Male gender Previous atrial fibrillation Mitral valve surgery Previous CHF
Renal failure	1%	Low postoperative CO Repeat cardiac surgery Valve surgery Age Diabetes

TIA, transient ischemic attack; PVD, peripheral vascular disease; CHF, congestive heart failure; CO, cardiac output.

are postoperative complications including sternal infection, respiratory failure, left ventricular failure, and death.

RISK ASSESSMENT MODELS

There are many risk assessment models for cardiac surgery published in the literature including the Parsonnet score, Higgins score, Tu score, French score, Bayes score, CARE (Cardiac Anesthesia Risk Evaluation) score, and EuroSCORE. All the scoring systems define preoperative variables associated with postoperative mortality either in hospital or at 30 days. Risk-scoring systems have allowed a greater appreciation of the factors that contribute to adverse events in cardiac surgery. Such systems have allowed for the comparison of different patient groups over time and between centers; they have also been used to adjust for direct comparisons of outcome and resource utilization between institutions. Unfortunately, the risk-scoring system has some inherent limitations that may lead to its inappropriate use, which could lead to erroneous conclusions. A primary drawback of scoring systems is the geographic variability that occurs between institutions, especially the ones that are geographically and/or politically distinct, which may not have the same risk factors for their cardiac surgery program (see Table 1-3).

The EuroSCORE has been widely used in risk assessment and in stratification for patients who have undergone cardiac surgery. The EuroSCORE is derived from three major risk-related factors: patient-related, cardiac-related, and operation-related factors. A EuroSCORE of 1 to 2, 3 to 5, and ≥6 defines the low-risk, medium-risk, and high-risk group, respectively.

The risk-adjusted prediction of outcome after cardiac surgery has been preferentially assessed by multifactorial risk indexes. These scores are obtained from multiple regression logistic analysis, which allows for identification of risk factors of morbidity, mortality, or both. Recently, a simple and reliable performance of CARE score was introduced to predict the duration of stay in the hospital, morbidity, and mortality after cardiac surgery. In contrast to multifactorial risk indexes, the CARE score is an intuitive risk, ranking similar to the American Society of Anesthesiologists (ASA) physician status classification. The scoring system was constructed on clinical judgment and three classic risk factors: comorbidity, surgical complexity, and operative priority. Although simple, the CARE score has a predictive performance similar to three popular multifactorial risk indexes (see Table 1-4).

PREOPERATIVE EVALUATION

The Preadmission Clinic

More than 70% of university hospital surgeries are performed on same-day admit (SDA) patients. Most cardiac programs are still striving to meet this level. This "one-time shopping" plan of preoperative evaluation must be done in a very predictable manner so that a surgery does not get cancelled on the decided date, and the plan must also ensure patient satisfaction and optimum medical outcomes.

Many health care personnel are involved with an SDA program: clerk, laboratory technicians, nurses, nurse practitioners, house staff, and physicians (medical, surgical,

▶ **TABLE 1-3** Multifactorial Risk Indexes for the Prediction of Outcome after Cardiac Surgery

Parsonnet Score		Tu Score		EuroSCORE	
Age (y)	Score	Age (y)	Score	Patient-related Factors Age >60 y	Score
70–74	7	65–74	2	Sex–Female	1
75–79	12	≥75	3	COPD	1
≥80	20			Extracardiac arteriopathy	2
Emergency surgery following heart cath[a]	10	Emergency within 24 h	4	Neurologic dysfunction	2
		Urgent	1	Re-do	3
LV function		LV function		Serum creatinine >200	2
EF 30%–49%	2	EF 35%–50%	1	μm/L	
EF <30%	4	EF 20%–34%	2	Active endocarditis	3
		EF <20%	3	Critical preoperative state (unstable)	3
Surgical characteristics		Surgical characteristics		Cardiac-related factors	
MVR or AVR	5	Single valve	2	Unstable angina	2
CABG+valve	2	Complex	3	LVEF 30%–50%	1
Reoperation 1st	5	Reoperation	2	Poor or LVEF <30	3
2nd	10			Recent MI (<90 d)	2
				Pulmonary hypertension	2
				Operation-related factors	
Female gender	1	Female gender	1		
Dialysis dependency	10			Emergency	2
Systolic PAP >60 mm Hg	8			Other than isolated CABG	2
Diabetes (any type)	3			Surgery on thoracic aorta	3
Morbid obesity	3			Postinfarct septal rupture	4
A-V gradient >120 mm Hg	7				
Perioperative IABP	2				
Ventricular aneurysm	5				
Hypertension	3				
Catastrophic states	10–50				
Rare circumstances	2–10				

COPD, chronic obstructive pulmonary disease; LV, left ventricle; EF, ejection fraction; MVR, mitral valve replacement; AVR, aortic valve replacement; PAP, Pulmonary Artery Pressure; CABG, coronary artery bypass graft; LVEF, left ventricle ejection fraction; MI, myocardial infarction; IABP, intra-aortic balloon pump.
[a]Emergency: surgery as soon as diagnosis is made and operating room is available.

and anesthesia). It has been proposed that anesthesiologists should be the "perioperative specialists" because of the extent and quality of their comprehensive approach to the patient who has undergone surgery.

Medical History and Physical Examination

The general inquiry should include the following symptoms of cardiac disease: chest pain, dyspnea, fatigue, hemoptysis, syncope, palpitation, peripheral edema, and cyanosis.

▶ TABLE 1-4 Cardiac Anesthesia Risk Evaluation Score

1. Patient with stable cardiac disease and no other medical problem. A noncomplex surgery is undertaken.
2. Patient with stable cardiac disease and one or more controlled medical problems. A noncomplex surgery is undertaken.
3. Patient with any uncontrolled medical problem or patient in whom a complex surgery is undertaken.
4. Patient with any uncontrolled medical problem and in whom a complex surgery is undertaken.
5. Patient with chronic or advanced cardiac disease for whom cardiac surgery is undertaken as a last hope to save or improve life.

The degree of physical disability that cardiac symptoms cause is expressed by the functional classification of the New York Heart Association:

Class I: No symptoms during ordinary physical activities.
Class II: No symptoms at rest; ordinary activities provoke symptoms.
Class III: No symptoms at rest; mild activities provoke symptoms.
Class IV: Symptoms at rest or during any activity.

The severity of angina pectoris is graded by the classification of the Canadian Cardiovascular Society:

Class I: Only very strenuous physical activity causes angina.
Class II: Moderate physical activity causes angina (e.g., walking more than two blocks on the level or climbing more than one flight of stairs at normal pace provokes pain).
Class III: Mild physical activity causes angina (e.g., walking one block on the level or one flight of stairs at normal pace provokes pain).
Class IV: Any physical activity causes pain.

Past History
- Previous operations such as thoracotomy, saphenous vein stripping/ligation, and peripheral vascular surgery including carotid endarterectomy.
- Allergies to drugs and other agents.
- Medications such as anticoagulants, antiarrhythmics, antiplatelet agents, angiotensin-converting enzyme (ACE) inhibitors, diuretics, and others.
- Review of recent medical consultations and the "old chart" wherever possible.

Review of Systems
- Central nervous system: Transient ischemic attacks or previous stroke requires a full neurologic workup.
- Respiratory system: If chronic obstructive lung disease is suspected, spirometry, pulse oximetry, and arterial blood gases should be obtained before surgery. Airway assessment about the likelihood of an easy tracheal intubation and the presence of

goiter or surgical scars should be noted. Documentation of dentures, caps, wires, bridges, and loose teeth should also be done.

- Endocrine system: Diabetes and its complications should be recorded in the chart.
- Hematologic system: All patients should be asked about bleeding disorders. In addition, patients of African origin should be checked for sickle cell trait.
- Renal system: Impaired renal function and renal dialysis increase the risk of perioperative complications. Renal transplant recipients seem to do well if renal function is normal, but the Renal Transplant Service should manage the medication and should follow up the patient perioperatively.
- Gastrointestinal system: Active peptic ulcer disease, active hepatitis, cirrhosis, and other gastrointestinal problems can seriously affect the outcome of cardiac surgery and must be evaluated preoperatively.
- Peripheral vascular system: The presence of venous and arterial disease should be noted. Aortic-iliac occlusive disease may prevent the insertion of an intra-aortic balloon pump through a femoral artery.
- Genitourinary system: It may be difficult to insert a Foley catheter in patients with prostatic problems.
- Musculoskeletal system: Major skeletal deformities or active arthritic conditions may interfere with ambulation and recovery.

Family and Social History

Family history of coronary artery disease, congenital heart disease, Marfan syndrome, malignant hyperthermia, and other hereditary disorders should be recorded. Marital status and living conditions should be considered in the discharge planning.

Physical Examination

Height, weight, and vital signs must be obtained on admission and recorded. Examination of the eyes, mouth, neck, chest, and abdomen should be performed, and all findings should be recorded. Pelvic and rectal examinations do not have to be done unless indicated. All peripheral pulses must be checked. The carotid and subclavian arteries should be auscultated for bruits. In patients undergoing coronary artery bypass, the Allen test must be performed in case a radial artery is used as bypass conduit.

Informed Consent

Perioperative anesthetic/surgical cares and risks, including blood transfusion, autologous blood predonation, and regional anesthesia, should be discussed. Requirements for postoperative care should also be established.

Preoperative Tests

- Blood tests: Complete blood count (CBC); prothrombin time; and levels of electrolytes, glucose, blood, urea, nitrogen (BUN), and creatinine should be obtained in all patients. Specific blood tests may also be appropriate for those with comorbid conditions.

- Urinalysis: A simple test to detect urinary tract and renal disease should be routinely done.
- Chest x-ray: Posteroanterior and lateral view chest x-rays should also be routinely obtained and displayed in the operating room, particularly in reoperations because the lateral view can indicate the site of the heart and the ascending aorta in relation to the sternum.
- Electrocardiogram: This is an indispensable test to diagnose heart rhythm abnormalities and myocardial ischemia.

PREOPERATIVE MEDICAL ORDER

1. Cardiac Medications
   All regular cardiac medications should be continued on the day of surgery. This includes nitroglycerin patches. However, stopping ACE inhibitors 24 hours before surgery is controversial. There is a small risk of these drugs causing hypotension perioperatively.
2. Anticoagulants
   - Coumadin: Coumadin should be stopped 4 to 5 days before surgery. If the patient is at high risk of thrombosis, he/she must be admitted and started on intravenous heparin.
   - Heparin: Intravenous heparin should be stopped 2 to 3 hours before surgery (unless the patient is on an intra-aortal balloon pump [IABP]).
   - ASA/Ticlopidine/nonsteroidal anti-inflammatory drugs (NSAIDs) should be stopped 7 to 10 days before the operation if possible.
   - Glycoprotein (GP) IIb/IIIa inhibitors: Abciximab—if possible, emergency or urgent CABG should be delayed for 12 hours, and platelet transfusion may be required during the operation.
   - Eptifibatide or Tirofiban: In emergency or urgent CABG, delay of medication administration is not necessary, but with an elective CABG, administration of medication should be delayed for 2 to 4 hours.
3. Psychotropic drugs
   - Monoamine oxidase (MAO): Long-acting inhibitors should be discontinued 2 weeks before surgery and short-acting inhibitors should be discontinued 1 week before surgery.
4. Others
   - Steroids and antirejection drugs (patients undergoing transplantation) must be continued.
5. Preoperative sedation should be given for same-day admission.
   - Lorazepam (Ativan): 1 to 2 mg sublingually.
   - Narcotics: Usually not required; intramuscular (IM) narcotics may be given in appropriate surgical holding areas.

SUGGESTED READINGS

Dupuis JY, Wang F, Nathan H, et al. The cardiac anesthesia risk evaluation score: a clinically useful predictor of mortality and morbidity after cardiac surgery. *Anesthesiology.* 2001;94:194–204.

Ferguson T Jr, Hammill B, Peterson E, et al. A decade of change-risk profiles and outcomes for isolated coronary artery bypass grating procedures, 1990–1999. A report from the STS

National Database Committee and the Duke Clinical Research Institute. *Ann Thorac Surg.* 2002; 73:480–489.

Immer F, Habicht J, Nessensohn K, et al. Prospective evaluation of 3 risk stratification scores in cardiac surgery. *Thorac Cardiovasc Surg.* 2000;48:134–139.

Nashef SA, Rogues F, Michel P, et al. European system for cardiac operative risk evaluation (EuroSCORE). *Eur J Cardiothorac Surg.* 1999;16:9–13.

Weightman WM, Gibbs NM, Sheminant MR, et al. Risk prediction in coronary artery surgery: a comparison of four risk scores. *Med J Aust.* 1997;166:408–411.

Wong D, Cheng D, Kustra R, et al. Risk factors of delayed extubation, prolonged length of stay in the intensive care unit, and mortality in patients undergoing CABG with fast tract cardiac anesthesia: a new cardiac risk score. *Anesthesiology.* 1999;91:936–944.

Anesthesia and Cardiopulmonary Bypass Management

Fast-track Cardiac Anesthesia Management in On-pump and Off-pump Coronary Artery Bypass Surgery

Davy C. H. Cheng and Daniel Bainbridge

Intensive care unit (ICU) costs rank second only to operating room costs, and, therefore, it is economically appealing for early extubation to facilitate earlier ICU and hospital discharge of patients who have undergone cardiac surgery. It is now feasible to accomplish early tracheal extubation because of improvement in perioperative anesthesia management, coupled with the advancement in surgical myocardial protection and tepid cardiopulmonary bypass (CPB) techniques.

Perioperative anesthetic management that facilitates early tracheal extubation coupled with the process of recovery is a successful key element of such a program. Fast-track cardiac anesthesia (FTCA) with tracheal extubation within 1 to 6 hours of arrival to the cardiac surgery recovery unit (CSRU) has been demonstrated to increase postoperative cardiorespiratory morbidity, sympathoadrenal stress, or mortality, and to reduce costs considerably and improve resource utilization.

Many cardiac surgical centers have embraced the philosophy of FTCA over the last decade. Given the known cost benefits of FTCA techniques, there would appear to be no compelling reason to persist with high-dose opioid regimens in routine cardiac surgical practice. The commonly adopted postoperative multimodal analgesia consists of nurse-administered narcotic analgesics, patient-controlled narcotic analgesics, and nonsteroidal anti-inflammatory drugs (NSAIDs).

Regional analgesia using intrathecal (IT) narcotics and thoracic epidural analgesia (TEA) has been advocated for immediate operating-room extubation and for facilitating postoperative recovery in these patients. When applying regional analgesia or block, we must carefully consider the potential risks and benefits associated with such practice. The optimal dose of intrathecal morphine (ITM) in terms of safety and efficacy in cardiac surgery has not yet been well-defined. Low-dose ITM (2.5 to 5 μg/kg) is found to be effective for postoperative analgesia with minimal side effects, but it is not consistently effective for earlier extubation time, and it is not effective for early hospital discharge.

For the analgesic efficacy of regional analgesia in cardiac surgery, TEA and ITM generally reduce the visual analog scale (VAS) pain score range in conventional multimodal analgesia from 4 to 6, to 0 to 2, and 2 to 4, respectively. TEA and ITM may facilitate but are not prerequisites for immediate extubation. FTCA with multimodal analgesia is as effective as TEA and ITM in achieving the same goal. Furthermore, regional analgesia has not been shown to reduce ICU and hospital length of stay (LOS). It is the FTCA management and postoperative process of care that play a more important role in determining the extubation time and hospital discharge.

FAST-TRACK CARDIAC SURGERY PROGRAM

This clinical pathway is a process of care including a multidisciplinary approach aimed at facilitating the recovery and discharge of patients who have undergone cardiac surgery. Early extubation anesthesia (1 to 6 hours postoperation) is a major key to the success of a fast-track cardiac surgery program. The program includes preoperative patient education, same-day admission surgery, expeditious and meticulous surgical management, early extubation anesthetic technique, horizontal integration of ICU and step-down unit as CSRU, dedicated medical coverage, flexibility in nursing practices, and supportive services.

Communication among cardiac patient management teams (i.e., cardiovascular surgeon, cardiac anesthesiologist, ICU staff, nurses, respiratory therapists, physiotherapists, and social workers) is vital to the success of the early extubation and a fast-track cardiac program. Nursing management needs to support single-day recovery and transfer, changes to analgesia and sedation practice, accelerated weaning and tracheal extubation of patients, early mobilization of patients and walking on postoperative day 1, early resumption of regular diet and chest tube removal, and hospital discharge on postoperative day 4 or 5.

Postoperative morbidity such as bleeding and atrial arrhythmia is potentially preventable, and care should be taken to avoid these complications. Antifibrinolytics, with close monitoring of coagulation, and careful dosing of heparin and protamine should be done to avoid coagulopathy. β-blockers, amiodarone, or sotalol should be administered, when indicated, to reduce perioperative arrhythmias (see Chapter 42).

Although it is imperative to include preoperative, intraoperative, and postoperative predictors as essential components of a cardiac surgery risk-scoring system, it is the intraoperative and postoperative morbidity that ultimately determine the feasibility of early extubation and ICU LOS. Therefore, every patient should be considered as a candidate for early extubation (see Table 2-1).

▶ **TABLE 2-1** Independent Predictive Factors of Delayed Extubation, Prolonged ICU LOS, and Hospital Mortality in Patients Who Have Undergone Cardiac Surgery Post–Early Extubation Anesthesia

	Preoperative	*Intraoperative*	*Postoperative*
Delayed extubation >10 h	Age Female		Excessive bleeding IABP Inotropes Atrial arrhythmia
ICU LOS >48 h	Age MI <1 wk Female		Renal dysfunction IABP Inotropes Arrhythmia Excessive bleeding
Hospital mortality	Inotropes Female MI <1 wk	Inotropes IABP CPB >120 min	

ICU LOS, intensive care unit length of stay; IABP, intra-aortal balloon pump; MI, myocardial infarction; CPB, cardiopulmonary bypass.
Adapted from Wong DT, Cheng DC, Kustra R, et al. Risk factors of delayed extubation, prolonged length of stay in the intensive care unit, and mortality in patients undergoing coronary artery bypass graft (CABG) with fast-track cardiac anesthesia: a new cardiac risk score. *Anesthesiology.* 1999;91:936–944.

Medical and Economic Implications

There is no increase in postoperative cardiorespiratory sympathoadrenal stress, morbidity, or mortality outcome in FTCA management both in index hospital stay and up to 1 year postoperation.

■ Cardiovascular: There was no major difference in postoperative myocardial ischemia incidence and ischemia burden between the early- and late-extubated patients; more importantly, there was no increase in creatine kinase isoenzyme fraction (CK-MB) levels or myocardial infarction (MI) rate.

■ Sympathoadrenal stress: Early extubation anesthetic adequately suppresses the stress response of the perioperative catecholamines (e.g., norepinephrine, epinephrine, and cortisol).

■ Respiratory: The first hour postextubation is most crucial in respiratory care, as reflected by the apnea index in either early or late extubation (see Table 2-2). The tidal volume and central respiratory drive also improved progressively. Postextubation oxygen saturation, respiratory rate, labored breath index, and apnea characteristics were similar between both groups. In addition, early extubation improved intrapulmonary shunt fraction by 30% to 40% post–coronary artery bypass graft (CABG) surgery.

■ Neurologic: Early extubated patients performed better and returned to baseline level earlier in the Mini-Mental State Examination (MMSE). This allows earlier chest tube removal, mobilization, and oral intake of food in the early extubated patients, resulting in reduced ICU LOS in the hospital.

■ Mortality: Early extubation does not increase mortality rate.

■ Costs: Early extubation anesthesia drugs do not increase perioperative anesthetic drug costs. It allows cost shifting from the high costs of the ICU to the lower costs of the ward. It reduces ICU LOS by earlier mobilization, leading to earlier hospital

▌ **TABLE 2-2** Postextubation Apnea

Extubation	Early	Conventional
Incidence	27.5% (14/51)	33.3% (17/51)
Duration (sec)	17.7 ± 23.0	15.7 ± 28.6
Index (rate/h)		
1 h	13	15
2 h	4	8
3 h	2	9
4 h	2	8

Reprinted with permission Cheng DCH, Karski J, Peniston C, et al. Morbidity outcome in early versus conventional tracheal extubation following coronary artery bypass graft (CABG) surgery: a prospective randomized controlled trial. *J Thorac Cardiovasc Surg.* 1996;112:755–764.

discharge. Including all complications in the cost analysis, early extubation anesthesia and management further reduces ICU (52.7%) and total CABG costs (25%) when compared with late extubation.

- Utilization: Other cost savings can be achieved by fewer cardiac surgery cancellations due to backlog of ICU beds, leading to a loss in operating room time and associated staffing and hospital costs.

PERIOPERATIVE MANAGEMENT OF PATIENTS TREATED WITH ANTIPLATELET DRUGS

There is increasing widespread use of potent antiplatelet drugs in patients with coronary artery disease and in patients who have undergone a high-risk coronary interventional procedure. Many patients who present to the operating room have been recently exposed to these drugs that substantially impair platelet function (see Appendix J).

Aspirin:
- Irreversibly inhibits platelet cyclo-oxygenase (COX).
- Inhibits thromboxane A_2 production.
- Results in impaired platelet activation.
- Increases bleeding and transfusions in patients who have undergone cardiac surgery, especially in "hyper-responders."
- Implications: desirable to discontinue if possible, but not necessary, especially in patients with CABG, because it reduces complications of angina, MI, transient ischemic attack (TIA), atrial fibrillation (AF), and stroke. Consider use of aprotinin, and in case of excess bleeding following protamine administration, transfuse platelets.

Ticlopidine (Ticlid) and Clopidogrel (Plavix):
- Irreversibly inhibit adenosine diphosphate (ADP)-mediated aggregation, thereby inhibiting activation of the glycoprotein (GP) IIb/IIIa receptor complex.
- Oral use only; biotransforms to active metabolite, which persists in serum.
- Ticlopidine associates with serious neutropenia 2.4%.

■ Implications: Delay surgery by 4 to 6 days if possible. Be careful if the patient has received an acute loading dose of clopidogrel (300 mg) for cardiac catheterization. Consider using aprotinin and transfuse platelets, as necessary, for excessive bleeding.

Abciximab (ReoPro), Tirofiban (Aggrastat), Eptifibatide (Integrilin):
■ Inhibits platelet membrane glycoprotein IIb/IIIa receptor.
■ Duration of platelet inhibition is 24 to 48 hours, 4 to 8 hours, and 2 to 4 hours for abciximab, tirofiban, and eptifibatide, respectively.
■ Abciximab: if possible, delay emergency or urgent CABG for 12 hours or elective CABG for 1 to 2 days. Prophylactic or antecedent platelet transfusion is required. Full loading and maintenance heparin doses are required for CPB; abciximab prolongs the activated clotting time (ACT) by 35 to 85 seconds. Use hemoconcentration during CPB to help eliminate abciximab. Transfuse platelet if excessive bleeding is present after protamine reversal.
■ Tirofiban and eptifibatide: No delay in emergency or urgent CABG is necessary. Delay elective surgery by 2 to 4 hours. No prophylactic platelet transfusion is necessary.

INTRAOPERATIVE ANESTHESIA CONSIDERATION AND MANAGEMENT

There are generally three anesthetic approaches in cardiac surgery:
1. General anesthesia with controlled ventilation: balanced narcotic-inhalational anesthesia or total intravenous anesthesia (TIVA).
2. Combined general anesthesia and regional analgesia with controlled ventilation: TEA or ITM (see Chapter 11).
3. Awake regional anesthesia with spontaneous ventilation: TEA. The safety and efficacy of this technique is not yet confirmed; only the feasibility of this technique has been confirmed.

Anesthesia induction and maintenance: Commonly, FTCA technique employs an induction dose of propofol (0.5 to 1.5 mg/kg) with low doses of narcotic and balanced concentration of inhalational agent.
■ Inhalational agent:
  ● No one agent has been shown to be superior to others. Shorter-acting agents may be beneficial (e.g., sevoflurane and desflurane), especially with ultra-fast-track anesthesia with operating room (OR) extubation as the goal.
■ Narcotic:
  ● No benefit has been seen with the use of one agent over another. Remifentanil, sufentanil, and fentanyl are all effective.
  ● Remifentanil: Loading induction infusion dose is 0.5 μg/kg/minute to 1 μg/kg/minute. Maintenance infusion dose is 0.5 μg/kg/minute to 1 μg/kg/minute.
  ● Sufentanil: Loading induction and total maintenance dose is 1 to 3 μg/kg.
  ● Fentanyl: Loading induction and total maintenance dose is 5 to 10 μg/kg.
■ Neuromuscular blockade:
  ● Shorter-acting neuromuscular blockers are likely to be of more benefit compared to long-acting agents.
  ● Rocuronium 0.5 to 1 mg/kg on induction, with intermittent boluses of 0.1 to 0.5 mg/kg to maintain neuromuscular blockade.

- Vecuronium 0.1 to 0.2 mg/kg on induction, with intermittent boluses of 0.05 to 0.1 mg/kg to maintain neuromuscular blockade.
- When pancuronium is employed, care should be taken to avoid intermittent re-bolus during the case, and neuromuscular blockade should be reversed before extubation.

PREBYPASS AND CARDIOPULMONARY BYPASS MANAGEMENT IN ON-PUMP CORONARY ARTERY BYPASS GRAFT

- Patient's blood pressure is typically maintained at a mean of 60 to 80 mm Hg.
- Blood tests are typically performed, including arterial blood gases (ABG), and levels of electrolytes (i.e., Na, K, Ca^{2+}, and Mg^{2+}), glucose, and baseline activated clotting time (ACT).
- Ventilation is adjusted to maintain a normal Pco_2 (35 to 45 mm Hg) and saturations above 95%.
- Heparin is given at a dose of 300 to 500 U/mL to maintain the ACT at >450 seconds in patients with CPB. Heparin resistance is common, especially in patients presenting to the OR with heparin infusions. Usually, because of reductions in antithrombin III, which necessitates increased doses of heparin, antithrombin III is administered, or in rare circumstances, fresh frozen plasma is transfused.
- Maintain normoglycemia (details in Chapter 10).
- Maintain hemoglobin levels at >70 mg/dL: In situations where blood volume is high, the patient may benefit from ultrafiltration during the bypass period to hemoconcentrate (details in Chapters 17 and 18).
- Electrolyte abnormalities during CPB: Hyperkalemia due to the cardioplegic solution—may require treatment with diuretics, calcium, or β_2 agonists. Hypocalcemia, may be treated at the end of CPB with 1 g of calcium chloride intravenously. Hypomagnesemia is typically managed by infusing 1 to 2 g of magnesium chloride.
- Blood pressure: Blood flow on bypass usually ranges from 2.2 to 2.5 L/m². Reductions in flow may lead to transient hypotension. In cases where pump flow is adequate, intermittent doses of phenylephrine may be administered (200 to 400 μg) to maintain mean pressures >50 mm Hg. Patients who fail to respond may require the addition of norepinephrine or vasopressin.

ANESTHESIA CONSIDERATION AND MANAGEMENT IN OFF-PUMP CORONARY ARTERY BYPASS SURGERY

- Monitoring: 5-lead electrocardiogram (ECG) (see Fig. 2-1), arterial line, pulmonary artery (PA) catheter, transesophageal echocardiography (TEE), thermoregulation.
- Carbon dioxide (CO_2) blower maintained at <5 L/minute to reduce direct endothelial injury and air emboli to distal vessel.
- Epicardial pacing readiness for bradycardia during posterior descending artery (PDA) or right coronary artery (RCA) anastomoses.
- Communication between anesthesia and surgical team: positioning for coronary anastomoses, ischemic preconditioning, and coronary shunt.
- Heparin dose of 300 to 400 U/kg to maintain ACT over 400 seconds.

- Three possible mechanisms are available in causing hemodynamic instability (see Fig. 2-1):
  - Vertical displacement of the heart (diastolic dysfunction predominantly).
  - Cardiac compression from myocardial stabilizer.
  - Myocardial ischemia during coronary artery occlusion for anastomosis.
- Treatment of hypotension: The goal is to maintain blood pressure (BP) >110/60 mm Hg, with mean pressures >70 mm Hg.
  - Reverse Trendelenburg position aids in surgical exposure and in filling of the heart.
  - Fluid boluses of crystalloid/colloid are used to maintain pulmonary capillary wedge pressure (PCWP)/central venous pressure (CVP).
  - Vasopressors: Phenylephrine/norepinephrine are used to maintain blood pressure during displacement/artery occlusion.
  - Milrinone: Used in patients with poor left ventricular (LV) function to improve myocardial relaxation/contractility.
- Ischemia:
  - Ischemia following completion of grafting should be managed by ensuring adequate graft flow. Addition of nitroglycerin/β-blocker may be employed if ischemia persists despite adequate graft flow. (Nitroglycerin is also beneficial to lower blood pressure during placement of the partial aortic clamp.) Calcium channel

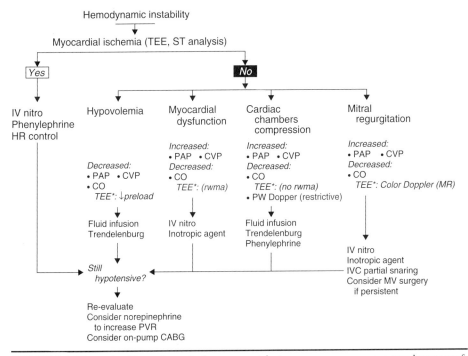

FIGURE 2-1. Diagnosis of hemodynamic derangement during on-pump coronary artery bypass graft (OP-CABG): simplified approach. (Reprinted with permission from Couture P, Denault A, Limoges P, et al. Mechanisms of hemodynamic changes during off-pump coronary artery bypass surgery. *Can J Anesth.* 2002;49:835–859.) IV, intravenous; HR, heart rate; PAP, pulmonary artery pressure; CO, cardiac output; CVP, central venous pressure; TEE transesophageal echocardiography; PVR, pulmonary vascular resistance; CABG, coronary artery bypass grafting; IVC, inferior vena cava; MV, mitral value.

blockers (e.g., diltiazem 5 to 10 mg/hour) are sometimes employed to prevent postoperative vasospasm, especially when multiple arterial grafts are used.

POSTOPERATIVE TRANSFER TO CARDIAC SURGERY RECOVERY UNIT

- Sedation and pain medication (e.g., propofol 50 to 100 μg/kg/minute and morphine 0.1 to 0.2 mg/kg/hour) should be provided on postoperative transfer to cardiac surgery recovery unit. Parasternal block and local anesthetic infiltration of the sternotomy wound and mediastinal tube sites can be a useful analgesic adjunct. Use nonselective NSAIDs in patients without renal dysfunction and ulcer disease or in patients <70 years (diclofenac or indomethacin 50 to 100 mg pr before extubation). Aim for early tracheal extubation in the OR for select patients or shortly after stabilization at CSRU (see Chapter 40).
- Antihypertensive agents may be used (e.g., metoprolol 1 to 5 mg intravenously in divided boluses, esmolol 50 to 300 μg/kg/minute infusion, or nitroglycerin 0.5 to 3 μg/kg/minute).

MORTALITY, MORBIDITY, AND RESOURCE UTILIZATION OUTCOMES IN OFF-PUMP CORONARY ARTERY BYPASS SURGERY

- In patients at low risk for off-pump coronary artery bypass (OPCAB), level I evidence has demonstrated that mortality, stroke, MI, and renal failure are not reduced when compared to conventional CAB surgery. However, OPCAB surgery may improve selected 30-day clinical outcomes (i.e., AF, inotropic requirement, respiratory infection, and blood transfusion) and resource utilization (i.e., ventilation time, ICU, and hospital LOS).
- In selected patients with high-risk OPCAB, level II evidence has suggested potential improvement in the major clinical morbidity outcomes.

SUGGESTED READINGS

Cheng DC, Bainbridge D, Martin JE, et al. Does off-pump coronary artery bypass reduce mortality, morbidity and resource utilization when compared to conventional coronary artery bypass or percutaneous coronary intervention? A meta-analysis of randomized trials. *Anesthesiology.* 2005;102:188–203.

Cheng DK, Jackevicius CA, Seidelin P, et al. Safety of glycoprotein IIb/IIIa inhibitors in urgent or emergency coronary artery bypass graft surgery. *Can J Cardiol.* 2004;20:223–228.

Cheng DCH, Karski J, Peniston C, et al. Morbidity outcome in early versus conventional tracheal extubation following coronary artery bypass graft (CABG) surgery: a prospective randomized controlled trial. *J Thorac Cardiovasc Surg.* 1996;112:755–764.

Cheng DCH, Wall C, Djaiani G, et al. A randomized assessment of resource utilization in fast-track cardiac surgery one-year after hospital discharge. *Anesthesiology.* 2003;98:651–657.

Couture P, Denault A, Limoges P, et al. Mechanisms of hemodynamic changes during off-pump coronary artery bypass surgery. *Can J Anesth.* 2002;49:835–859.

McDonald S, Jacobsohn E, Kopacz D, et al. Parasternal block and local anesthetic infiltration with levobupivacaine after cardiac surgery with desflurane. *Anesth Analg.* 2005;100:25–32.

Wong DT, Cheng DC, Kustra R, et al. Risk factors of delayed extubation, prolonged length of stay in the intensive care unit, and mortality in patients undergoing coronary artery bypass graft with fast-track cardiac anesthesia: a new cardiac risk score. *Anesthesiology.* 1999;91:936–944.

Anesthetic Management in Valvular Heart Surgery

Rita Katznelson and Patricia Murphy

AORTIC VALVE

Aortic Stenosis

Aortic stenosis (AS) may occur at three levels: valvular, subvalvular, and supravalvular.

- Valvular AS has three main causes:
  1. Calcification and fibrosis of normal trileaflet aortic valve (AV) (very common).
  2. Calcification and fibrosis of a congenitally bicuspid AV.
  3. Rheumatic valve (RV) disease (uncommon since the advent of antibiotics).
- Subvalvular AS is caused by an obstruction proximal to AV, and the possible etiologies include subaortic membrane, hypertrophic cardiomyopathy, tunnel subaortic obstruction, and upper septal bulge.
- Supravalvular AS occurs in congenital conditions such as William syndrome.
- The AV area is reduced to approximately 1 cm^2 before hemodynamic significance occurs, except in the presence of left ventricular (LV) dysfunction. Normal LV function and severe AS have a mean pressure gradient (PG) of >50, whereas poor LV function and severe AS have a PG of <50.

Pathophysiology

- Chronic pressure overload of the LV.
- Concentric left ventricle hypertrophy (LVH) is a compensatory mechanism to reduce LV wall stress.
- LVH causes reduced diastolic compliance, impaired coronary blood flow, and imbalance of the myocardial oxygen supply and demand.

- Low diastolic compliance elevates left ventricle end diastolic pressure (LVEDP) and left ventricle end diastolic volume (LVEDV).
- Myocardial ischemia occurs because of increased oxygen demands of hypertrophied muscle and because of increased wall stress, coupled with a reduced diastolic coronary perfusion pressure and a low coronary flow reserve.

Hemodynamic Goals

- Sinus rhythm is crucial. Supraventricular tachycardia (SVT) can severely reduce cardiac output (CO) and can increase myocardial oxygen demands. Prompt conversion to sinus rhythm is essential.
- Optimal heart rate is 60 to 80 beats per minute (bpm). Tachycardia may cause ischemia and ventricular ectopy. Bradycardia can decrease CO due to fixed stroke volume (SV).
- Adequate preload is essential to maintain CO, but this may be difficult to predict. High filling pressures in AS may reflect low LV compliance and diastolic dysfunction and not the true LVEDP. Transesophageal echocardiography (TEE) is beneficial for optimal preload.
- The use of vasodilators should be avoided and fixed afterload should be maintained. The treatment of hypotension must be immediate and must include maintenance of intravascular volume, Trendelenburg position, and the use of α-adrenergic agonists such as phenylephrine (40 to 80 μg).
- Contractility should be maintained. Myocardial depressants should be avoided.

Anesthetic Management
Premedication

- The young and anxious patients are premedicated with benzodiazepine, and the frail and elderly patients are premedicated with a reduced dose of benzodiazepine or no premedication at all.

Intraoperative Management

- A large-bore intravenous (IV) catheter, preferably of 14 gauge, and an arterial catheter are placed before induction. If considerable LV dysfunction or left main (LM) coronary stenosis is present, femoral arterial access (wire or catheter) is preferred before induction.
- The surgeon and perfusionist must be ready for emergency use of cardiopulmonary bypass (CPB).
- Narcotic-based anesthetic technique has few adverse hemodynamic effects.
- The choice of muscle relaxant depends on the resting heart rate. Pancuronium is used when bradycardia is present; vecuronium is used if tachycardia is present.

Weaning from Cardiopulmonary Bypass

- The thick, hypertrophied LV can be difficult to protect during a CPB; therefore, myocardial damage can occur. "Stone heart" is still seen (rarely).
- Noncompliant LV is dependent on a stable rhythm for adequate filling.
- Inotropic support may be required to wean from CPB, especially with LV dysfunction or with incomplete myocardial revascularization.

- Patients with severe LVH can develop dynamic subaortic or cavitary obstruction after aortic valve replacement (AVR). Inotropic agents will worsen left ventricular outflow tract (LVOT) obstruction. The treatment is volume replacements/administration and β-blockers. If the obstruction is intractable, a myectomy should be considered. The diagnosis of the obstruction is only possible intraoperatively using TEE.

Monitoring

- Standard electrocardiogram (ECG), with continuous monitoring of leads II and modified V_5 with ST analysis, provides optimal information on rhythm and ischemia.
- Use of a central venous catheter is best suited for administration of vasoactive drugs.
- A pulmonary artery catheter (PAC) is beneficial for hemodynamic management post-CPB. The PAC is positioned in the right atrium (RA) initially until the aortic cannula is inserted before CPB. Once the aortic cannula is in place, the PAC can be floated into PA.
- TEE is essential for the optimal management of hemodynamics and LV filling.

Aortic Regurgitation

Aortic regurgitation (AR) results from the inadequate coaptation of the AV leaflets during diastole.

The etiology includes the following:

1. Aortic root dilatation (hypertension [HTN], ascending aortic dissection, cystic medial necrosis, Marfan syndrome, syphilitic aortitis, ankylosing spondylitis, osteogenesis imperfecta).
2. Deformity and thickening of the leaflets (rheumatic disease, infective endocarditis [IE], and bicuspid AV).
3. Cusp prolapse (due to aortic dissection or abnormality of commissural support).

Pathophysiology of Aortic Regurgitation
Chronic Aortic Regurgitation

- Individuals with chronic AR will be asymptomatic for many years because of LV compensation.
- LV volume and pressure overload occurs.
- LV maintains systolic function by dilation and by increasing compliance.
- LV decompensates at later stages, and LVEDP and LVEDV rise.
- As systolic function declines, congestive heart failure (CHF), arrthymias, and sudden death can occur.
- Subendocardial ischemia develops because of an imbalance between increased oxygen demands of the "overloaded" ventricle and reduced diastolic perfusion pressure.

Acute Aortic Regurgitation

- In case of individuals with acute AR, the LV is unable to dilate acutely and LV volume overload occurs.

- LVEDV and LVEDP rise quickly, resulting in acute pulmonary edema.
- Urgent/emergent surgical intervention is usually required.

Hemodynamic Goals

- Optimal heart rate is 90 bpm; bradycardia will increase regurgitation.
- High afterload should be avoided. Low systemic vasodilators response (SVR) increases forward flow.
- Arterial vasodilators (sodium nitroprusside) are preferred over venodilators.
- Acute AR requires a positive inotropic agent and/or vasodilator/inodilator.
- Intra-aortic balloon counterpulsation is contraindicated.

Anesthetic Management

- The patient is premedicated with benzodiazepines.
- Monitoring is by routine ECG, arterial line, and central venous pressure (CVP) and PAC.
- TEE is beneficial to guide fluid and inotropic management.
- Anesthetic technique:
  - Regional or general techniques are favorable with normal LV.
  - A narcotic-based regimen is preferable with impaired LV.
  - Acute AR is often an emergency procedure in the operating room (OR). Ketamine and succinylcholine may be appropriate in unstable patients if rapid sequence induction is required.
- Weaning from bypass may require inotropic agents or vasodilator/inodilator therapy in presence of LV dysfunction or acute AR.
- TEE is beneficial for hemodynamic therapy.

MITRAL VALVE

Mitral Stenosis

- Mitral stenosis (MS) is usually rheumatic in origin and is characterized by thickening, calcification, and fusion of the valve leaflets and commissures. MS is often combined with mitral regurgitation (MR) and AR.
- Surgery is indicated when the mitral valve area (MVA) is <1 cm^2, the patient develops New York Heart Association (NYHA) Class III or IV dyspnea, or an embolus occurs.

Pathophysiology

- MS causes a PG between the left atrium (LA) and LV and prevents the filling of LV.
- Pulmonary HTN develops as the left atrial pressure (LAP) rises.
- Elevated LAP induces LA enlargement.
- Atrial arrhythmias, especially atrial fibrillation, are very common and occur because of increased LA size.
- RV dysfunction occurs with severe pulmonary HTN. RV dilation often results in tricuspid regurgitation (TR). Tricuspid valve repair is often concomitant with mitral valve surgery.

- LV dysfunction is uncommon and is usually caused by concomitant ischemic heart disease (IHD).

Hemodynamic Goals

- To preserve sinus rhythm (if present) and avoid tachycardia. Tachycardia reduces the time for diastolic filling of LV, thereby worsening MS.
- To maintain preload to preserve LV filling.
- To avoid factors that exacerbate pulmonary HTN, such as hypercarbia, acidosis, hypothermia, sympathetic nervous system activation, and hypoxia.

Anesthetic Management
Premedication

- Oral benzodiazepine premedication is preferred to prevent anxiety and tachycardia. Mild premedication should be used for patients with severe MS and for frail and elderly patients.
- Patients with concomitant pulmonary HTN will benefit from supplemental oxygen, with premedication to prevent hypoxia, which may worsen pulmonary HTN.
- Medications to control heart rate, such as digoxin, calcium channel blockers, β-blockers, or amiodarone, should be taken on the morning of surgery.
- It is preferable to avoid diuretics preoperatively on the day of surgery.

Intraoperative Management

- Narcotic-based induction technique is preferred for hemodynamic stability.
- Low-dose inhalational agents can be used with preserved LV and RV function.
- Nitrous oxide (N_2O) is avoided because of its effects on pulmonary HTN.
- The choice of muscle relaxant depends on the resting heart rate.

Weaning from Cardiopulmonary Bypass

- Mitral valve replacement (MVR) resolves the obstruction to LV filling; therefore, in the post-bypass period, the hemodynamic status usually improves.
- Usually, PA pressures and pulmonary vascular resistance (PVR) will decrease. In cases of severe pulmonary HTN and RV dysfunction preoperatively, the PA pressures may not decrease after CPB.
- Phosphodiesterase inhibitors (e.g., amrinone and milrinone), which produce inotropy and vasodilation, are beneficial with pulmonary HTN and RV dysfunction.
- Nitric oxide (NO) at a concentration of 5 to 40 parts per million (ppm) may be used for severe pulmonary HTN and RV dysfunction.

Monitoring

- Monitoring by ECG, arterial line, CVP, and PAC are recommended.
- TEE is recommended for RV/LV function, hemodynamic manipulation, and for avoiding surgical complications of MVR.

Mitral Regurgitation

MR is more common than MS and can be due to a variety of possible etiologies.
- Myxomatous degeneration is the most common cause of MR.
- Ischemic (functional) MR occurs because of papillary muscle dysfunction, annular dilatation, or left ventricular dysfunction.

Pathophysiology
- Progressive volume loading of the LV, with LV and LA dilation.
- Compliance of the LA is preserved, and this chamber can massively dilate.
- Atrial arrhythmias occur due to increase in LA size.
- Dilated LV decompensates at later stages and LVEDP rise.

Hemodynamic Goals
There are three factors that determine the severity of MR:

1. The PG between the LA and LV.
2. The size of the regurgitant orifice.
3. The duration of ventricular systole.

Manipulation of any of these factors can reduce the severity of MR.
- A reduction in the afterload with vasodilators can reduce the regurgitant fraction by improving forward CO.
- A fast heart rate must be maintained to increase the time for ventricular ejection.
- Contractility must also be maintained to ensure optimal forward flow.

Anesthetic Management
Premedication
- Oral benzodiazepines are recommended.
- Patients with concomitant pulmonary HTN will benefit from supplemental oxygen along with premedication to prevent hypoxia, which may worsen pulmonary HTN.
- Medications to control heart rate, such as digoxin, calcium channel blockers, β-blockers or amiodarone, should be taken in the morning of surgery.
- It is preferable to avoid diuretics preoperatively on the day of surgery.

Intraoperative Management
- A narcotic-based anesthetic technique is preferable for hemodynamic stability.
- Nitrous oxide is usually avoided because of its myocardial depressant effects.
- Inhalational agents can be tolerated in small doses.
- Muscle relaxation is generally accomplished with pancuronium or vecuronium.

Weaning from Cardiopulmonary Bypass
- LV dysfunction is "unmasked" after MV surgery because the LV cannot offload into the LA. LV failure may occur, necessitating inotropes and vasodilators. Phosphodiesterase inhibitors (e.g., milrinone and amrinone) are beneficial.

- Use of an intra-aortic balloon pump can reduce afterload and can improve CO.
- TEE is useful to guide adequacy of valve repair/replacement, detect surgical complications, and manage hemodynamics.

TRICUSPID VALVE
Tricuspid Regurgitation

- TR may be a primary valvular disease caused by rheumatic heart disease, IE, carcinoid syndrome, Epstein (congenital) anomaly, or trauma.
- Functional TR secondary to chronic RV dilatation is more common than primary pathology. It often exists with long-standing mitral valve disease.

Pathophysiology
- RV and right atrium (RA) are overloaded and dilated.
- RA is very compliant, whereas RA pressure only rises in end-stage TR.
- Pulmonary HTN due to left heart lesion increases RV afterload and worsens TR.
- RV volume overload and dilation causes paradoxical motion and shifts the intraventricular septum toward LV, impairing LV filling and compliance.
- Right heart failure occurs as the RA pressure rises, causing hepatomegaly and ascites.

Hemodynamic Goals
- If TR is secondary to other valve pathology (e.g., MV disease), hemodynamic goals for left heart lesions should be considered.
- Pulmonary hypertension (PHT) and high PVR should be avoided.
- Normal to high preload is important for the RV stroke volume.
- Cautious titration of vasodilators in combination with volume loading can optimize RV forward flow.
- Hypotension should be treated with inotropes and volume, not with vasoconstrictors, which will worsen pulmonary HTN.

Anesthetic Management
Premedication
Mild benzodiazepine premedication is indicated with RV dysfunction and pulmonary HTN.

Intraoperative Management
Choice of anesthetic technique depends on the underlying pathology, ventricular function, and presence of PHT. Narcotic-based anesthetic technique is more hemodynamically stable.

Monitoring
- Monitoring by ECG, arterial line, and CVP are essential; PAC is useful with pulmonary HTN and MV pathology.

- Thermodilution CO may be overestimated with severe TR.
- TEE should be used for optimal fluid and hemodynamic management.

Weaning from Cardiopulmonary Bypass

- The RV/LV dysfunction requires inotropes, vasodilators, and NO post-CPB.
- Patients with IE usually do not require inotropes post-CPB.
- TEE is essential for fluid and hemodynamic management.

SUGGESTED READINGS

Bonov RO, Carabello B, de Leon AC Jr, et al. ACC/AHA guidelines for the management of patients with valvular heart disease: executive summary. A report of the American College of Cardiology/American Heart Association Task Force on Practice Guidelines (Committee on Management of Patients with Valvular Disease). *Circulation.* 1998;98:1949–1984.

Braunwald E. *Heart disease. A textbook of cardiovascular medicine.* 6th ed. Philadelphia, PA: WB Saunders, 2001.

Perrino AC Jr, Reeves ST. *A practical approach to transesophageal echocardiography.* Philadelphia, PA: Lippincott Williams & Wilkins; 2003.

Chapter 4

Anesthetic Management in Robotic Cardiac Surgery

Wojciech Dobkowski

Robotically enhanced telemanipulation is a new method, which has expanded the possibilities for cardiac surgeons to perform minimally invasive surgeries. This new technology has been used for both extracardiac and intracardiac operations. Presently, many cardiac procedures can be performed with the total or partial use of the robotic system. These procedures include robotically assisted vision-enhanced coronary artery bypass (RAVECAB), minimally invasive robotically assisted mitral valve repair (MIRAMVR), aortic valve replacement, patent ductus arteriosus closure, atrial septal defect closure, and pulmonary vein ablation.

Minimally invasive cardiac surgery is currently using two robotic telemanipulation systems, which are the ZEUS robotic system (Computer Motion Inc., Goleta, California) and the da Vinci Robotic System (Intuitive Surgical Inc., Mountain View, California). The advantages of the da Vinci system are three-dimensional visualization and a robotic "wrist," which provides articulated motion with 7-degrees of freedom inside the chest cavity. For surgical details, see Chapters 24 and 28.

ROBOTICALLY ASSISTED VISION-ENHANCED CORONARY ARTERY BYPASS AND MINIMALLY INVASIVE ROBOTICALLY ASSISTED MITRAL VALVE REPAIR

Extracardiac procedures such as RAVECAB are performed on a beating heart, whereas intracardiac partially robotic surgeries such as MIRAMVR require the implementation of cardiopulmonary bypass (CPB). Both techniques not only present some similarities in the preparation of the patients and in the intraoperative management but also present many different challenges for the anesthesiologist.

Anesthesia—General Considerations

- Selection of the patient is very important to avoid intraoperative and postoperative complications.
- Prolonged one-lung ventilation and incomplete revascularization in hybrid procedures should be considered.
- Noncardioplegic myocardial protection must be provided.
- Risk of arrhythmias should be considered while providing anesthesia.
- Unexpected bleeding may occur.
- Limited access for rapid intervention with the closed chest poses a challenge to the anesthesiologist involved in these cardiac surgeries.
- The use of regional analgesia has been an important part of robotic cardiac surgery, such as in minithoracotomy.
- Transesophageal echocardiography (TEE) has been one of the most important monitors during robotic heart surgery.

Preoperative Assessment: *RAVECAB and MIRAMVR*

- Prolonged one-lung ventilation and the potential risk of this technique for respiratory and cardiovascular instability during surgery, the choice of regional anesthesia, and the possibility of incomplete revascularization should be taken into consideration before surgery. The patient is assessed and prepared at the preadmission clinic by the anesthesiologist.

Airway and Respiratory System: RAVECAB, MIRAMVR

- Airway and chest anatomy assessment should be undertaken for one-lung ventilation.
- Patients with chronic lung diseases, such as hypercarbia, hypoxia, active bronchospasm, emphysema, or emphysematous bullae, and patients who are morbidly obese will not tolerate prolonged one-lung ventilation. Patients who may be optimized before surgery, especially those with mild chronic obstructive lung disease, should be assessed by the chest medicine specialist.

Cardiovascular System: RAVECAB, MIRAMVR

- Physiology of prolonged one-lung anesthesia and insufflations of carbon dioxide (CO_2) to the right or left side of the chest during robotic heart surgery will increase pulmonary artery pressure; pulmonary vascular resistance may cause hypoxia and hypercarbia and, subsequently, dysfunction of the right ventricle and decreased cardiac output.
- Patients should continue to be treated with β-blockers, calcium channel blockers, and nitrates. Aspirin should not be taken for at least 5 days before surgery, and antiplatelet agents or coumarin should be discontinued adequately well before the day of the procedure. Patients undergoing treatment with continuous infusion of

heparin will have increased risk of bleeding from the lungs and should not be considered as candidates for robotic operation.

■ Metabolic stability should be maintained before surgery, especially in respect to electrolytes such as potassium, magnesium, and calcium, for the prophylaxis of arrhythmias and to enhance myocardial contractility during surgery.

Anesthesia Management: *RAVECAB, MIRAMVR*

■ The combined techniques of general and regional anesthesia have been the most commonly used procedures in partially robotic and totally robotic heart surgeries.

■ A number of different regional blocks have been implemented for these operations. The most common blocks are continuous blockade of multiple intercostal nerves (ICB), percutaneous paravertebral block (PVB), thoracic epidural analgesia (TEA), and intrathecal opioid injection (ITM). The duration of pain following these procedures usually is 48 hours. Continuous catheter analgesia technique will provide smooth transition to postoperative analgesia.

■ With ICB technique, local anesthetic toxicity, infection, pneumothorax, and Horner syndrome have been documented. With TEA, the risk of neuroaxial injury due to hematoma, although statistically low, may preclude the use of this technique. Intrathecal opioid injection may cause postoperative sedation and, in some patients, respiratory depression.

■ In our institution we have been using the PVB technique for the last 6 years. The PVB block is initiated in the operating room before surgery, with the patient awake, in the lateral position. The superior aspect of the spine of T4 is marked. After skin infiltration, a 17-gauge needle is inserted until the transverse process of the T5 vertebra is contacted. The needle is "walked" off the superior aspect of the transverse process, puncturing the superior costotransverse ligament with a distinct "pop," and is advanced farther by 1.5 cm. The space is distended with 4 to 5 mL of 1.5% lidocaine with epinephrine, and an epidural catheter is inserted 13 cm into the skin. A loading dose of 0.4% ropivacaine, 20 mL, is given, and after 2 hours, an infusion of 0.2% ropivacaine, 6 to 8 mL/hour, is started and is maintained for 48 hours.

■ The general anesthesia is induced with a small dose of fentanyl, 3 to 5 μg/kg; propofol, 0.5 to 1 mg/kg; and rocuronium, 1 mg/kg. Anesthesia is maintained with sevoflurane, 1% to 2%; air and oxygen; and a continuous infusion of rocuronium to ensure absolute patient immobility during robotic manipulation inside the chest and during myocardial stabilizer placement until anastomosis is completed.

Specific Considerations

Patient Positioning and Monitoring: RAVECAB, MIRAMVR

The patients are positioned in the lateral tilt position, with the left or right arm being left free—draped to facilitate robotic arm movements. Careful positioning of the arm is essential to avoid neurologic injury, especially to the brachial plexus. Patients are draped, with the thorax, abdomen, both groins, and one limb being exposed for surgical access. This positioning gives the anesthesiologist access to only one arm for arterial pressure monitoring and for intravenous access.

Cardiovascular System: RAVECAB

- A five-lead electrocardiogram (ECG) is mandatory, but surgical incision on the left side of the chest, anteriorly, between the fourth and fifth intercostal space and ports in the midaxillary line preclude proper positioning of the lateral chest leads V_5 and V_6 and complicate ischemia monitoring. Multiple modalities should be implemented for ischemia monitoring. ST segment should be continuously monitored using at least two leads—lead II and the lateral chest lead. TEE is routinely used to detect intraoperative ischemia. Continuous mixed venous saturation using an oxymetric pulmonary artery catheter provides information about peripheral oxygen delivery in the presence of induced pneumothorax, hypoxemia, and changes in cardiac output during one-lung ventilation.
- External defibrillator pads are applied before induction of anesthesia. Right coronary artery bypass by right minithoracotomy has been related to perioperative bradycardia; atrioventricular conduction blocks and the insertion of the pacemaker lead through the pulmonary catheter should be considered.
- RAVECAB is performed on a normothermic beating heart. Noncardioplegic myocardial protection becomes an important part of this procedure. Ischemic preconditioning has been used when coronary vessels are not totally occluded. Intracoronary shunts have been used by surgeons to provide myocardial protection in both partially and totally robotic procedures. Dilation of the poststenotic epicardial vessel, maintenance of coronary filling pressure, and reduction of myocardial contractility and irritability optimize myocardial oxygen demand. This optimization can be achieved by pharmacologic protection of the myocardium with β-blockers, calcium channel blockers, nitrates, and magnesium. Infusion of nitroglycerin may help control ST segment changes or pulmonary capillary wedge pressure (PCWP) elevation. Also, infusion of magnesium (2 to 4 g) and/or lidocaine during the procedure may reduce ventricular irritability. Calcium channel blockers inhibit excitation–contraction coupling, reduce afterload, increase coronary vasodilatation, improve collateral blood flow, and prevent reperfusion-induced arrhythmias. Nicardipine is a potent calcium channel blocker, which provides myocardial protection and has antianginal effects and spasmolytic effects in arteries. It does not have an effect on A-V conduction or myocardial contractility. Diltiazem is also a possible choice to optimize myocardial oxygen demand. It is more cardioselective and cardiodepressive than nicardipine. Magnesium has also been shown to exert a protective effect when given before an ischemic period.
- One of the most important aspects of exerting a protective effect on the myocardium is the maintenance of a mean arterial pressure above 50 mm Hg in order to provide adequate coronary perfusion pressure. The protocol for conversion to sternotomy or CPB should include a mean arterial pressure below 50 mm Hg, mixed venous oxygen saturation (SvO_2) <60%, arrhythmia, and ST segment changes above 4 mm, which do not respond to pharmacologic treatment.

Respiratory System: RAVECAB

- A left-sided double lumen tube or a single lumen tube with bronchial blocker (Univent) can be used to provide one-lung ventilation. We usually apply continuous positive airway pressure (CPAP) to the collapsed lung. This technique improves oxygenation and reduces shunt fraction. One-lung ventilation with induced pneumothorax by carbon dioxide insufflation can increase pulmonary artery pressure and pulmonary artery resistance, produce hypoxia and hypercarbia, and cause hemodynamic instability with low cardiac output. A pleural pressure of 5 to 10 mm Hg is well tolerated. This pressure should be monitored closely to avoid unnecessary administration of vasoactive medications or inotropic agents.

- Frequent communication between the surgical team and the anesthesiologist is essential. Continuous monitoring of ventilatory parameters and/or spirometry is mandatory.
- At the end of the surgery, the double lumen tube should be changed to a single lumen endotracheal tube, which requires a deeper level of anesthesia and a proper dose of muscle relaxant.

Fluid and Temperature Management: *RAVECAB*

- Because of the length of the surgery (4 to 6 hours), a patient may experience hypothermia if not properly protected. We use an upper body warming blanket, which is attached to the patient's shoulders and neck, and a lower body warming blanket, which covers one leg. All intravenous fluids are warmed. Warmer ambient air can be used, in addition to positioning the hose under the drapes around the patient's head. Temperature is monitored using the oropharyngeal and pulmonary catheter. Hypothermia should be avoided so that the risk of shivering during the postoperative period is decreased and extubation is delayed.
- Fluid management during these procedures is important. During prolonged controlled ventilation and one-lung anesthesia with progressively increasing pulmonary artery pressure, increased levels of antidiuretic hormone (ADH) and decreased levels of atrial natriuretic peptide have been observed. These changes lead to reduced glomerular filtration rate and low urine output during the procedure. In this situation, proper fluid balance monitoring will help avoid fluid overload, with possible increased interstitial lung water and postoperative hypoxemia.
- RAVECAB surgery requires adequate intravascular volume status for hemodynamic stability and organ perfusion. We attempt to titrate fluid therapy to maintain PCWP at 12 to 15 mm Hg. TEE has been used routinely to verify the preload in the left side and the right side of the heart. When conversion to CPB is required, the addition of pump prime solution may result in fluid overload. Communication between the anesthesiologist and the perfusionist is important, and possible ultrafiltration should be instituted.

Anticoagulation: *RAVECAB*

- At our institution, we use heparin at a dose of 15,000 to 25,000 IU to maintain an activated clotting time (ACT) >400 seconds. Coagulation function is better maintained at the end of surgery because CPB has been avoided.
- When a hybrid procedure is planned, after robotic coronary revascularization is completed, heparin is reversed using adequate dose of protamine, and the patient is given antiplatelet medication (clopidogrel) through a nasogastric tube 45 minutes

before stenting of the coronary artery. An additional dose of heparin 5,000 IU is administered before the procedure. This approach may cause coagulation disturbance and, consequently, bleeding in the postoperative period. Our experience in six cases of hybrid procedures showed one case of bleeding, which required transfusion of blood and blood products.

Specific Anesthetic Consideration for *MIRAMVR*

Every case of MIRAMVR should undergo routine intraoperative TEE. In addition to evaluating mitral valvular pathology, aortic valve, and left ventricular function, the intraoperative TEE should evaluate intraluminal aortic atherosclerotic pathology, coronary sinus cardioplegia catheter placement, femoral venous cannula positioning, endoaortic catheter positioning (when used), and residual intracardiac air at the end of the procedure and the surgical result and postoperative cardiac function.

Postoperative Management: *RAVECAB, MIRAMVR*

All our robotic heart surgeries are extubated in the cardiac surgery recovery unit (CSRU). One-lung ventilation requires very close monitoring of respiratory function. Like other patients with cardiac disorders, the patients undergoing this surgery are monitored for anastomotic potency, myocardial ischemia and infarction, arrhythmia, and postoperative bleeding. PVB is reassessed when the patient is awake and, if needed, modifications of the dose and rate of infusion of local anesthetic are ordered. Patient-controlled analgesia is ordered when PVB does not provide adequate pain relief. All patients are in a fast-tracking recovery pathway.

CONCLUSION

- Robotic-assisted cardiac surgery showed advantages in a select group of patients, such as reduction of wound infection, preservation of stable thorax, excellent cosmetic result, shorter hospital stay, and lower incidence of cognitive dysfunction compared with the patients undergoing conventional coronary artery bypass graft (CABG).
- Anesthesia management of these patients is challenging when cardiovascular and respiratory systems may be compromised in a closed-chest system. Pharmacologic protection of myocardium is an additional challenge. TEE is crucial for continuous monitoring of cardiac function and necessary for proper placement of cannulas during intracardiac procedures and for assessment of mitral valve after repair.

SUGGESTED READINGS

Awad H, Wolf RK, Gravlee GP. The future of robotic cardiac surgery. *J Cardiothorac Vasc Anesth.* 2002;16:395–396.

Boyd WD, Rayman R, Desai ND, et al. Closed-chest coronary artery bypass grafting on the beating heart with the use of a computer-enhanced surgical robotic system. *J Thorac Cardiovasc Surg.* 2000;120:807–809.

Czibik G, D'Ancona G, Donias HW, et al. Robotic cardiac surgery: present and future applications. *J Cardiothorac Vasc Anesth.* 2002;16:502–507.

D'Attelis N, Loulmet D, Carpantier A, et al. Robotic assisted cardiac surgery: anesthetic and postoperative considerations. *J Cardiothorac Vasc Anesth.* 2002;16:397–400.

Dogan S, Aybek T, Andresen E, et al. Totally endoscopic coronary artery bypass grafting on cardiopulmonary bypass with robotically enhanced telemanipulation: report of forty-five cases. *J Thorac Cardiovasc Surg.* 2002;86:845–857.

Ganapathy S, Murkin JM, Boyd WD, et al. Continuous percutaneous paravertebral block for minimally invasive cardiac surgery. *J Cardiothorac Vasc Anesth.* 1999;13:594–596.

Mehta N, Goswami S, Argenziano M, et al. Anesthesia for robotic repair of the mitral valve: a report of two cases. *Anesth Analg.* 2003;10:96–97.

Chapter 5

Circulatory Arrest and Neuroprotection

Ivan Iglesias and John M. Murkin

Surgical reconstruction of the distal ascending aorta and aortic arch requires a clearly visible, blood-free field, necessitating interruption of perfusion to the great vessels of the head. Techniques must therefore be employed to maintain cerebral perfusion or to protect the brain during such interruptions in blood flow. Currently, three approaches are used for cerebral protection, all based on the premise that metabolic inhibition induced by brain cooling will improve tolerance to ischemia. The first involves profound cooling and a period of hypothermic circulatory arrest (HCA). The second combines HCA with retrograde cerebral perfusion (RCP) via superior vena cava (SVC), while the third technique involves HCA with selective antegrade cerebral perfusion (SACP) using selective cannulation of the epiaortic vessels.

CLINICAL PRESENTATION

- The two main pathologies found in adult patients requiring HCA for reconstruction of the aortic arch are aortic dissection and degenerative aneurysm, which may often be coexistent.
- Such patients are at high risk because they frequently present emergently, often with an abrupt onset of pain and with varying degrees of hemodynamic compromise.
- Aortic dissection may extend to involve the innominate or carotid arteries, coronary arteries, and aortic valve or may rupture into the pericardial sac.
- Intraoperative transesophageal echocardiography is of particular benefit to identify the site of the intimal tear and potential secondary extensions.

- Patients are often older, have a higher incidence of significant comorbidities, and generally evidence more advanced and diffused atherosclerotic processes than other patients who have undergone surgery.
- Operative mortality in aortic arch surgery is 5% to 10%, and the poor outcome is related to emergency surgery, advanced patient age, poor preoperative functional status, and aortic cross clamp and circulatory arrest times.
- In addition to a higher perioperative mortality, massive bleeding, stroke, respiratory insufficiency, and renal failure are not infrequent accompaniments.

CARDIOPULMONARY BYPASS

- Monitoring and control of temperature is of paramount importance. Core temperature should be evaluated with either rectal or bladder thermistry, whereas brain temperature must be monitored specifically using nasopharyngeal or tympanic or, less commonly, retrograde jugular bulb thermistor.
- Anticoagulation with heparin, 300 to 400 IU/kg intravenously (IV), to produce activated clotting time (ACT) >450 seconds before cardiopulmonary bypass (CPB) is done. An additional bolus of heparin, 150 IU/kg, may be administered immediately before HCA.
- Aortic dissection generally necessitates arterial inflow cannulation via femoral artery or axillary artery.
- Aortic arch, or descending aorta, is utilized for arterial cannulation for aneurysm repair depending on the type of procedure and the clinical circumstances.
- Venous drainage is preferably via the right atrium or, alternatively, from the femoral vein.
- With systemic cooling, the heart will spontaneously fibrillate as temperatures approach 25°C. Insertion of a vent line via the superior pulmonary vein will minimize distention of the left ventricle.
- Secondary aortic insufficiency may necessitate manual decompression of the heart to prevent distention and to facilitate systemic perfusion.
- Generally a 30- to 45-minute CPB is required to achieve sufficient cooling, after which HCA is commenced. The CPB machine is stopped, the ascending aorta is opened and evaluated, and the distal anastomosis of the prosthetic graft to aorta or arch is commenced.
- During HCA, a brain protection strategy is employed until completion of the distal aortic anastomosis.
- With completion of the distal anastomosis, the arterial inflow cannula is repositioned into the graft, and antegrade perfusion is commenced.

HYPOTHERMIC CEREBRAL PROTECTION

- Hypothermia is the mainstay of cerebral protection. Before commencing HCA, systemic cooling to a minimum brain temperature (nasopharyngeal, jugular bulb, or tympanic) of 18°C is recommended.
- Homogeneity of brain cooling is of paramount importance, and, therefore, the additional endpoints that are to be met before commencing HCA include onset of

isoelectric electroencephalograph activity, increase and plateau in jugular oxygen saturation, or increase and plateau in cerebral oxygen saturation measured via noninvasive near infrared spectroscopy (NIRS).

- External ice packs should be applied circumferentially to the head before HCA to minimize ambient rewarming. Coverage of any applied NIRS or bispectral index (BIS) monitoring pads and connections with a transparent adhesive occlusive dressing are recommended before application of ice packs because water leakage frequently prevents signal generation.
- Antegrade perfusion should commence as soon as possible, with a minimum 5-minute interval of cold reperfusion before active rewarming begins.
- During rewarming, arterial blood inflow temperature must be closely monitored and should never exceed 37°C because brain temperature is directly related to perfusate temperature. Even mild cerebral hyperthermia has been demonstrated to increase the extent and severity of ischemic brain injury.

RETROGRADE AND SELECTIVE ANTEGRADE CEREBRAL PERFUSION

- For RCP, a cannula is placed in the SVC and arterial blood at 10°C to 12°C is perfused retrograde at a rate of flow of 250 to 500 mL/minute.
- Inferior vena caval occlusion may be employed as a supplemental technique to enhance delivery of RCP blood to the cerebral circulation.
- To minimize cerebral hemorrhagic complications, RCP line pressure is monitored continuously and is generally maintained at 15 to 20 mm Hg and should not exceed 26 mm Hg.
- Because of venous valves and plexuses, a relatively minimum quantity of RCP blood from SVC actually perfuses the brain. This occurs largely by way of retrograde flow via epidural veins.
- Although it is insufficient to provide adequate metabolic substrate to the brain, RCP is of some benefit for minimization and flushing of cerebral emboli and provides an effective means of maintaining cerebral hypothermia.
- For continuous cerebral perfusion, SACP via selective cannulation of the carotid artery employs arterial blood at 10°C to 12°C using flow rates of 250 to 500 mL/minute at line pressures of 50 to 70 mm Hg.
- Adequacy of cerebral perfusion with SACP is predicated upon the presence of an intact circle of Willis and carries some embolic risk in the presence of carotid atheromata.
- Although many centers employ RCP for HCA of <30-minute duration, evidence increasingly favors SACP for HCA of longer duration. SACP has been associated with a lower risk of transient neurologic syndromes and decreased incidence of cognitive dysfunction versus RCP.
- An advantage of perfusing the brain with cold blood (10°C to 12°C) via either RCP or SACP is its ability to maintain systemic temperatures at moderate hypothermia (25°C to 28°C). By avoiding profound systemic hypothermia, in addition to shortened rewarming and total CPB times, this may better preserve coagulation status and may lessen perioperative bleeding.

pH MANAGEMENT

- Clinical studies and experimental evidence points to some overall benefit of pH-stat management in infants and children undergoing HCA. Efficiency and homogeneity of cerebral cooling appears to be better with pH-stat rather than alpha-stat.
- In adult CPB patients, alpha-stat has been associated with decreased cerebral embolization and with preservation of cerebral autoregulation.
- For adults undergoing moderate hypothermic CPB, clinical outcomes from at least three separate prospective randomized clinical trials support alpha-stat management over pH-stat.
- Given the current absence of the data of specific outcomes, the best practice for HCA in adults would include alpha-stat during initial CPB, pH-stat only during profound cerebral cooling, and alpha-stat during HCA with continuous RCP or SACP, and, again, alpha-stat during reperfusion and rewarming.
- An important adjunct therapy is carbon dioxide (CO_2) insufflation into the graft and open-chambers of the heart during deairing maneuvers before reperfusion. CO_2 will displace nitrogen (N_2) from any air-containing cavities, and because the solubility of CO_2 is much greater than N_2, the size and time course of any gaseous emboli will be significantly decreased.

GLUCOSE MANAGEMENT

- All glucose-containing intravenous, cardioplegic, and pump-priming solutions should be avoided. Ringer lactate or a starch-based colloid are preferable to glucose-containing solutions.
- In addition to the suppression of leukocyte function and an enhanced susceptibility to perioperative infections, hyperglycemia considerably exacerbates cerebral injury after focal and global ischemic episodes, as may occur during HCA.
- Hyperglycemia is common during CPB even in patients without diabetes and is a function of insulin suppression, decreased insulin responsiveness, and gluconeogenesis, which is responsible for the release of CPB-induced stress hormone.
- Blood glucose concentration should be monitored frequently both during CPB and throughout the perioperative period, especially in the presence of catecholamine inotropic infusions.
- Enhanced awareness and treatment of catecholamine-induced hyperglycemia and aggressive insulin dosing strategies are advocated.

RENAL PROTECTION

- To ensure a brisk diuresis before and following cessation of systemic perfusion is an important goal.
- Administration of a bolus of 1 g/kg of 20% mannitol before circulatory arrest generally ensures a diuresis and may provide additional antioxidant protection.
- Recent evidence shows that low-dose dopamine therapy does not protect the kidney. There is not enough evidence yet on the role of fenoldopam and *N*-acetyl cysteine in protecting renal function.

BLEEDING AND COAGULATION

- To minimize excessive bleeding and to decrease blood product utilization, administration of an antifibrinolytic, either 0.05 to 0.10 g/kg tranexamic acid or 6 M kallikrein inhibitory unit (KIU) aprotinin, is recommended as soon as possible, ideally before initial skin incision but certainly before the institution of CPB.
- As a serine protease inactivator, anti-inflammatory benefit and a decrease in perioperative stroke have additionally been associated with full-dose aprotinin.
- Availability of blood products, specifically platelets, fresh frozen plasma, and cryoprecipitate, in addition to packed red blood cells, must be ensured before separation from CPB.
- After separation from CPB, residual circulating heparin can be estimated on the basis of 100-minute half-life and neutralized with protamine accordingly.

SUGGESTED READINGS

DiEusanio M, Wesselink RM, Morshuis WJ, et al. Deep hypothermic circulatory arrest and antegrade selective cerebral perfusion during ascending aorta-hemiarch replacement: a retrospective comparative study. *J Thorac Cardiovasc Surg.* 2003;125:849–854.

Fleck TM, Czerny M, Hutschala D. The incidence of transient neurologic dysfunction after ascending aortic replacement with circulatory arrest. *Ann Thorac Surg.* 2003;76:1198–1202.

Kazui T, Yamashita K, Washiyama N. Usefulness of antegrade selective cerebral perfusion during aortic arch operations. *Ann Thorac Surg.* 2002;74:S1806–S1809.

Murkin JM. Retrograde cerebral perfusion: More risk than benefit. *J Thorac Cardiovasc Surg.* 2003;126(3):631-633.

Neri E, Sassi C, Barabesi L. Cerebral autoregulation after hypothermic circulatory arrest in operations on the aortic arch. *Ann Thorac Surg.* 2004;77:72–79.

Sakamoto T, Zurakowski D, Duebener LF. Interaction of temperature with hematocrit level and pH determines safe duration of hypothermic circulatory arrest. *J Thorac Cardiovasc Surg.* 2004;128:220–232.

Spielvogel D, Strauch JT, Minanov OP. Aortic arch replacement using a trifurcated graft and selective cerebral antegrade perfusion. *Ann Thorac Surg.* 2002;74:S1810–S1814.

Chapter 6

Anesthesia for Combined Cardiac and Thoracic Surgery

Peter Slinger

CONTROVERSIES

There is no complete agreement about the surgical management of patients who are found to have both cardiac and thoracic surgical lesions.

- The one-stage combined procedure:
  - Avoids a second anesthetic and surgical incision.
  - May reduce hospital stay and may have economic benefits.
- The two-stage procedure:
  - May be associated with less blood loss than with pulmonary resection in patients who are heparinized.
  - May allow better operative exposure and staging of mediastinal nodes for malignant lung lesions.
  - May be associated with better long-term survival because of the immunologic consequences of cardiopulmonary bypass (CPB).
- Suggested management:
  - Preferred management at our institution is a one-stage combined procedure because of the documented comparable long-term survival with a low incidence of short-term morbidity and mortality.
  - Most cardiac operations can be combined with thoracic procedures either for malignant or for benign disease.

PRESENTATION

- Patients with combined surgical lesions present in one of the following three patterns:
  1. An asymptomatic lung lesion is found during evaluation for cardiac surgery.
  2. A patient being investigated for lung pathology is found to have significant cardiac disease.
  3. A previously undetected lung lesion is found intraoperatively after sternotomy.

- In scenarios 1 or 2, adequate pulmonary assessment can be arranged preoperatively to guide perioperative anesthetic management. In scenario 3, anesthetic management will be more *ad hoc*. However, most of these "surprise" lesions are benign (i.e., granulomas or bullae) and require only simple wedge resection without intraoperative lung isolation or loss of postoperative pulmonary function.

PREOPERATIVE EVALUATION

Respiratory function is assessed in three related areas: lung mechanics, pulmonary parenchymal function, and cardiorespiratory reserve (see Fig. 6-1).

- Respiratory function
  1. Mechanics:
     - The most valid test of lung mechanics is spirometry, which is specifically the use of the forced expiratory volume in one second as a percentage of normal ($FEV_{1\%}$) to derive the predicted postoperative (ppo) $FEV_{1\%}$ on the basis of the amount of functioning lung that is resected. A ppo-$FEV_{1\%}$ <40% is associated with increased respiratory complications; ppo-$FEV_{1\%}$ <30% may require prolonged weaning from mechanical ventilation.
  2. Cardiorespiratory reserve:
     - The most valid tests—maximal oxygen consumption (Vo_2 max), exercise tolerance, and oximetry—will not be applicable in most patients with cardiac disease.
     - Useful indirect tests are the echocardiogram or cardiac catheterization to show left and right ventricular function.
  3. Lung parenchyma:
     - The diffusing capacity of the lung for carbon monoxide (D_{LCO}) is a noninvasive test performed at the time of spirometry. A ppo-D_{LCO} that is <40% increases the risk of respiratory complications.
     - Arterial blood gases partial pressure of oxygen (Pao_2) <60 mm Hg and partial pressure of carbon dioxide ($PaCo_2$) >45 mm Hg also increase risk of respiratory complications.

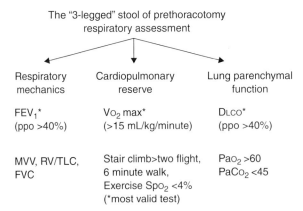

FIGURE 6-1. The "three-legged" stool of prethoracotomy respiratory assessment. D_{LCO}, diffusing capacity of the lung for carbon monoxide; FEV_1, forced expiratory volume in 1 second; FVC, forced vital capacity; MVV, maximal voluntary ventilation; ppo, predicted postoperative; RV/TLC, residual volume/total lung capacity; Vo_2 max, maximal oxygen consumption.

- Chronic obstructive pulmonary disease (COPD): A large proportion of the adult thoracic surgical population has COPD, particularly those with a >20 pack/year history of smoking. Severity of COPD is graded according to the degree of airflow obstruction—severe: FEV_1 <35%; moderate: 35% to 60%; mild: 60% to 80%. Anesthetic considerations in COPD include:
  - Bullae/blebs: There exists a possibility of rupture occurring during positive pressure ventilation, resulting in a pneumothorax or bronchopleural fistula. Lung isolation is considered and nitrous oxide is avoided.
  - Hypercapnia: Patients with moderate or severe COPD may be "carbon dioxide (CO_2)-retainers" who will develop an increased respiratory dead space when supplemental oxygen is administered and will subsequently retain more CO_2 during spontaneous ventilation. The fraction of inspired oxygen (FIO_2) must be titrated with care postoperatively, keeping the oxyhemoglobin saturation as low as is clinically acceptable to aid weaning from mechanical ventilation.
  - Bronchodilators must be continued perioperatively.
- Lung cancer: Preanesthetic assessment of patients with lung cancer should consider the "4-Ms":
  - Mass effects: obstructive pneumonitis, superior vena cava (SVC) syndrome, Pancoast syndrome, and so on.
  - Metabolic effects: Eaton-Lambert syndrome, syndrome of inappropriate antidiuretic hormone secretion (SIADH), hypercalcemia, and so on.
  - Metastases: Specifically brain, bone, liver, and adrenal glands.
  - Medications: Chemotherapy with bleomycin, doxorubicin corticosteroids, and so on.
- Smoking:
  - Stopping smoking for <8 weeks preoperatively has not been shown to benefit patients undergoing cardiac surgery.
  - Stopping smoking for any period preoperatively decreases the risk of respiratory complications in patients undergoing thoracic surgery.
  - Patients should be advised to stop smoking.
- Chest radiography and computerized tomography (CT) scan: Most abnormalities of the tracheobronchial tree, which cause problems for lung isolation, can be appreciated from the assessment of the preoperative chest x-ray and CT scan. Often these abnormalities will not be described in a written or verbal report. The anesthesiologist must examine the radiograph before induction.
- Mediastinoscopy:
  - Because of the difficulty in assessing subcarinal nodes for staging by a sternotomy, all patients known to have lung cancer should have a mediastinoscopy done as the first step of a combined procedure.
  - Because of the risk of brachiocephalic artery compression during mediastinoscopy, the circulation in the right arm (e.g., right-sided radial arterial line or pulse oximeter) is monitored.
  - Surgical access to the suprasternal notch should be allowed after central line placement.

ANESTHETIC TECHNIQUE

- To decrease the risk of bronchospasm, intubate patients having COPD and reactive airway disease during deep general anesthesia.
- Consider the possibility of surgical clamping of an *in situ* posteroanterior catheter during lung resection.
- Placement of a transesophageal echocardiogram (TEE) probe with an *in situ* double-lumen tube can be done safely.
- *If a pulmonary procedure is performed before CPB during a single anesthetic, it is important to perform fiberoptic bronchoscopy to clear the airways before weaning from CPB.*
- Lung isolation techniques:
  - Three basic options: double-lumen endobronchial tubes, single-lumen endobronchial tube, or bronchial blockers (see Fig. 6-2).
  - Left-sided double-lumen tubes are the optimal choice because they offer continuous access to both mainstem bronchi for suction, fiberoscopy, application of continuous positive airway pressure (CPAP), and they are more stable intraoperatively than bronchial blockers.
  - Because of their limited versatility, double-lumen tubes are often not practical in patients with abnormal tracheobronchial anatomy.
  - In patients with abnormal anatomy or when the need for lung isolation is not foreseen, a bronchial blocker is passed intraluminally through an *in situ* single-lumen tube for one-lung isolation.
  - An 8-French Fogarty venous embolectomy catheter with a 10-mL balloon is useful as a bronchial blocker; it can be passed together with a 4-mm fiberoptic bronchoscope through a single-lumen tube of >7-mm internal diameter. Two bronchial blockers (Arndt and Cohen, *Cook Critical Care,* Bloomington, Indiana), specifically designed to be placed through standard endotracheal tubes, are available.

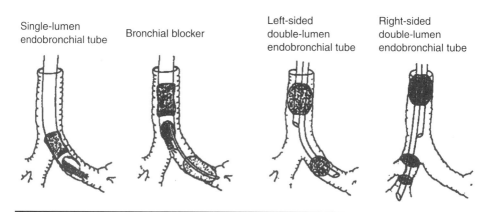

Single-lumen endobronchial tube   Bronchial blocker   Left-sided double-lumen endobronchial tube   Right-sided double-lumen endobronchial tube

FIGURE 6-2. Three basic options: double-lumen endobronchial tubes (right- or left-sided), single-lumen endobronchial tube, or bronchial blockers.

- The position of all endobronchial tubes and blockers with fiberoptic bronchoscopy is confirmed.
- Hypoxemia during one-lung ventilation (OLV):
  - Hypoxemia occurs in a few patients during OLV. This hypoxemia is largely due to intrapulmonary shunt in the nonventilated lung, which may not be adequately compensated by hypoxic pulmonary vasoconstriction.
  - Patients who are more likely to develop hypoxemia during OLV are those with increased alveolar–arterial oxygen gradients during two-lung ventilation, good preoperative spirometry, and right-sided surgery, and those who are receiving vasodilators.
  - Maneuvers to prevent hypoxemia during OLV are by the use of high FIO_2 and a sustained vital capacity inflation of the ventilated lung to recruit atelectatic areas just before OLV.
  - Treatment of hypoxemia: Oxygen at a CPAP of 2 to 3 cm H_2O after reinflation of the nonventilated lung is the most useful therapy.
  - Other treatments of hypoxemia: application of positive end expiratory pressure (PEEP) to the ventilated lung is of benefit in few patients. Similarly, individual patients may benefit from a larger (14 mL/kg) or smaller (7 mL/kg) than usual (10 mL/kg) tidal volume during OLV.

COMBINED PROCEDURES

- Cardiac valvular surgery:
  - Because of the risk of contamination of the operative field from an open bronchus, it is recommended to complete the cardiac procedure, wean from CPB, and close the pericardium before the pulmonary resection.
  - Lung isolation and OLV are necessary for lung resection in these cases.
  - A double-lumen endobronchial tube that is placed at induction is an optimal airway management.
- Aortocoronary bypass (and other cardiac procedures):
  - These procedures can be performed during CPB, whereas lung isolation and OLV may not be necessary.
  - It is optimal to perform the pulmonary resection at the end of CPB after the aortic cross-clamp is removed.
  - For cases where difficulty in weaning from CPB is anticipated, optimal management is to wean from CPB and stabilize and then perform the pulmonary resection. Lung isolation will aid in these cases.
  - Because problems in weaning from CPB are not always predictable, a double-lumen tube should be used.
- CPB management:
  - Because of the increased incidence of phrenic nerve injury and diaphragmatic paralysis associated with topical cooling (slush) of the heart during CPB, topical cooling is not advised during combined cardiac–thoracic procedures.

POSTOPERATIVE ANALGESIA

- Thoracic epidural infusion analgesia with a combination of local anesthetic and opioid provides better postoperative pulmonary function in high-risk thoracic surgical patients.
- Because of concerns about the risk of epidural hematoma formation with anticoagulation, and the generally improved pulmonary function and pain control after sternotomy versus thoracotomy incisions, epidural analgesia is not widely used for cardiac surgery in North America.
- For select patients having combined cardiac–thoracic procedures with poor respiratory function, placement of an epidural catheter 12 to 24 hours preoperatively is a useful option.

SUGGESTED READINGS

Brutel de la Riviere A, Kuaepen P, VanSwieten H, et al. Concomitant open-heart surgery and pulmonary resection for lung cancer. *Eur J Cardiothorac Surg.* 1995;9:310–314.

Kaplan J, Slinger P. *Thoracic anesthesia.* 3rd ed. Philadelphia, PA: Churchill Livingston; 2003.

Rao V, Todd TRS, Weisel RD, et al. Results of combined pulmonary resection and cardiac operation. *Ann Thorac Surg.* 1996;62:342–347.

Ulicny KS Jr, Schmelzer V, Flege JB, et al. Concomitant cardiac and pulmonary operation: the role of cardiopulmonary bypass. *Ann Thorac Surg.* 1992;54:289–295.

Chapter 7

Anesthesia for Intrathoracic Transplantation

Karen McRae

INTRODUCTION

Intrathoracic transplantation involves the care of high-risk patients with end-stage cardiac or pulmonary disease and limited survival without transplant. Transplant surgery is performed as an emergency procedure dependent on the availability of a compatible donor, who may be far away from the recipient. Successful management of the patient undergoing heart, lung, or heart–lung transplant (HLT) requires planning, skill, and collaboration of a perioperative team with a sound knowledge of all the aspects of the procedure.

Planning Transplantation

- Clear communication about the timing of induction of anesthesia to the patient who is to undergo transplantation is vital. Although an early start would seem desirable, allowing surgical dissection to proceed and having the recipient ready for organ implantation as soon as the allograft is available, and thereby minimizing ischemic time, the procedure is always at risk of cancellation until the allograft is fully assessed by the donor team.

■ The predicted cross-clamp time of the donor aorta, the estimated duration of travel of the allograft from the donor site, and the difficulty of the removal of the native organ should all be considered in the choice of the induction time of anesthesia. Clinically, the duration of allograft preservation of <6 hours is sought in donor heart and lungs, although improved preservation techniques have allowed successful longer ischemic times.

■ Prior thoracic surgery, adhesions or congenital anomalies may make dissection difficult. Knowledge of the recipient's condition permits optimal planning for all aspects of care.

■ The entire team must be present—surgeons, anesthesiologist, perfusionist, and nurses. The induction period of the patients who are critically ill is frequently eventful and may require an emergent response.

■ The immunosuppressed state of transplant recipients requires strict adherence to sterile techniques during the placement of catheters.

Donor Management

■ Management of multiorgan donors requires some compromise because of competing interests for different organs. For example, the copious hydration that is advocated for maintaining urine output may lead to right heart distention and pulmonary edema that are deleterious to the heart and lung grafts. Resuscitation of the donor yields a greater number of transplantable organs; guidelines for donor stabilization are outlined in Table 7-1.

■ Correction of anemia, acidosis, and electrolyte disturbances and adjustment of fluids and inotropes to maintain intravascular volume, cardiac output (CO), and perfusion pressure ensure adequate delivery of oxygen to all organ tissues. Autonomic instability and hypotension occur in approximately 80% of donors. Fluid administration and the use of inotropes are tempered by avoiding fluid overload and tachycardia. Metabolic resuscitation is an area of ongoing investigation.

  ● After brainstem death, vasodilatory hypotension often occurs, which can be due to vasopressin deficiency even in the absence of signs of diabetes insipidus. A continuous infusion of low-dose vasopressin can increase systemic blood pressure and allow weaning from catecholamine vasopressors.

  ● In the many donors who do exhibit diabetes insipidus after brain death, desmopressin (Desamino-D-Arginine-Vasopressin [DDAVP] 4 μg intravenously [IV]) has traditionally been administered. DDAVP may not be needed after initiation of vasopressin.

  ● The use of high-dose steroids (methylprednisolone 1 g IV) in donors is widely accepted to result in increased proportion of lungs that are suitable for transplantation.

■ Preservation solutions are organ specific. Donor hearts are flushed with approximately 2 L of crystalloid solution (Celsior). Lungs are flushed with approximately 4 L of low potassium dextran solution (Perfadex) supplemented with prostaglandin E1, while inflated with a fraction of inspired oxygen (F_{IO_2}) of 0.5. Both the donor hearts and lungs are maintained at 4°C.

▌ **TABLE 7-1** Donor Management Guidelines

1. **Airway management**
   - Aspiration precautions
   - Frequent suctioning and bronchoscopy
   - Albuterol therapy for wheezing (may improve lung fluid clearance)
2. **Mechanical ventilation**
   Adequate oxygenation
   - $PaO_2 > 100$ mm Hg, $FIO_2 = 0.40$ or O_2 saturation $>95\%$
   Adequate ventilation
   - Maintain tidal volume 10–12 mL/kg
   - Maintain minimum PEEP of 5 cm H_2O
   - Maintain peak airway pressures <30 cm H_2O
   - Maintain slight respiratory alkalosis (pH 7.35–7.45, pCO_2 30–35 mm Hg)
3. **Monitoring**
   - Central venous line
   - Arterial line and pulse oximetry
   - Pulmonary artery catheter desirable for rational use of inotropes, pressors, and fluids
4. **Fluid management**
   Judicious fluid resuscitation to achieve the lowest CVP/PCWP consistent with adequate urine out-put and blood pressure to ensure end-organ perfusion (*euvolemia not hypervolemia*)
   - Maintain CVP 6–8 mm Hg, PCWP 8–12 mm Hg
   - Urine output 1 mL/kg/hr
   - Hemoglobin >10 g/dL or HCT $\geq 30\%$
   Electrolytes
   - Maintain $Na^+ <150$ mEq/dL
   - Maintain $K^+ >4.0$ mEq/dL
   - Correct acidosis with sodium bicarbonate and mild to moderate hyperventilation ($PaCO_2$ 30–35 mm Hg)
5. **Hemodynamic management goals**
   - Blood pressure ≥ 90 mm Hg or MAP ≥ 60 mm Hg
   - SVR $800 - 1,200$ dynes/s/cm^2
   - Cardiac index 2.4 L/min/m^2
   - Dopamine or dobutamine dose <10 μg/kg/min
   - Arginine vasopressin: 1 unit bolus $+$ infusion up to 0.04 unit/kg/h
   - Norepinephrine titrate to blood pressure
6. **Hormonal resuscitation**
   - Methylprednisolone: 15 mg/kg bolus (Repeat q24h PRN)
   - Arginine vasopressin: titrate infusion to blood pressure (up to 0.04 unit/kg/h)
   - Insulin: start infusion at rate of 1 unit/h then titrate blood glucose to 6–9 mmol/L
   - Tri-iodothyronine (T3): 4 mcg bolus; 3 μg/h continuous infusion
7. **Early echocardiogram for all cardiac donors—with insertion of PA catheter for patients with LVEF $>45\%$ or on high dose inotropes.**
   - If LVEF $>45\%$ to optimize hemodynamic and hormonal management, then reassess

FIO_2, fraction of inspired oxygen; PEEP, positive end expiratory pressure; PA, pulmonary artery; CVP, central venous pressure; PCWP, pulmonary capillary wedge pressure; HCT, hematocrit; SVR, systemic vascular resistance; MAP, mean arterial pressure; PRN, as needed; LVEF, left ventricular ejection fraction.
Adapted from D'Ovidio F, McRitchie D, Keshavjee S. Care of the multiorgan donor. In: Hall JB, Schmidt GA, eds. *Principles and practice of critical care.* 3rd edition. New York: McGraw-Hill; 2004.

HEART TRANSPLANTATION

Recipient Characteristics

Typically, patients have end-stage biventricular failure, with ongoing treatment with multiple drugs. Nonpharmacologic therapy may include synchronized pacing and ventricular assist devices both percutaneous (intra-aortic balloon pump [IABP]) and implanted (left ventricle assist device [LVAD] +/− right ventricle assist device [RVAD]). The International Society of Heart and Lung Transplantation (ISHLT) registry of heart transplants performed during 2000 to 2003 lists the etiology of recipient heart failure as:

- Ischemic cardiomyopathy (45%).
- Idiopathic cardiomyopathy (46%).
- Congenital heart disease: valvular (3%) or complex congenital (2%), which may have had prior palliative or corrective surgery.
- Retransplantation (2%).

Preoperative Recipient Management

- Ongoing therapy, which may include digoxin, diuretics, vasodilation with hydralazine and β-blocker as tolerated, neurohumoral blockade with angiotensin converting enzyme (ACE) inhibitor or angiotensin receptor blocker, and nitrates in patients with ongoing ischemia, is to be continued. Patients who are critically ill may be dependent on intravenous inotropes, which have to be maintained until cardiopulmonary bypass (CPB) is achieved.
- Most patients will have elevated pulmonary artery (PA) pressures. Irreversible pulmonary hypertension may preclude heart transplantation. Although no absolute rule exists, guidelines for maximally acceptable PA pressures include:
  - Systolic PA pressure <45 mm Hg.
  - Systolic PA pressure, which is 50% of the systemic pressure or less (if systemic pressure is >80 mm Hg).
  - Transpulmonary gradient = mean PA pressure − mean pulmonary capillary wedge pressure (PCWP) <15 mm Hg.
  - Pulmonary vascular resistance <6 wood units (<460 dynes/second/cm^5). Pulmonary vascular resistance = transpulmonary gradient/CO.

The need to obtain current hemodynamic measurements requires that transplant recipients be urgently admitted to the coronary care unit (CCU) for PA catheter placement when a suitable donor is found. Some patients with pulmonary vascular resistance (PVR) exceeding the guidelines will respond to acute diuresis and vasodilators.

- Many patients will have experienced life-threatening arrhythmias related to their end-stage heart disease; chronic amiodarone therapy increases perioperative risk. Patients may have pacemakers or implanted defibrillators.
- LVAD (+/−RVAD) is increasingly being used as a bridge to transplantation. The complexity of surgery is increased by the need for removal of an assist device, the formation of adhesions, chronic anticoagulation, and patient exposure to multiple blood products with attendant antibody production. The patient care team should be aware of the risk of recent exposure to aprotinin during LVAD placement.

- Routine premedication is not recommended. Antacid prophylaxis, H_2 blockers, and gastric prepulsants may be indicated for a full stomach.

Monitors/Lines

- Five lead electrocardiogram (ECG), noninvasive blood pressure cuff, pulse oximeter, nasopharyngeal temperature probe, and urinary catheter are all needed.
- Large-bore intravenous access is required. The radial arterial line and PA catheter are preferably placed in the left internal jugular vein because the right internal jugular is routinely used for postoperative myocardial surveillance biopsies. The PA catheter is withdrawn during heart engraftment; a long sterile sleeve should be used.
- Transesophageal echocardiography (TEE) is used during cardiac transplantation for identification of ventricular dysfunction and assessment of filling pressures.

Anesthetic Technique

- A modified rapid sequence induction is performed if the patient is unfasted. A variety of induction agents such as fentanyl, sufentanil, etomidate, ketamine, and midazolam have been used successfully for induction of anesthesia.
- An induction and maintenance regimen that is suitable for early extubation (detailed in Chapter 2) is used with dosing that is modified for a prolonged circulation time and reduced volume of distribution associated with low CO. Nitrous oxide is not used because its use may increase PVR and will increase the size of any gas emboli entrapped in the graft. Inhalational anesthetics reduce myocardial contractility in a dose-dependent fashion; maintenance of a propofol infusion is better tolerated by most patients.
- The primary anesthetic objective is to ensure amnesia while maintaining end-organ perfusion, such as kidney and brain, within the autoregulatory range. To maintain adequate systemic perfusion pressure, inotropes and vasopressors (dopamine, epinephrine, norepinephrine) are frequently required, often in high doses. Cardioprotection is not a priority pre-CPB because the recipient's native heart will be discarded. Recipients have usually been carefully diuresed preoperatively, and hypotensive episodes before CPB are treated with *inotropes and not with fluid*. Excess infused fluid will contribute to pulmonary hypertension and right heart failure.

Cardiopulmonary Bypass

- Anticoagulation and anesthesia maintenance are as for routine CPB.
- The need for femoral–femoral cannulation and partial bypass (possibly pre-induction) for patients at particular risk of bleeding or vascular damage at sternotomy should be considered.
- Preparation for a long CPB run is warranted as there may be:
  - Difficulty in removing the native heart.
  - A delay in the arrival of the donor heart.

- Difficult anastomosis.
- Difficulty in weaning from CPB.

Ultrafiltration/hemoconcentration on CPB should be considered, particularly when patients are volume-overloaded.

The Physiology of the Transplanted Heart (Acute Effects)

- During transplantation, the cardiac plexus is interrupted. The recipient atrium remains innervated but is hemodynamically unimportant; the donor atrium is denervated and is the source of the electrophysiologic response of the transplanted heart. The ECG often contains two P waves. The denervated heart loses efferent and afferent sympathetic and parasympathetic innervation:
  - The vagus nerve will no longer influence the sinus and atrioventricular (AV) nodes.
  - The sinus node will have an increased refractory period, atrial conduction may be prolonged, and first degree AV block is common.
  - Indirect sympathomimetic agents will have no effect on the transplanted heart (Table 7-2).
  - Chemosensitive and mechanosensitive afferents from the left ventricle are lost.
- Intrinsic control mechanisms are retained including normal α- and β-adrenoreceptor responses to circulating catecholamines. The denervated heart cannot respond to acute hypotension or hypovolemia with reflex tachycardia and relies entirely on the intact Frank–Starling mechanism to increase CO by increased stroke volume (strength of contraction is proportional to end-diastolic volume). The transplanted heart is therefore *preload dependent*.
- Potential hemodynamic complications after reperfusion include the following:
  - RV dysfunction: caused by incomplete myocardial protection, which is worsened if the recipients have increased pulmonary resistance. Transient dysfunction is common; treatment is with inotropes and afterload reduction of PA pressures.
  - LV dysfunction: caused by prolonged ischemic time, poor myocardial preservation.
  - Decreased systemic vascular resistance (SVR) (vasodilatory hypotension): can be worsened by long-term amiodarone exposure. This vasoplegia may only respond to high doses of catecholamines.

▌ **TABLE 7-2 Response to Drugs of the Transplanted Heart**

Drugs	Action	Normal HR	Normal BP	Denervated HR	Denervated BP
Anticholinergics	Indirect	↑	∅	∅	∅
Anticholinesterases	Indirect	↓	∅	∅	∅
Pancuronium	Indirect	↑	∅	∅	∅
Propranolol	Direct	↓	∅	↓	∅
Verapamil	Direct	↓	↓	↓	↓
Ephedrine	Both	↑	↑	± ↑	↑
Phenylephrine	Both	↓	↑	∅	↑

Weaning from Cardiopulmonary Bypass

A strategy for weaning from CPB must include treatment that is specific to the physiologic compromise of the newly transplanted heart.

- Many patients will be bradycardic. Although pacing is effective for heart rate (HR) support, isoproterenol (1 mg/250 mL D5W), administered by infusion at a rate titrated to maintain a HR of 90 to 110 bpm also improves RV function.
- RV failure (or biventricular failure) is treated with inotropes: Dopamine, dobutamine, milrinone, epinephrine, and norepinephrine doses are titrated to effect.
- Pulmonary hypertension is treated with vasodilators:
  - Inhaled nitrous oxide (NO) has supplanted nitroglycerin and nitroprusside for this purpose.
  - Prostaglandin E_1 0.01 to 0.1 μg/kg/minute.
- Systemic hypotension due to low SVR (vasodilatory hypotension):
  - Norepinephrine infusion dose is titrated to effect.
  - Vasopressin, 1 to 4 units/hour IV infusion, if not responsive to increasing doses of norepinephrine.
- Patient management must be individualized; however, dopamine and isoproterenol are routinely used at the Toronto General Hospital (TGH) followed by milrinone and norepinephrine, and NO is used as second-line therapy. A randomized comparison of inhaled NO versus prostaglandin E_1 in heart transplantation reported greater reduction in PVR and more patients successfully weaned from CPB when NO was used. Inhaled NO is a selective pulmonary vasodilator, given that NO has strong physiologic properties, reducing PA pressure with minimal reduction of SVR. There is general consensus that NO is helpful in the post-CPB period. There is no evidence that NO improves long-term outcome. In patients with life-threatening primary graft failure that is unresponsive to pharmacologic therapy, placement of an LVAD/RVAD is possible and may permit some graft recovery.

Hematology and Fluid Management

- Fluid management continues to require careful attention: While LV output is preload-dependent, the RV is easily overloaded, and a central venous pressure (CVP) and PCWP <10 mm Hg may improve RV function. Sparing use of crystalloid and hemofiltration of excessive intravascular volume on CPB may facilitate infusion of large volumes of blood products that are frequently required.
- Risk of coagulopathy increases with long CPB duration, perioperative liver dysfunction secondary to right heart failure, and preoperative anticoagulation (warfarin). Early and aggressive intervention is required as surgical re-exploration for bleeding is often poorly tolerated. Infusion of fresh frozen plasma (FFP), platelets, and cryoprecipitate is frequently required. At TGH, 65% of the heart recipients received one or more units of red blood cells (RBCs), 85% received FFP, and 61% received platelets. A mean of 8 ± 8 RBC units (median 6), 6 ± 6 FFP units, and 10 ± 10 units platelets were transfused per case performed during the period 1999 to 2004. Desmopressin (DDAVP 20 μg) may be helpful. After separation from CPB, the operating room and infused fluids should be warmed to avoid patient cooling and the resulting coagulopathy.

- The use of aprotinin is warranted for antifibrinolytic and possibly anti-inflammatory properties: 2×10^6 units before CPB, 2×10^6 units in the CPB circuit, and 2×10^6 units after CPB by an infusion of 0.5×10^6 units/hour.

Postoperative Care

- Prophylaxis against organisms infecting the skin is required in the immediate perioperative period using cefazolin 1 g IV q6–8h.
- There is no specific reason why stable recipients of heart transplants should not be extubated shortly after the surgery; however, immune-mediated injury can worsen over hours during the postoperative period, and bleeding remains a major risk.
- A period of careful observation (4 to 8 hours) is warranted. Patients with pulmonary hypertension, RV failure, or hemodynamic instability require continued hemodynamic and respiratory support as described in the preceding text.

LUNG TRANSPLANTATION

Recipient Characteristics

The management of patients receiving a lung transplant requires consideration of the physiologic derangement specific to their underlying pulmonary disease. The list of disease frequency reflects patients recorded in the ISHLT registry from 1995 to 2004.

- *Airway disease*: Chronic obstructive pulmonary disease (39%), emphysema caused by α-1-antitrypsin deficiency (9%), cystic fibrosis (16%), bronchiectasis (2.5%), bronchiolitis obliterans (1.9%, including retransplantation). Patients with airway disease:
  - Have hyperinflation and may have bronchospasm.
  - Are at risk of life-threatening gas trapping with positive pressure ventilation, which responds to increased expiratory time.
  - Often have right ventricular dysfunction.
- *Pulmonary vascular disease*: Pulmonary arterial hypertension (PAH) caused by primary pulmonary hypertension (4.2%), patients with PAH secondary to congenital heart disease (Eisenmenger syndrome) (1.1%) in whom transplantation is combined with cardiac repair, and, rarely, PAH secondary to chronic thromboembolism that is not amenable to pulmonary endarterectomy. In patients with pulmonary vascular disease:
  - High systemic PA pressures and minimally responsive PVR are observed.
  - In case of severe right ventricular failure, one-lung ventilation is not attempted.
  - There is little tolerance for myocardial depression or increased PVR—anesthetics, hypercarbia, and hypoxemia may produce cardiovascular collapse.
  - May be anticoagulated, requiring reversal before or during transplantation.
- *Diseases destructive of pulmonary parenchyma*: Idiopathic pulmonary fibrosis (IPF) (17%), sarcoidosis (2.6%), lymphangiomyomatosis (1.1%) or secondary to collagen vascular disease, eosinophilic granulomatoses, histiocytosis, and so on (approximately 2%). Patients with diseases that destruct the pulmonary parenchyma:
  - Have reduced gas exchange apparatus, are difficult to ventilate, and are prone to hypoxia and hypercarbia.

- Have a small chest cavity, making surgical dissection difficult; hemodynamic tolerance to mediastinal manipulation may be particularly poor.

Preoperative Recipient Management

Transplant recipients should continue to take medications that optimize their overall condition until surgery.

- Patients responsive to bronchodilators should use these medications before the transplantation; patients with copious secretions should undergo chest physiotherapy (in case of cystic fibrosis).
- Patients should continue chronic oxygen therapy or noninvasive ventilation.
- Patients taking antiarrhythmic, antihypertensive, or pulmonary vasodilator medication should continue to do so. Of note, continuous pulmonary vasodilator therapy such as intravenous prostaglandin PGI_2, epoprostenol (Flolan) or inhaled nitric oxide should be maintained until the patient is on CPB to avoid catastrophic increases in PA pressure.
- Many patients with chronic lung disease are taking medication for gastroesophageal reflux, H_2 blockers, proton pump inhibitors, and gastric prepulsant; medication which should be continued. Many transplant recipients should have eaten in the 8 hours before the surgery and should be considered to have full stomachs. Antacid prophylaxis may be beneficial.
- Routine sedative premedication is not recommended; judicious monitored sedation may be used in the operating room.

Monitors/Lines

- Five-lead ECG, noninvasive blood pressure cuff, pulse oximeter, nasopharyngeal temperature probe, and urine catheter are required.
- Large-bore intravenous access is required. An arterial line and PA catheter are both placed before induction in patients who are at extreme risk of hemodynamic instability on induction. The PA catheter is left in the pulmonary vasculature throughout the procedure whenever possible; surgeons should be reminded to palpate the PA for the presence of the Swan–Ganz catheter before clamping or stapling the artery.
- TEE is increasingly used to monitor right ventricular function, biventricular filling, and pulmonary venous blood flow.
- A forced air-warming blanket is used, and intravenous fluids are warmed.

Anesthetic Technique

- A true rapid sequence induction is not ideal because of the patient's overall condition; induction may be modified with the application of cricoid pressure. Induction with propofol, pentothal, midazolam, and ketamine have been used at the TGH in combination with narcotic analgesics, often 10 to 15 μg/kg of fentanyl or an equivalent dose of sufentanil. Centers outside Canada report successful use of etomidate for induction.

- Pancuronium is the most frequently used relaxant; the duration of surgery is typically 5 hours for single lung transplant (SLT) and 8 hours for bilateral lung transplant (BLT).
- Patients are ventilated with oxygen and air mixtures, but never with nitrous oxide, because nitrous oxide increases PVR and expands intravascular gas emboli, which may be entrapped in the graft. Inhaled isoflurane or sevoflurane are often used initially for maintenance of anesthesia, particularly during the early stages of surgery, however, they tend to be less well tolerated as patients become more hemodynamically unstable because of mediastinal manipulation and vasodilatory hypotension.
- A propofol infusion at a dosage of 50 μg/kg/minute is started, and it ensures amnesia (younger patients with cystic fibrosis are at particular risk for intraoperative awareness) and allows prompt extubation in the postoperative period if the patient's condition warrants. Supplemental narcotic analgesic (fentanyl, approximately 5 μg/kg) is administered every 2 to 3 hours as needed.
- Analgesia is an integral part of the anesthetic plan. Although preoperative epidural placement and use of short-acting balanced general anesthetic by infusion has been described to facilitate immediate postoperative extubation, routine practice at the TGH is to assess the allograft function and the stability of the patient immediately after the procedure and to proceed with epidural placement in suitable patients to facilitate extubation early during the stay in the intensive care unit (ICU).

The Role of Cardiopulmonary Bypass

- CPB is used at the TGH during lung transplantation not as a routine but when indicated; approximately 35% of cases require CPB for hemodynamic instability and for inability to oxygenate/ventilate. The need for CPB was anticipated in one third and was unanticipated in the remainder of patients. CPB is anticipated in patients with a reduced pulmonary vascular bed, PAH, and in those undergoing lobar lung transplantations. Patients with IPF also have an increased need for CPB support.
- When CPB is used, the patient is anticoagulated with heparin, 300 to 400 units/kg, for activated clotting time (ACT) >460.
- During CPB without heart surgery, the heart remains warm and beating, and no aortic cross clamp is required.
- During CPB, the heart is arrested and is moderately cooled when concomitant cardiac repair (atrial septal defect [ASD],ventricular septal defect [VSD]) is performed.

Advantages of CPB:
- Right side of the heart is unloaded (decreased afterload).
- The procedure provides greater hemodynamic stability in some patients.

Disadvantages of CPB:
- Obligate infusion of crystalloid.
- Heparinization with resultant bleeding from raw surfaces.
- RBC trauma (hemolysis) which is worse with long CPB.
- Coagulopathy caused by dilution, platelet dysfunction, and activation of fibrinolysis.
- Activation of complement, neutrophil activation, and systemic inflammatory response may contribute to allograft injury at reperfusion.

Ventilation

Separation of ventilation, usually through a double-lumen tube (DLT), is required in almost all cases (exception is SLT performed on CPB).

■ Patients with severe *obstructive airway disease* and *parenchymal lung disease* require:
  ● High peak airway pressures to maintain gas exchange. A high gas flow ventilator such as an ICU ventilator is frequently required.
  ● Patients may start with severe but compensated hypercapnia; pH is a better determinant of the inability to ventilate than $Paco_2$.
  ● Permissive hypercapnia that is usually well tolerated is required; progressive hypercarbia/acidosis (pH persistently <7.20 with hemodynamic instability) or hypoxia on one-lung ventilation (OLV) may require CPB.
■ Additionally, patients with *obstructive airway disease* may need:
  ● Increased expiratory time, to minimize gas trapping.
  ● Treatment of bronchospasm.
  ● Frequent suctioning of secretions (e.g., in case of cystic fibrosis and bronchiectasis).
■ Patients with *pulmonary vascular disease* require:
  ● Avoidance of hypoxemic and hypercapnic episodes, and, in severe pulmonary hypertension, one-lung ventilation is not attempted.
  ● Avoidance of atelectasis and excessive pulmonary distension—both increase PVR.

Significant Intraoperative Physiologic Events

■ Hypoxia is common during OLV (intrapulmonary shunt in the nonventilated lung) and improves considerably when contralateral PA is clamped.
■ A period of particular risk occurs immediately after reperfusion of the lung that is transplanted first: Ventilation may go preferentially to the compliant allograft, and perfusion is predominantly to the diseased native lung because the vasculature of the allograft is initially vasoconstricted. Differential ventilation may be helpful. In BLT, surgical clamping of the PA of the native lung may avoid CPB during OLV of the allograft.
■ Clamping of the native PA forces the CO through the new allograft and may worsen reperfusion syndrome, necessitating CPB. Inhaled NO may contribute to the avoidance of CPB in some cases.

Hemodynamic Management

■ Hemodynamic derangement commonly occurring during lung transplantation is systemic hypotension caused by mediastinal manipulation and vasodilatory hypotension, and right ventricular dysfunction caused by intermittent single-lung perfusion. Specific treatments are as follows:
  ● Systemic hypotension due to low SVR (vasodilatory hypotension) is treated with:
    ▲ Norepinephrine infusion IV started at a dosage of 0.05 μg/kg/minute and titrated to effect.
    ▲ Vasopressin 1 to 4 units/hour IV if blood pressure is not responsive to increasing doses of norepinephrine.

- Pulmonary hypertension is treated with vasodilators:
  - ▲ Inhaled NO (5 to 40 ppm) has largely supplanted nitroglycerin and nitroprusside for this purpose and has the advantage of selective pulmonary vasodilation.
  - ▲ Prostaglandin E_1 0.01 to 0.1 μg/kg/minute is used much less with NO; however, it may be helpful with NO in severe ischemia-reperfusion injury.
- RV failure is treated with inotropes:
  - ▲ Milrinone loading dose 50 μg/kg followed by 0.5 μg/kg/minute.
  - ▲ Dopamine, dobutamine, and epinephrine are titrated to effect.
- Poor perfusion of the lung may contribute to gas exchange abnormalities during the transplant and the postoperative period; if hypoxia occurs in the presence of hypotension, improving the hemodynamic profile may result in improved gas exchange.
- Arrhythmias are common; the onset of sustained atrial fibrillation during surgical manipulation is usually poorly tolerated, requiring cardioversion. Nonsustained ventricular tachycardia is frequently observed, and sustained ventricular tachycardia is usually a result of acute electrolyte abnormalities or systemic air embolism from the allograft released after anastomosis of pulmonary veins to the left atrium and should be treated aggressively. During prolonged surgery with hypercapnic acidosis and decreased urine output, insidious, progressive hyperkalemia should be treated with glucose, insulin, and calcium. Magnesium supplementation may limit some arrhythmias, and, additionally, calcineurin inhibitors are magnesium wasting.

Hematology and Fluid Management

- In principle, it is desirable to keep transplant recipients "dry" to minimize pulmonary edema in a newly reperfused allograft. However, fluid underreplacement contributes to hemodynamic instability during mediastinal manipulation. The fluid balance may be several liters positive despite clinical euvolemia. Third space loss is likely to diffuse because of a systemic inflammatory response to surgery and transplant.
- Recent review of blood loss and transfusion requirement at the TGH has revealed that recipient pulmonary pathology was not a reliable predictor of intraoperative blood loss, which ranged from 300 mL to >10 L. Sixty-six percent of patients received RBC transfusion, with a mean of 2.4 ± 3.0 units transfused, with a range of 0 to 24 units to maintain a target hematocrit of 0.25. Additionally, 25% of patients received intraoperative FFP (mean 4.4 ± 3.0 units), and 16% received platelets (mean 6.5 ± 2.9 units).
- Patients who required CPB received aprotinin: 2×10^6 units before CPB, 2×10^6 units in the CPB circuit, and an infusion of 0.5×10^6 units/hour after CPB. It is unclear whether antifibrinolytic therapy in recipients who do not need CPB is beneficial (by anti-inflammatory action) or is potentially detrimental (intravascular thrombosis occurs in primary graft failure).

Antibiotics

- Patients with colonization of the respiratory tract with multiresistant bacteria (as is the case in cystic fibrosis and bronchiectasis) receive a predetermined antibiotic regiment to cover known pathogens.

- Other patients receive a second-generation cephalosporin (e.g., cefuroxime 1.5 g IV) prophylaxis against organisms normally colonizing in the respiratory tract.

Postoperative Care

Early extubation is dependent on allograft function, the patient's overall condition, and on a reversible general anesthetic technique and adequate analgesia.

- Ischemia-reperfusion injury is a common cause of early allograft dysfunction, manifest as impaired gas exchange, decreased pulmonary compliance, and noncardiogenic pulmonary edema. Radiologic findings include reticular interstitial disease and air space disease, frequently asymmetric, the first transplanted lung being worse. Treatment is supportive mechanical ventilation with increased positive end expiratory pressure (PEEP). Inhaled NO used prophylactically at reperfusion has been shown not to decrease the incidence of injury in humans.
- Immunologically mediated injury presents and worsens several hours after the operative period. Together, ischemia-reperfusion and immunologic injury comprise primary graft dysfunction, which compromises oxygenation. Mild injury is common; the incidence of severe life-threatening disease is approximately 15%. Treatment includes ventilatory and hemodynamic support using the same principles as during the operation. Immunologic injury may respond to plasmapheresis. In patients with life-threatening primary graft dysfunction, extracorporeal oxygenation (ECMO) may temporarily support oxygenation to permit some graft recovery.
- Other aspects of patient condition that influence the timing of extubation include the absence of ongoing hemorrhage, the resolution of upper airway edema that may occur during prolonged surgery, and the maintenance of adequate ventilation, particularly in patients who were severely hypercapnic before surgery and, therefore, more prone to carbon dioxide (CO_2) narcosis.

HEART–LUNG TRANSPLANTATION

Heart–lung transplantation is offered to suitable patients with both end-stage cardiac and pulmonary disease, including patients with heart disease and irreversible pulmonary hypertension. Care for these patients incorporates the many considerations for heart transplantation (the denervated heart) and lung transplantation (reperfusion syndrome). Ventilation occurs through a single-lumen endotracheal tube, which may need to be pulled back during the tracheal anastomosis.

IMMUNOLOGIC CONSIDERATIONS FOR INTRATHORACIC TRANSPLANTATION

- Human leukocyte antigen (HLA) matching is not performed in heart and lung transplantation because of the effort to minimize ischemic periods and small donor and recipient numbers. Often, donor/recipient crossmatches are available only postoperatively. The presence of recipient preformed antibodies against the donor is the cause of acute allograft failure due to hyperacute rejection. A positive crossmatch may not always be present. Urgent plasmapheresis is an established treatment in cardiac transplantation and is increasingly used in lung transplantation for abrupt allograft deterioration of unknown etiology.

■ Prophylactic perioperative plasmapheresis may be used in patients with known increased T-cell panel reactive antibody (PRA) and can be accomplished during CPB, or perioperatively using a dialysis catheter. Recipient plasma should be replaced with autologous FFP rather than albumin to avoid dilutional coagulopathy.

■ Triple immunosuppression with cyclosporin, azathioprine, and steroids ushered the modern era of transplantation 25 years ago. Transplant drug regimens continue to be based on the same suppressive principle—the targeting of T-cell activation and clonal expansion.

  ● Calcineurin inhibitors, cyclosporin and tacrolimus, inhibit T-cell interleukin-2 production.

  ● Antiproliferative agents, azathioprine and mycophenolate mofetil, inhibit Deoxyribo nucleic acid (DNA) synthesis, thereby preventing the proliferation of all activated T and B cells.

  ● Corticosteroids are nonspecific anti-inflammatory agents, and they inhibit cytokine production by T cells and macrophages.

■ Induction immunosuppression involves the additional administration of potent anti–T-cell antibody preparations: either polyclonal antilymphocyte antibodies (antithymocyte globulin), monoclonal anti-CD3 antibodies (OKT3), or interleukin-2 receptor blockade (basiliximab).

Perioperative regimen for heart transplantation at the Toronto General Hospital:
■ Methylprednisolone 1 g IV on induction, 500 mg on cross clamp removal.
■ Mycophenolate mofetil 1 g IV on induction.
■ Thymoglobulin 75 mg or basiliximab 20 mg after CPB.

Postoperatively:
■ Cyclosporine PO adjusted to peak (C2) levels of 1,200 ng/mL, trough levels of 300 to 400 ng/mL.
■ Mycophenolate mofetil 1 to 1.5 g IV/PO bid.
■ Methylprednisolone 0.25 mg/kg q6h for 48 hours; prednisone 0.5 mg/kg/day in a tapering dose, achieving 0.1 mg/kg/day by 6 months.

Perioperative regimen for lung transplantation at the Toronto General Hospital:
■ Cyclosporine 5 mg/kg PO immediately before surgery.
■ Methylprednisolone 1 g IV on induction.

Postoperatively:
■ Cyclosporine 5 mg/kg/day PO to achieve level 250 to 300 ng/mL.
■ Prednisone 0.5 mg/kg/day PO.
■ Azathioprine 1.5 to 2.0 mg/kg/day PO.

SPECIFIC CHALLENGES IN TRANSPLANTATION

Transplantation is a relatively new field of medicine and is constantly evolving. Randomized, controlled trials are hampered by the small number of cases in most centers and differences in regional practice for both donor and recipient management. The area of greatest variation is in lung transplantation: the choice of operation, SLT versus DLT or HLT, and use of CPB. Allograft function is affected by organ preservation, mechanical injury, and immunologic effects. Most trials have involved immunomodulation and choice of immunosuppression; to date no aspect of perioperative anesthetic care has been unequivocally established to prolong allograft and, therefore, patient survival.

SUGGESTED READINGS

Cheng DCH, Day F. Heart transplantation and subsequent non-cardiac surgery. In: Fun-Sun Y, ed. *Anesthesiology, problem-oriented patient management*. 5th ed. Philadelphia, PA: Lippincott Williams & Wilkins; 2003:409–423.

Marczin N, Royston D, Yacoub M, et al. Pro: Lung transplantation should be routinely performed with cardiopulmonary bypass. *J Cardiothorac Vasc Anesth.* 2000;14:739–745.

McRae K. Anesthesia for pulmonary transplantation. *Curr Opin Anesthesiol.* 2000;13:53–59.

McRae K. Con: Lung transplantation should be routinely performed with cardiopulmonary bypass. *J Cardiothorac Basc Anesth.* 2000;14:746–750.

Meade MO, Granton JT, Matte-Martyn A, et al. A randomized trial of inhaled nitric oxide to prevent ischemia-reperfusion injury after lung transplantation. *Am J Respir Crit Care Med.* 2003; 167:1483–1489.

Myles PS. Pulmonary transplantation. In: Kaplan JA, Slinger PD, eds. *Thoracic anesthesia.* 3rd ed. Philadelphia, PA: Harcourt Inc; 2003:295–314.

Rajek A, Pernerstorfer T, Kastner J, et al. Inhaled nitric oxide reduces pulmonary vascular resistance more than prostaglandin E(1) during heart transplantation. *Anesth Analg.* 2000;90:523–530.

Chapter 8

Anesthesia for Patients with Ventricular Assist Devices

Jacek M. Karski

Heart disease is one of the leading causes of death in Canada and the United States. Approximately 18,000 patients could benefit from heart transplantation, but in 2002, only 2,400 transplantations were performed in these countries. A lack of donors has kept the number of transplantations low over the last few years. New developments in temporary and permanent left ventricular and biventricular support devices (left ventricle assist device [LVAD], biventricle assist device [BIVAD]) have increased their use in patients with end-stage heart failure (ESHF). The growing number of LVAD implantation procedures and longer survival of the patient with these devices (1-year survival—52%—versus medical therapy—25%) presents new challenges for anesthesiologists and medical teams taking care of these patients.

INDICATION FOR USE OF LEFT VENTRICLE ASSIST DEVICE

- Emergency:
  - Patients who cannot be weaned from cardiopulmonary bypass (CPB) (although semi-implantable/pericorporeal devices may be more effective for patient stabilization before LVAD placement).
  - Patients with heart failure in whom acute decompensation does not respond to medical therapy.
  - Acute heart failure due to myocarditis.

- Scheduled:
  - Candidates who have not had a transplantation (i.e., >65 years or relative contraindications to transplantation such as amyloidosis or severe diabetes).
  - Candidates undergoing heart transplantation who are too ill to survive the waiting period for cardiac transplantation (patients with blood type O or positive reactive antibody titer).

CONTRAINDICATION TO LEFT VENTRICLE ASSIST DEVICE/BIVENTRICLE ASSIST DEVICE IMPLANTATION

- Severe aortic sclerosis.
- Severe obstructive or restrictive pulmonary disease (forced expiratory volume in 1 second [FEV_1] <30% predicted).
- Recent pulmonary embolism with infarction.
- Fixed pulmonary hypertension (pulmonary vascular resistance >8 Woods units).
- Acute anuric renal failure.
- Severe liver disease with coma or coagulopathy.
- Severe gastrointestinal malabsorption.
- Bleeding ulcer disease.
- Sepsis.
- Long-term high dose steroid therapy.
- Metastatic terminal cancer.
- Body surface area <1.5 m^2.

TYPES OF LEFT VENTRICLE ASSIST DEVICES

- Counter pulsation.
  - Intra-aortic balloon pump (IABP).
- Extracorporeal kinetic displacement: Various centrifugal devices commonly used in CPB machine can be used for temporary left or right ventricular support with or without an oxygenator. Their use is limited to a few days because of the necessity of full heparinization and destruction of platelets and red blood cells.
- Pulsatile pumps: These are the second-generation of LVADs. These pumps all provide pulsatile flow and are able to sustain full cardiac output of 4 to 6 L/minute. They can be divided into two categories:
  1. Extracorporeal: Extracorporeal pumps provide short to medium (30 days) support for left, right, or both ventricles in case of acute ventricular failure. They require long-term systemic anticoagulation with heparin. The ABIOMED BVS 500 (ABIOMED, Inc., Danvers, Massachusetts) and Thoratec (Thoratec Corporation, Pleasanton, California) are examples. ABIOMED can be used as single ventricle or biventricular support device. Thoratec is a biventricular device, which can be used for longer periods in small-sized (<1.6 m^2) patients.
  2. Implantable: Implantable pulsatile LVADs, including Novacor (World Heart Corporation, Oakland, California) and a pneumatic and vented electric HeartMates (Thoratec Corporation, Pleasanton, California) are implanted in the abdomen.

Blood is taken from the apex of the LV and returned by the pump to the patient's aorta using a flexible graft. Both LVADs contain two one-way cardiac tissue valves and drive lines exiting through the patient's skin. Implantable LVADs can be used as a bridge to transplantation or as a destination treatment of end-stage left ventricular failure (LVF).

- Nonpulsatile pumps: Electrically powered, the newest LVADS produce axial nonpulsatile flow. The Jarvik 2000 (Jarvik Heart, Inc., New York, New York) is an intraventricular device and the DeBakey VAD (MicroMed, Inc., Houston, Texas) is an extra cardiac support device. They can support the failing heart or provide full cardiac output.

LEFT VENTRICLE ASSIST DEVICE PERIOPERATIVE CONSIDERATIONS

- Preoperative evaluation: Temporary LVADs are implanted if it is not possible to separate the patient from CPB in the operating room on an emergency basis. However, most LVADs are implanted in scheduled operations and require careful preparation of the patient for surgery. The cardiologist in the coronary care unit (CCU) usually stabilizes and prepares the patient for the surgery. The anesthesiologist's visit will be a part of routine patient assessment before cardiac surgery. Some of the patients will have invasive monitoring instituted in the CCU and will be supported with inotropes, vasopressors, and IABP. Recent laboratory results and assessment of the physical status of patients are mandatory. Patients should be cross-matched for 4 units of blood.

- Anesthesia: Invasive monitoring (if not *in situ*) should be instituted before induction to anesthesia. Routine cardiac drugs are also prepared. Induction should be performed in a manner that will not depress myocardial function and does not produce vasodilatation because these patients have fixed limited cardiac output. Any drop in systemic blood pressures and cardiac output should be treated promptly to prevent injury to the end organs.

    Separation from CPB requires adequate volume loading of LVAD and pharmacologic support of the right ventricle (RV) (LVAD flow is volume dependent). Maintaining adequate preload is also necessary to prevent low cardiac output (below 3 L/minute to prevent risk of LVAD thrombosis). Nitric oxide can be used to reduce pulmonary vascular resistance and to support the RV. Not infrequently, patients with good RV function will require control of hypertension in the postoperative period. Usually, the most serious problem is postoperative bleeding, and this needs to be addressed in the manner described in Chapter 17. Patients are prophylactically treated with a high dose of aprotinin infusion or a high dose of tranexamic acid.

- Transesophageal echocardiography (TEE): Use of TEE preoperatively and postoperatively is necessary to evaluate the intra-atrial septum for atrial septal defect (ASD) or patent foramen ovale (PFO) because after left ventricular decompression by LVAD, any shunt will be directed from the right to the left side, thereby inducing hypoxia. Also, aortic valve evaluation is important to exclude major aortic valve insufficiency that prevents proper functioning of LVAD. After surgery, the position of the cannulas and de-airing are assessed, and emptying of the LV is monitored by TEE. RV filling and function can also be monitored.

- Postoperative period: Insertion of the LVAD that is functioning properly will usually require a few days of patient stay in the intensive care unit to stabilize the patient homodynamically. RV arrhythmias are poorly tolerated and some centers pretreat the patients with amiodarone to prevent their occurrence. External massage of the heart is not an option in treatment of cardiac arrest in these patients. The question for the need of anticoagulation is still open, but most centers do not use warfarin in patients with LVADs. In the long-term, improvement in the end-organ function is seen. Remodeling of the left ventricle can follow and in some cases will result in return of proper LV function and explantation of the LVAD device. Most commonly, the patient will proceed to heart transplantation or will be discharged home with the device as a destination therapy.

COMPLICATIONS OF LEFT VENTRICLE ASSIST DEVICE IMPLANTATION

- Early complications:
  - RV failure.
  - Air embolization.
  - Bleeding.
  - Kinking of the cannulas.
  - Arrhythmias.
  - Stroke.

- Late complications:
  - Infections (fungal and bacteria).
  - Thrombosis, embolization.
  - Electrical failure of LVAD.
  - Mechanical failure of the LVAD valves.

ANESTHESIA FOR PATIENT WITH LEFT VENTRICLE ASSIST DEVICE FOR REDO OR NONCARDIAC SURGERY

Most of the experience in this new field has been gained during induction of patients with LVAD for heart transplantation. There is not much experience in anesthetizing patients with LVADs for noncardiac surgery. Logically, the principles of monitoring, anesthesia, and maintenance of hemodynamic stability in these patients are the same as during the recovery phase of device implantation. TEE monitoring of RV function and preload may be useful. Strict adherence to sterility and use of prophylactic antibiotics is mandatory. The presence of staff who are familiar with the technical aspects of the functioning of the console and LVAD device and the presence of backup equipment are mandatory. Placement of adhesive defibrillator pads will facilitate defibrillation or cardioversion without bridging sterility of the operating field. Postoperative care in cardiovascular intensive care will provide additional safety for patients with LVAD who are undergoing noncardiac surgery.

SUMMARY

In the future, an increased number of patients will benefit from LVAD implantation as a bridge to recovery or transplantation, or as a destination therapy for ESHF. LVAD implantation has been proven to be a better treatment of ESHF and improves the patient's quality of life, thereby reducing the cost of medical care of these patients. A limited number of donors will necessitate the future development of LVADs as the destination therapy for patients with ESHF.

SUGGESTED READINGS

Heath M, Dickestein M. Perioperative management of the left ventricular assist device recipient. *Prog Cardiovasc Dis.* 2000;43:47–54.

Mason V, Konicki A. Left ventricular assist devices as destination therapy. AACN Clin Issues. 2003;14:488–497.

Mets B. Anesthesia for left ventricular assist device placement. *J Cardiothorac Vasc Anesth.* 2000; 14(3):316–326.

Radovancevic B, Vrtovec B, Frazier O. Left ventricular assist devices: an alternative to medical therapy for end-stage heart failure. *Curr Opin Cardiol.* 2003;18:210–214.

Stone ME, Soong W, Krol M, et al. The anesthetic considerations in patients with ventricular assist devices presenting for noncardiac surgery. *Anesth Analg.* 2002;95:42–49.

Chapter 9

Anesthesia and Congenital Heart Disease

Helen M. K. Holtby

Congenital heart disease (CHD) is one of the more frequent birth defects with an occurrence of approximately 8 per 1,000 live births (not counting patent ductus arteriosus [PDA] or bicuspid aortic valve).

- Common lesions:
  - Ventricular septal defect (VSD).
  - Atrial septal defect (ASD).
  - Tetralogy of Fallot (TOF).
  - Pulmonary stenosis (PS).
- CHD has a diverse etiology with genetic (e.g., chromosomal abnormalities and syndromes), environmental (e.g., infections and toxins), and maternal factors (e.g., diabetes).
- Associated extracardiac anomalies occur in 25% of affected infants.
- Lesions can be broadly categorized:
  - Shunt (e.g., ASD, VSD).
  - Obstruction (e.g., PS).
  - Complex (e.g., TOF, transposition of the great arteries [TGA]).
- The pathophysiology of CHD is highly diverse, complex, and varies with age; therefore, the management also varies. PDA is a "simple" lesion, yet its management varies with the age of the patient:
  - Premature infant: surgical ligation by thoracotomy.
  - Older child or adult with a small PDA: transvenous device closure in the cardiac catheterization laboratory treated as a day case.

- Older child or adult with a large PDA: pulmonary hypertension is a major risk factor and/or cardiopulmonary bypass (CPB) *may* be required.
- There is now a significant cohort of adults with palliated or repaired CHD.
- The anatomy should be determined, the pathophysiology should be worked out, the psychology of the patient must be analyzed (e.g., teens and compliance, parental anxiety) and an anesthetic plan developed.

PATHOPHYSIOLOGY

- The pulmonary circulation and right ventricle (RV) are very important in CHD.
- RV hypertrophy and RV failure are much more common; however, isolated left ventricular (LV) failure is relatively rare.
- Right-to-left (R-L) shunts, complete mixing, or inadequate pulmonary blood flow result in cyanosis (e.g., TOF, TGA, and pulmonary atresia). R-L shunts may cause:
  - Polycythemia.
  - Coagulation abnormalities.
  - Development of collaterals.
  - Risk of stroke.
- Left-to right (L-R) shunts cause congestive heart failure (CHF) (e.g., ASD, VSD, endocardial cushion defects). L-R shunts may also cause:
  - Pulmonary congestion and frequent chest infections.
  - Increased pulmonary vascular resistance (PVR).
  - LV volume overload.
  - Malnutrition and failure to thrive (FTT).
  - Anemia.
  - Pulmonary hypertension.
- Obstructive lesions cause ventricular hypertrophy and diastolic dysfunction.
  - Global subendocardial ischemia is often not recognized in children.
- Complex lesions have variable pathophysiology.
  - Single ventricle: cyanosis, coronary ischemia, and volume overload.
  - Pulmonary atresia and intact ventricular septum: RV-dependent coronary circulation.
  - Obstructed total anomalous pulmonary venous drainage: pulmonary edema and pulmonary hypertension.
- Cardiopulmonary interactions can be significant.
  - Positive pressure ventilation markedly *reduces* cardiac output (CO) and leads to RV failure.
  - Positive pressure ventilation is *therapeutic* for LV failure.
- Hemodynamic management should be tailored to the specific diagnosis (see Table 9-1).

Repaired Congenital Heart Disease

- Most children are repaired or palliated within the first 3 years of life.
  - 30% are repaired as neonates, 50% within the first year of life.

▌**TABLE 9-1 Synopsis of Common Congenital Heart Disease**

Anatomy	Prevalence (% CHD)	Pathophysiology	Treatment	Other
ASD Primum Secundum Sinus venosus	7% 1:2 M:F	L-R atrial shunt RV volume loaded High PA pressure in adults	Transcatheter device closure Surgical closure	Low risk of endo-carditis No prophylaxis 6 mo after closure
VSD Perimembranous Muscular Subarterial Juxtatricuspid	20%–50%	Restrictive: Biventricular volume load Unrestrictive: RV volume and pressure load CHF and FTT PVR is high Eisenmenger syndrome	Transcatheter device closure Surgical closure of defects >80% aortic valve size at <1 y 50% of small defects close spontaneously	Late outflow tract obstruction, AI Heart block (RBBB) Pulmonary hypertension
PS Critical PS Valve Supravalve	10% 80% typical 20% dysplastic	Neonates: RVH, cyanosis, tricuspid anomalies Patients >2 y RV/PA >50 mm Hg	PGE$_1$ and balloon dilation BT shunt Balloon dilation Surgical treatment	Preload dependent, stiff RV with diastolic dysfunction RV infarction RV hypertrophy
TOF VSD, PS, aortic override, RVH	6% 25% with associated anomalies	Displaced infundibu-lar septum: RVH, R-L shunt	Primary repair in infancy Pulmonary insufficiency postoperatively Arrhythmias Late sudden death	Treatment of hyper-cyanotic spells involves β-blocker, O$_2$, and phenylephrine Stiff RV with diastolic dysfunction or dilat-ed RV with PI
DTGA	4% 2:1 M:F	Preoperative mixing via ASD or VSD usually hemodynamically stable.	PGE$_1$+balloon sep-tostomy then primary repair as neonate	Late PS Sudden death from coronary artery events

CHD, congenital heart disease; ASD, atrial septal defect; M:F, male-to-female; L-R, left-to-right; RV, right ventri-cle; PA, pulmonary artery; VSD, ventricular septal defect; CHF, congestive heart failure; FTT, failure to thrive; PVR; pulmonary vascular resistance; RBBB, right bundle branch block; PS, pulmonary stenosis; BT, Blalock-Taussig; TOF, Tetralogy of Fallot; RVH, right ventricular hypertrophy; PGE$_1$, prostaglandin E$_1$; DTGA, D-transpo-sition of the great arteries; PI, pulmonary incompetence.

- Note that only ASD II, simple VSD, and PDA are "cured"—all other lesions have some residua even if minor (e.g., risk of endocarditis).
- Common problems after repair:
  - Ventricular dysfunction.
  - Arrhythmias (usually supraventricular).
  - Heart block.
  - Residual lesions.
  - Respiratory complications.
  - Neurologic deficit.

Palliated Congenital Heart Disease

- The American Society of Anesthesiology (ASA) and the New York Heart Association (NYHA) classification of physical status is the best guide to anesthetic risk.
- The most common major palliative procedure is Fontan, which is the final procedure for most single ventricle lesions.
- Single ventricle palliation:
  - Hypoplastic left heart syndrome (HLHS) is the archetype (but other complex CHD can be similar).
  - PDA or shunt to the pulmonary arteries (PA) *plus* unrestrictive ASD is imperative along with no outflow obstruction (i.e., Norwood operation).
  - It is important to keep PVR relatively high to avoid coronary ischemia, heart failure, and inadequate systemic perfusion.
  - O_2 delivery depends on CO *and* balance between systemic vascular resistance (SVR) and PVR.
  - Saturation alone is a poor guide to shunt flow (Qp/Qs).
  - These babies are at risk of sudden death.
- Bidirectional cavopulmonary shunt (bidirectional Glenn):
  - This procedure provides interim palliation as part of staged approach to Fontan.
  - Superior vena cava (SVC) is implanted into the PA and a Blalock-Taussig (BT) shunt is ligated.
  - This procedure reduces volume load on a single ventricle and *may* improve oxygenation.
  - It is increasingly used to prepare patients for a transcatheter Fontan procedure.
- Fontan procedure:
  - Superior and inferior vena cava (IVC) are directly connected to the PA using a variety of techniques; there is no pumping chamber to the PA.
  - CO depends on:
    - ▲ Preload.
    - ▲ Low PVR and normal pulmonary vasculature.
    - ▲ Good ventricular function.
    - ▲ Absence of outflow tract obstruction.
    - ▲ Absence of atrioventricular (AV) valve regurgitation.
    - ▲ Spontaneous ventilation or at least low intrathoracic pressures.
    - ▲ Sinus rhythm (risk of atrial arrhythmias increases over time).

The anesthetic management of any procedure in these patients must be planned with these considerations in mind.

PREOPERATIVE ASSESSMENT AND PREPARATION FOR PROCEDURES REQUIRING CARDIOPULMONARY BYPASS

Assessment

- Most patients are assessed through a history, physical examination, electrocardiogram (ECG), and transthoracic echocardiography.
  - Sedation/sleep is required for many children for diagnostic studies.
  - Transesophageal echocardiography (TEE) in small patients (<20 kg) needs general endotracheal anesthesia (big probe, small airway).
- Cardiac catheterization is required in select cases only:
  - Hemodynamic evaluation (e.g., before cavopulmonary shunt or Fontan).
  - Transcatheter intervention (>50% cases involved intervention in 2004).
- Magnetic resonance imaging (MRI) and computerized tomography have growing roles in defining anatomy and physiology.
- Infants and children need sedation or general anesthesia for investigations and catheterization; adolescents also need sedation or general anesthesia for electrophysiologic studies.
- Anesthetic considerations for diagnostic procedures.
  - All the usual patient considerations apply (e.g., neonates, other anomalies, psychosocial issues, fasting interval).
  - "Sedation" is *in no way* safer than general anesthesia.
  - All anesthetic drugs have hemodynamic effects.
  - Blood must be made immediately available during interventional cardiac catheterization.
    - ▲ Hemodynamic instability is common but usually transient.
    - ▲ Overall risk of death is <0.05%, but there is a 5% risk of serious complications if the patient is <14 months old (7 deaths per 5,000 cases in 1998 series).
  - An MRI is usually done in a remote site, monitoring is difficult, and apnea is sometimes needed for specific images.
  - Keeping small patients (<10 kg) warm can be difficult.

Preoperative Preparation

- Neonates are usually inpatients; many infants and older children may be admitted on the day of surgery.
- PDA-dependent lesions (e.g., HLHS, critical PS, coarctation) are maintained on prostaglandin E_1 (PGE_1) 0.03 to 0.1 μ/kg/minute.
- Immediate preoperative evaluation includes physical examination to rule out intercurrent illness, chest x-ray (CXR), ECG, blood count, electrolyte levels, and coagulation screen.
- Other tests done on an individual basis are chromosomal analysis for T21 or DiGeorge, renal function in VACTERL, thyroid function testing, and so on.

- The physician should discuss fasting and fluid intake, anesthetic plan, premedication, monitoring, special techniques, and blood transfusion with parents and children.
- Cardiac drugs should be continued up to surgery, with the exception of digoxin and acetyl salicylic acid (ASA).
  - The physician should be aware of drug interactions especially with drugs that reduce afterload.
- Routine fasting:
  - 6 to 8 hours for solids and formula.
  - 4 hours for breast milk.
  - 2 hours for clear fluids.
- Age-appropriate conversation with a child is important.
  - Children 4 years and older need a "special nap," the mask needs to be shown to them, and cooperation with premedication is necessary.
  - Older children may prefer or dislike either the mask or needles and might have more detailed questions.
  - Adolescents often need reassurance about awareness, pain management, and survival.
- Be aware of the different laws and cultural beliefs around consent (e.g., there is no age of consent in Ontario). Competent individuals should give their own consent.
- Clear communication between *everyone* involved (i.e., parents, patient, cardiologist, surgeon, anesthetist, and critical care staff) is imperative.
- Premedication should be given to every patient:
  - who is aware of the planned procedure.
  - who will be upset by separation from caregivers.
- Midazolam 0.5 to 0.75 mg/kg by mouth (PO) (to a maximum of 20 mg) has rapid onset of action (10 to 20 minutes), is safe, and is effective for infants and children.
- Lorazepam 0.1 mg/kg PO or sublingually given 60 minutes before the surgery is useful for adolescents and can be supplemented with midazolam.
- Intramuscular injections are to be avoided.

INTRAOPERATIVE MANAGEMENT

Patient Considerations

Neonates have unique physiology in every system.

- Cardiovascular:
  - Noncompliant ventricles with less contractile elements.
  - Neonatal myocardium tolerates hypoxia better.
  - Extracellular Ca^{2+} is important.
  - Prone to bradycardia (high vagal tone).
  - Have high PVR.
- Neurologic:
  - Immature blood–brain barrier and intracranial vasculature.
  - Loss of cerebral autoregulation in infants with birth asphyxia.
  - Intraventricular hemorrhage.
  - Seizures are a common manifestation of perioperative central nervous system (CNS) injury but are often difficult to diagnose clinically.

- Respiratory:
  - Minute ventilation and O_2 consumption are twice as high as adult values.
  - Anatomic differences in the upper airway mean obstruction is more likely and desaturation occurs rapidly.
  - Effect of complications (e.g., vocal cord palsy and phrenic nerve injury) is more profound.
- Hematologic:
  - Hemoglobin F is quantitatively and qualitatively different.
  - Coagulation system is maturing and so factor levels are different from adults.
  - Cyanotic CHD is associated with platelet abnormalities and coagulopathy.
  - Dilutional coagulopathy is common during major surgery and is inevitable during CPB.
  - Citrate toxicity is also common during platelet or fresh frozen plasma (FFP) transfusion.
- Metabolic:
  - Small babies (<10 kg) become hypothermic very quickly if exposed on an operating room (OR) table (see vascular access).
  - Plasma protein levels are generally reduced and total body water is increased.
  - Hypocalcemia, hypoglycemia, and hyponatremia are quite common in critically ill neonates.
  - Glucose levels goes up on bypass due to the inflammatory response.
  - The pharmacokinetics and pharmacodynamics of most drugs are profoundly different for multiple reasons.
  - Renal impairment is common.
  - Neonates demonstrate a marked inflammatory response to CPB.
- Technical:
  - Choice of appropriate equipment, suitable ventilation, and so on can be an issue: Custom CPB equipment has been available only since the 1990s.
  - Most anesthetic monitoring equipment defaults to adult settings.
  - Vascular access can be very difficult; cutdowns are more frequent in children but are also technically demanding and not ideal.

CARE OF CHILDREN UNDERGOING CARDIOPULMONARY BYPASS

- Induction:
  - The goal is to induce coma without psychological or cardiovascular collapse.
  - Careful inhalation or intravenous induction is generally well tolerated: no one technique is preferable.
  - Suitable approaches include the following:
    - ▲ Sevoflurane in oxygen/air has been shown to be safe in CHD.
    - ▲ Fifty percent nitrous oxide for intravenous placement followed by thiopentone or propofol (but propofol *hurts*) are administered. Nitrous oxide is discontinued after induction because of the risk of air embolism.
    - ▲ Fentanyl 30 μg/kg ($\pm$ 1 to 2 mg/kg thiopentone or ketamine) is used for the very frail (e.g., patients who are undergoing heart transplantation).

- Muscle relaxation with pancuronium bromide is routine.
- The use of vapor or benzodiazepines is necessary to avoid awareness.
- It is imperative to make sure that the airway is secure and that the child is ventilated appropriately for his or her lesion (e.g., HLHS; truncus arteriosus may need hypercarbia and low oxygen concentration, whereas TOF with spells may need high levels of oxygen).
- Hemodynamics and temperature during placement of lines should be monitored with care: it is easy to focus on the procedure and forget about the patient.
- Children with CHF often present with low circulating volume and may need bolus fluids.
- Vascular access has to be decided: At least two sites of reliable intravenous access (which may be central) are required for primary procedures, along with an arterial line and Foley catheter.
- Redo surgery needs at least two large (for the patient) catheters and three sites of intravenous access.
- There is no evidence that any one site (e.g., internal jugular versus subclavian, femoral versus radial artery) is preferable.
- Potential complications of monitoring lines should be borne in mind and vigilance should be exercised.
- Monitoring: routine monitoring plus urinary, arterial, and central venous pressure (CVP) catheters.
- The use of electroencephalography, transcranial Doppler (TCD) and near infrared spectroscopy (NIRS) is increasing.
- Emergency drugs:
  - ▲ Atropine 10 μg/kg.
  - ▲ Phenylephrine 0.5 to 2 μg/kg.
  - ▲ Epinephrine 1 μg/kg.
  - ▲ Calcium chloride 10 mg/kg.
- Positioning:
  - Position supine for median sternotomy.
  - Make sure that patients are well padded: procedures can be long and hypothermia/low perfusion adds to risk of skin breakdown.
  - Make sure that stopcocks and intravenous (IV) lines are accessible.
- Pre-CPB:
  - Adjuvant drugs:
    - ▲ Heparin 350 units/kg before bypass: in some centers it is given by the surgeons. Heparin effect by point-of-care testing is routine.
    - ▲ Antifibrinolytics have been shown to be useful in CHD: tranexamic acid 50 to 100 mg/kg or aprotonin 3 to 5 $\times$ 10^4 KIU/kg.
    - ▲ Antibiotics are useful for wound prophylaxis: cefazolin 40 mg/kg every 4 hours of surgery.
    - ▲ Steroids reduce inflammatory markers in infants; methylprednisolone 10 mg/kg three times given pre- and intraoperatively.
  - Cannulation:
    - ▲ Cannulation can be accompanied by major hemodynamic upset, bleeding, arrhythmias, and ECG changes and, therefore, it is necessary to pay close attention.

- ▲ Cannulation often triggers hypercyanotic episodes in TOF: esmolol infusion (100 to 300 μg/kg/minute) is useful, plus phenylephrine bolus 2 μg/kg.
- ▲ The sites most commonly cannulated are aorta, SVC, and IVC, but it can vary depending on the anatomy and the procedure.
- ▲ Be aware of the variation in pump prime constituents if transfusion is from the pump (e.g., low concentration of Ca^{2+}).

- ■ CPB:
  - • Priming volumes vary: for neonates the volumes are often two to three times the circulating volume but are less for older children.
    - ▲ Major physiologic upheaval.
    - ▲ Possibility of abrupt changes in electrolyte levels, especially in glucose and sodium levels.
    - ▲ Drug levels fall abruptly, so additional dosage is necessary and awareness is a concern.
    - ▲ Dilution of plasma proteins, including coagulation factors.
    - ▲ Inflammatory response.
  - • Blood prime is commonly utilized to avoid dilutional anemia. Some centers use heparinized whole blood; constituent therapy is most common.
  - • "Ideal" flow rates and perfusion pressures are not known. There is some evidence that mean arterial pressure (MAP) <25 mm Hg may result in no cerebral perfusion in neonates.
  - • Deep hypothermia and circulatory arrest (DHCA).
    - ▲ The patient is cooled to a temperature ranging from 18°C to 20°C.
    - ▲ Vasodilator therapy is needed: vapor, nitroprusside, or phenoxybenzamine.
    - ▲ Profound neuromuscular blockade is important.
    - ▲ Application of ice on the head is effective (protect the skin).
    - ▲ Methylprednisolone 30 mg/kg and thiopentone 5 mg/kg are administered for "neuroprotection."
    - ▲ Alpha-stat pH management and a minimum hematocrit (HCT) value of 0.30 are advocated.
    - ▲ All DHCA reduces neurodevelopment scores and increases the risk of seizures.
    - ▲ Antegrade cerebral perfusion may reduce neurologic injury and facilitate aortic arch repair.
  - • Flow is through the innominate artery at the rate of 30 to 50 mL/kg.
  - • Right radial arterial line, NIRS, and TCD are useful but not imperative.
- ■ Separation from CPB.
  - • Completion of repair is confirmed.
  - • Assess and correct acid-base and electrolyte abnormalities. Check HCT level.
  - • Assess coagulation.
    - ▲ Platelet count and fibrinogen level.
    - ▲ Blood products are available.
  - • Adequate ventilation and reasonable lung compliance are checked.
  - • If pulmonary hypertension is a concern, then hyperventilation with 100% oxygen to a P_{CO_2} 30 mm Hg is, and the maintenance of pH at 7.5 is then reassessed; patients must be warm and well oxygenated, with optimum positive end expiratory pressure (PEEP), and deeply anesthetized. Nitric oxide is occasionally required.

- Norwood procedure: Weaning from CPB starts with 100% oxygen and Pco_2 40 mm Hg, and the patient is then reassessed: usually, high PVR is present for the first few hours and hypoxia predominates.
- Vasoactive drugs are started if indicated:
  - ▲ Most neonates.
  - ▲ Preoperative CHF or poor function.
  - ▲ Long (>60 minutes) aortic cross-clamp.
  - ▲ Poor myocardial protection.
  - ▲ Ventricular hypertrophy.
  - ▲ Hyper- or hypotension.
- Drug doses:
  - ▲ Milrinone 100 μg/kg bolus given on bypass, followed by 0.33 to 1 μg/kg/min.
  - ▲ Dopamine or dobutamine 5 to 15 μg/kg/minute.
  - ▲ Epinephrine 0.01 to 1 μg/kg/minute.
  - ▲ Vasopressin 0.0001 to 0.001 units/kg/minute.
- The flow from the pump is reduced under supervision, venous drainage is clamped, and the patient is transfused from the pump. The following should be assessed:
  - ▲ Adequate preload: transfuse 5 mL/kg aliquots if blood pressure (BP)/CVP is reasonable.
  - ▲ Heart rhythm: or treat arrhythmia or heart block.
  - ▲ Heart is not distended: it is very easy to overload neonates.
  - ▲ Reasonable BP.
  - ▲ End tidal CO_2 ($Etco_2$) trace (ventilation *and* CO *and* PA flow).
  - ▲ Arterial oxygen saturation (Sao_2) (perfusion *and* oxygenation).
  - ▲ Bleeding: suture deficiency is difficult to treat with blood products.
  - ▲ TEE to assess adequacy of repair and assessment of function (NOT done by individual giving the anesthetic).
- ■ Modified ultrafiltration:
  - Many centers use modified ultrafiltration in patients <10 kg. It involves controlled withdrawal of blood from the aorta with reinfusion via an atrial cannula.
  - The blood is passed across a semipermeable membrane to remove water and smaller molecules: the process removes interleukins, cytokines, tumor necrosis factor, and other molecules.
  - It increases HCT and plasma protein concentration.
  - The process generally results in improved hemodynamics; there is some evidence of improved lung compliance.
- ■ Post-CPB:
  - Once the repair is deemed adequate, surgical bleeding is under some control and the hemodynamic status is reasonable.
  - Protamine 2 to 4 mg/kg is given to reverse heparinization.
  - Indications for blood transfusion are as follows:
    - ▲ Platelets are transfused if the count is <100,00/μL and in case of bleeding: 1 U platelets per 5 kg raises the platelet count to approximately 50,000, but this is variable.
    - ▲ FFP/cryoprecipitate is transfused if the fibrinogen level is <1.

- ▲ Packed red blood cells (PRBC) 3 mL/kg increase hemoglobin concentration by 10 g/L.
- Coagulopathy: The patient should be kept warm.
- DDAVP 0.3 units/kg is sometimes helpful.
- The use of tranexamic acid 50 mg/kg repeat bolus has been reported.
- There are isolated case reports of the use of recombinant factor VIIa for severe coagulopathy (90 μg/kg).
- Hemodynamics, mixed venous saturation, and lactate levels should be frequently evaluated.
- It is easy for children to either overheat or get cold:
  - ▲ Hyperthermia is detrimental to the CNS.
  - ▲ This condition predisposes the patient to atrial tachycardia.
  - ▲ Hypothermia to <35°C causes coagulopathy.
- Closure of the sternum can be associated with cardiac compression and decreased cardiac output.
- Transport of patients requires adequate personnel, similar hemodynamic monitoring to the OR, appropriate means of ventilation, intravenous fluid and blood products, and resuscitation capabilities.

CARE OF CHILDREN UNDERGOING CLOSED PROCEDURES

- PDA ligation:
  - This is usually indicated for a premature infant who is ventilator-dependent.
  - Primary anesthetic issues relate to prematurity.
  - The simplest technique is fentanyl 30 μg/kg, pancuronium 0.1 mg/kg, and 0.2% to 0.5% isoflurane.
  - Lactated Ringer solution with 5% dextrose solution is administered as needed for maintaining BP.
  - It is imperative that blood level is checked and is immediately available.
- Coarctation of the aorta:
  - Usually neonates are on PGE_1. Patients with coarctation combined with an intracardiac lesion (eg., coarctation plus VSD) will have the entire surgery with CPB.
  - Left thoracotomy is performed in case of left aortic arch.
  - Arterial line in right arm is ideal (definitely not in left arm).
  - The baby is cooled to 35°C before aortic cross-clamp to minimize the risk of spinal cord injury.
  - Heparin is given at a dose of 100 units/kg.
  - Proximal hypertension during cross-clamp is usually managed with vasodilators.
  - When the cross-clamp is removed, observe the patient for hypotension and bleeding; there is a risk of cerebral hypoperfusion if this is not promptly managed.
  - Catheter-based therapy is more common in older patients with recurrent coarctation.
  - Blood should be made immediately available.
- Blalock-Taussig (BT) shunt:
  - BT shunt is done to palliate complex CHD that is not amenable to early repair (e.g., pulmonary atresia with small pulmonary arteries).

- Arterial line with or without CVP for monitoring may be useful.
- Maintain patient on PGE_1 during surgery: patients can be very desaturated (and worse when the pulmonary artery is clamped).
- The surgery can be done by thoracotomy or sternotomy; CPB may be needed.
- Usually, a tube graft is placed from the innominate or subclavian to the right pulmonary artery (RPA).
- Heparin is given as a bolus 100 μ/kg and then as a continuous infusion for the first 24 hours.

POSTOPERATIVE CARE

- Major concerns in the first 24 hours are pain, bleeding, and low CO.
- Pain needs multimodal treatment with narcotic analgesics, acetaminophen, and nonsteroidal analgesics.
  - Infiltration with local anesthetics may be helpful.
  - Neuraxial anesthesia has been reported but is highly controversial.
- Arrhythmias should be aggressively managed because they are often poorly tolerated.
  - Ventricular arrhythmias are relatively rare.
  - Atrial arrhythmias can be very significant.
- The nadir of function is 6 to 12 hours postoperatively.
- Positive pressure ventilation has a major negative effect on CO in TOF and Fontan.
- The incidence of perioperative neurologic complications ranges from 5% to 30%.
- Most patients with straightforward lesions stay 1 to 3 days in the intensive care unit (ICU) and 3 to 7 days in the hospital (not neonates).
- Difficulties in feeding are the most common cause of delayed discharge.

ADULT CONGENITAL HEART DISEASE: A GROWTH INDUSTRY

It is recommended that adult patients with CHD be treated in a specialist center (Canadian Cardiovascular Society Consensus, 2001).

Incidence

- It is estimated that there are 800,000 patients in the United States, and this number is rising because there is increased success with repairs and palliation.
- There are now more adults than children with CHD. Adults present for a variety of procedures:
  - Complications of CHD and surgery.
  - Degenerative disease unrelated to CHD.
  - Pregnancy and childbirth.
- Late complications of cardiac surgery are:
  - Arrhythmias: patients present for pacemaker or maze procedures.
  - Ventricular failure (e.g., late Mustard repair: the RV is structurally flawed to support the systemic circulation).

- Conduit failure: calcification and stenosis.
- Coronary artery disease superimposed on CHD.
- Failed Fontan with obstruction, thrombosis, poor function, protein-losing enteropathy, plastic bronchitis, and cyanosis.

■ Anesthetic considerations:
  - Patients with cyanosis have specific considerations and complications.
  - Pulmonary hypertension is a major independent risk factor.
  - Cardiac/noncardiac surgery:
    ▲ For noncardiac surgery, ASA/NYHA status is a good guide to assess patient risk.
  - Obstetrics.
  - Other pathology (e.g., chronic obstructive pulmonary disease [COPD], obesity).
  - Redo sternotomy and collaterals: bleeding can be very significant especially in cyanosed patients.

SUGGESTED READINGS

Andropoulos DB, Stayer SA, Russell IA, eds. *Anesthesia for congenital heart disease*. Malden, MA: Blackwell-Futura Publishing Co.; 2004.

Bissonnette B, Dalens BJ, eds. *Pediatric anesthesia: principles and practice*. New York: McGraw-Hill; 2001.

Canadian Adult Congenital Heart Network, 2005. Available at: http://www.cachnet.org/. Accessed 2005.

Freedom RM, Yoo SJ, Mikailian H, et al., eds. *The natural and modified history of congenital heart disease*. New York: Blackwell-Futura Publishing Co.; 2004.

Nichols DG, Cameron DE, eds. *Critical heart disease in infants and children*. St. Louis, MO: Mosby–Year Book; 1995.

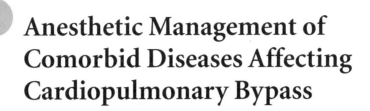

Anesthetic Management of Comorbid Diseases Affecting Cardiopulmonary Bypass

Neal H. Badner

This chapter presents a concise approach to the preoperative, intraoperative, and postoperative management of patients with comorbid diseases presenting for cardiopulmonary bypass (CPB).

DIABETES MELLITUS

The incidence of diabetes mellitus (DM) is steadily rising in North America, and it now affects approximately 2 million Canadians and 40 million Americans. It is a major risk factor for coronary artery disease and, therefore, is a common comorbidity in patients undergoing CPB.

- Most patients have type 2 DM. These patients produce insulin in insufficient quantities for normal control of glucose level. They are prone to develop hyperglycemia and potentially nonosmolar hypertonic coma.
- Less commonly, patients with type 1 DM can develop both hypo- or hyperglycemia, as well as diabetic ketoacidosis (DKA).

Preoperative Management

- Preoperative assessment should focus on the method of diabetic management, including diet, oral hypoglycemic agents, and any insulin requirements.

- Most patients with diabetes should keep a log of blood glucose measurements, and a review is warranted to determine how stable they have been.
- The goal from a preoperative perspective is to avoid hypoglycemia while fasting, and therefore, oral hypoglycemic agents are withheld on the day of surgery, while maintaining moderate glucose control, thereby avoiding hyperglycemia. For patients on insulin, who have a glucose level higher than 12 mmol/L or 200 mg/dL on the day of surgery, an intravenous (IV) infusion of dextrose-containing solution with regular Humulin (recombinant human insulin) is given, starting at 1 unit/hour (see Table 10-1). An alternative is to give IV dextrose combined with half of the normal insulin dose given in the morning. This approach is simpler but less responsive to changes in the glucose levels of the patient or the operating room schedules.

Intraoperative Management

- Long-term goals in diabetic management are to maintain as normal a glucose control as is possible to maintain renal and visual function.
- In general, when anesthetized, one is unaware of the warning symptoms of the impending hypoglycemia, and, therefore, the intraoperative management goals are loosened because undetected hypoglycemia can lead to cerebral ischemia.
- Intraoperative glucose control needs to be balanced with the knowledge that studies in nondiabetic patients undergoing neurosurgical procedures noted improved neurologic outcomes when hyperglycemia was avoided. Similar studies, however, in nondiabetic patients undergoing CPB have been unsuccessful in duplicating this finding.
- Lastly, studies have indicated that glucose–potassium–insulin infusions may improve cardiac function both in patients with and without diabetes by providing an energy substrate. This approach does have the potential of creating hyperglycemia.
- The accepted management, therefore, is to keep blood glucose levels lower than 12 mmol/L or 200 mg/dL. This requires repeated blood glucose sampling and insulin therapy given either as boluses or as an infusion (Table 10-1).
- Insulin requirements usually increase on CPB, especially if hypothermia is utilized because of decreased endogenous insulin secretion, and then will decrease following discontinuation of CPB.

▌ **TABLE 10-1** Insulin Sliding Scale as Boluses and Infusion

Glucose (mmol/L)	Glucose (mg/dL)	Insulin Bolus Dose (U)	Insulin Infusion Rate (Starting 1 U/h)
0–4	0–80	25 mL with 50% glucose	Stop insulin infusion
4–6	80–120	2	Decrease infusion rate by 0.25
6–10	120–180	4	No change
10–12	180–220	6	Increase infusion rate by 0.25
>12	>220	8	Increase infusion rate by 0.5

Postoperative Management

- The aim is to return the patients to their preoperative management as soon as possible.
- However, patients do not resume a normal diet immediately, and the stress response to surgery includes an endocrine surge, which increases blood glucose level through glycogenolysis and gluconeogenesis.
- Most patients will therefore need supplemental insulin for 48 hours (Table 10-1).
- Patients with diabetes are at increased risk for delayed wound healing and infection, the first sign of which may be insulin resistance.

CHRONIC RENAL FAILURE

The incidence of renal failure also continues to rise as a result of increasing incidences of diabetes and hypertension. Because diabetes and hypertension are both risk factors for coronary artery disease, an increasing number of patients (up to 5% of the adult population) with renal insufficiency (elevated creatinine levels higher than 2 mg/dL or 15 μmol/L due to <40% functioning nephrons), as well as chronic renal failure (presence of uremia due to <10% functioning nephrons), will be presenting for CPB.

Preoperative Management

- Detailed assessment of the patient's etiology of the renal failure, current renal function, method of dialysis (peritoneal or hemo), as well as secondary complications including anemia, hypertension, fluid, and electrolyte imbalances should be performed.
- Currently, most North American patients with renal failure receive recombinant erythropoietin, and anemia is therefore well controlled.
- Preoperative antihypertensive drugs should be continued on the day of surgery.
- Careful review of biochemical test results, including calcium, magnesium, and phosphate levels, is warranted.
- Efforts should be made to schedule hemodialysis the day before the surgery to optimize fluid and electrolyte balance.

Intraoperative Management

- Efforts to avoid utilizing drugs that require renal metabolism or excretion should be made. From an anesthetic perspective, this approach mostly involves the neuromuscular blockers pancuronium and, to a lesser extent, vecuronium and rocuronium; however, antibiotics and other medications may require renal excretion.
- CPB management requires attention to fluid and electrolytes. Excess fluid can be removed by hemofiltration or ultrafiltration. This process, whereby blood under pressure is passed through semipermeable hollow fibers, removes fluid and, passively, potassium with it.

- If, because of the large extent of cardioplegia, or other reasons, the potassium level becomes excessively high, hemodialysis can be performed in conjunction with CPB to actively lower the potassium level and remove wastes.

Postoperative Management

- Continued vigilance of fluid and electrolyte management is required.
- Extra hemodialysis or changes in peritoneal dialysis dialysates may be required until the patients return to their preoperative state and routine life.

SICKLE CELL DISEASE

Sickle cell disease is a genetic abnormality in the formation of the β chain of the hemoglobin molecule that occurs in the heterozygous form (sickle trait) in approximately 10% of the North American black population and in the homozygous form (sickle disease) in 0.25% of the same population. The abnormal hemoglobin (Hb S or Hb C) deforms when deoxygenated and leads to stasis. Patients with the sickle trait usually have small amounts of Hb S and require marked desaturation before the occurrence of sickling. Patients with the disease can have considerable amounts of Hb S or Hb C and can present with sickling crises or aplastic anemia.

Preoperative Management

- Determination of the presence of sickle cell disease is a simple test whereby a reducing agent is added to a blood sample.
- Quantification of the disease (i.e., trait versus disease and amount of Hb S/Hb C) requires hemoglobin electrophoresis.
- Presence of anemia usually indicates sickle cell disease unless another cause of anemia is also present.
- Past approaches to perioperative management advocated exchange transfusions to decrease Hb S/Hb C concentration to <40%; however, this approach has recently been discontinued for patients undergoing noncardiac surgery. Patients should consult a hematologist about the need to transfuse/exchange transfuse preoperatively on an individual basis.

Intraoperative Management

- Care should be undertaken to maintain normal temperature, hydration, and positioning to avoid blood stasis, thereby minimizing sickling.
- Red cell transfusion should be undertaken on the basis of normal CPB transfusion guidelines for patients with sickle cell trait and, in discussion with the consulting hematologist, for patients with sickle cell disease. The optimal intraoperative transfusion would be on an exchange basis during CPB using a circuit primed with blood. The removed blood can be centrifuged to allow the plasma with platelets and clotting factors to be returned.

- Although hypothermic CPB has been successfully utilized in patients with sickle cell disease, normothermic CPB is recommended.

Postoperative Management

- A continuation of the intraoperative approach is recommended postoperatively.

MALIGNANT HYPERTHERMIA

Malignant hyperthermia (MH), a rare autosomal disease of variable penetrance, is an abnormality of the skeletal muscle at the level of the sarcoplasmic reticulum whereby uncontrolled intracellular release of calcium occurs after the patient is exposed to succinylcholine or anesthetic vapors. This release of calcium causes sustained muscle contraction, and because the return of calcium to the sarcoplasmic reticulum is an energy-requiring process, this also leads to heat production (fever), hypoxemia, and hypercarbia. This process becomes futile and eventually leads to cell death with subsequent potassium release. If the process is not stopped, tachycardia, hypertension, arrhythmias, hyperkalemia, renal failure, and disseminated intravascular coagulation (DIC) can ensue. Dantrolene, a direct muscle inhibitor, blocks the calcium release. Diagnosis is made by a skeletal muscle biopsy and a halothane–caffeine contracture test.

Preoperative Management

- The key to management of MH is to obtain a thorough history to determine whether any abnormality occurred with the patient or a family member during previous anesthetic inductions.
- Ideally, muscle testing to confirm or exclude the diagnosis should be made preoperatively; however, because the biopsy technique leaves a major scar, many patients are reluctant to undergo the test.

Intraoperative Management

- The cornerstone of management of patients with MH is to avoid the triggering agents. This requires the use of either a specifically vapor-free machine or the flushing of a regular machine at high flows (>10 L/minute for at least 20 minutes) that also has a new circuit, hoses, a reservoir bag, and a CO_2 absorbent. Patients should also be scheduled as first case in the day in order to minimize exposure to trace amounts of vapor in the operating room (OR) air.
- Use of nondepolarizing neuromuscular blockers and propofol infusions with opioids provides a trigger-free anesthetic.
- Monitoring of both central and muscle (axilla) temperatures is recommended.
- An MH crisis is treated with IV dantrolene, in a dose of 2 to 3 mg/kg. This may require assistance because each 20-mg vial requires mixing with 60 mL sterile water. This dose may be repeated up to 10 mg/kg, if necessary, until the crisis is aborted.

■ Supportive therapy in terms of cooling, management of electrolyte imbalances (hyperkalemia), DIC, and maintaining urine output (dantrolene is provided with mannitol in the vial) is required.

■ Because patients undergoing CPB may have an unstable course because of the severity of their cardiovascular disease, one must maintain a higher index of suspicion of a crisis when patients have a known history and when they become unstable without an obvious cardiovascular cause.

Postoperative Management

■ Continued monitoring of temperature and suspicion of unexplained instability as evidence of a triggered MH crisis are warranted.

SUGGESTED READINGS

Gronert GA, Antognini JF, Pessah.IN. Malignant hyperthermia. In: Miller RD, ed. *Anesthesia*. Orlando, FL: Churchill Livingstone; 2000:1033–1050.
Lazar HL, Chipkin SR, Fitzgerald CA, et al. Tight glycemic control in diabetic coronary bypass graft patients improves perioperative outcomes and decreases recurrent ischemic events. *Circulation*. 2004;109:1497–1502.
Oliver WC, de Castro MA, Strickland RA. Uncommon diseases and cardiac anesthesia. In: Kaplan JA, Reich DL, Konstadt SN, eds. *Cardiac anesthesia*. Philadelphia, PA: WB Saunders; 1999:901–955.
Stoelting RK. Kidneys. *Pharmacology and physiology in anesthetic practise*. Philadelphia, PA: Lippincott Williams & Wilkins; 2003:722–735.
Stoelting RK, Dierdorf SF. Endocrine disease. *Anesthesia and co-existing disease*. New York: Churchill Livingstone; 1993:339–373.

Chapter 11

Regional Anesthesia Techniques and Management

George N. Djaiani

Regional anesthesia in cardiac surgery is claimed to produce superior pain control, shorter intubation times, earlier patient mobilization, and better preservation of respiratory function. Regional anesthesia techniques remain an essential part of many fast-track cardiac anesthesia protocols. In adult cardiac surgery, spinal anesthesia is used by 7.6% and epidural anesthesia is used by 7% of practicing cardiac anesthesiologists. Considering that >800,000 patients undergo cardiac surgery yearly worldwide, the neuraxial anesthesia is likely performed in thousands of patients each year.

BENEFITS AND RISKS OF REGIONAL ANESTHESIA IN CARDIAC SURGERY

Benefits of Regional Anesthesia

The claimed benefits of neuraxial anesthesia include reduction of myocardial infarction area, improved metabolic and functional myocardial recovery, and lower incidence of arrhythmias during myocardial ischemia. Patients with coronary artery disease seem to benefit from thoracic epidural anesthesia (TEA) through preferential redistribution of the coronary blood flow to endocardial layers, maintenance of hemodynamic stability, reduced incidence and duration of the ischemic episodes, improved left ventricular function, and reduced incidence of atrial arrhythmia.

Several reports have outlined a superior pain relief after cardiac surgery with both intrathecal and epidural analgesia.

Furthermore, patients receiving TEA appear to have lower incidence of respiratory tract infections after surgery and considerable reduction in perioperative renal dysfunction. In addition, patients managed with perioperative TEA seem to have reduced incidence of acute confusion and lower postoperative sedation scores.

Efficacy of Regional Anesthesia in Coronary Artery Bypass Graft Surgery: Meta-analysis Approach

An attempt to overcome the limitations of underpowered small studies have been used by Liu et al. and Djaiani et al. to determine the effects of regional anesthesia on clinically relevant outcomes in patients undergoing coronary bypass surgery. Although the selection methods of the available studies were slightly different, the general methodology of meta-analysis was applied in both reviews. Conclusions from these two studies are very similar in most but not all outcome variables.

Both TEA and intrathecal regional techniques resulted in lower in-hospital postoperative analog pain scores. Both reviews demonstrated that there was a significant reduction in perioperative atrial arrhythmia in the TEA group but not in the intrathecal group. Djaiani et al. assessed myocardial ischemia in seven studies (total of 377 patients) and myocardial infarction in 13 studies (total of 1,055 patients). The results of meta-analysis indicated a considerable reduction in myocardial ischemia and myocardial infarction with employment of neuraxial techniques. This was in contrast to the review by Liu et al., which could not demonstrate a reduction in myocardial infarction rates in the analysis. The methodologic differences and study selection may account for the different conclusions in this crucial outcome.

Both reviews found highly significant reduction in the duration of mechanical ventilation in patients managed with regional techniques, particularly with TEA. However, there was no demonstrable difference in the change in vital capacity in either spinal or epidural anesthesia. There were no differences in overall mortality between the neuraxial and conventional general anesthesia groups.

Potential Complications of Neuraxial Block

Most of the reports on the use of regional anesthesia in cardiac surgery have been limited to relatively low-risk patients in whom the potential risk of adverse postoperative events is expected to be minimal. As a consequence, most of these studies are underpowered to detect complication rates associated with regional techniques.

Using the principle of calculated estimate of epidural hematoma that was put forward by Ho et al., we can calculate the predicted maximal rate of any neurologic complication including epidural hematoma, abscess, and spinal cord infarction. The 99% confidence interval for overall incidence of these events would be 7/6,000 cases or 1 in 857 cases. The definitive test for the diagnosis of neurologic complications associated with neuraxial block is magnetic resonance imaging (MRI). Relatively high frequency of confusional states and the presence of pacemaker wires after cardiac surgery may render MRI tests more challenging in the immediate postoperative period. Complete neurologic recovery can be achieved if a surgical intervention (e.g., laminectomy) is performed within 8 hours, and permanent paralysis is more likely beyond 24 hours of the event.

Epidural Hematoma

The risk of paraplegia from a spinal hematoma in patients undergoing cardiac surgery was mathematically modeled to have a maximal risk of 1:3,600 for spinal anesthesia and 1:1,500 for TEA, a minimum risk of 1:220,000 for spinal anesthesia and 1:150,000 for TEA at the 95% confidence interval, and further increase in a maximum risk of 1:2,400 for spinal anesthesia and 1:1,100 for TEA at the 99% confidence interval.

The first report of epidural hematoma was described in a patient who had a thoracic epidural placed under general anesthesia preceding an aortic valve replacement. On the second postoperative day, this patient was anticoagulated and, in addition, received antithrombotic medication with the epidural catheter still being *in situ*. During ambulation, the patient experienced pain in his back, which coincided with the appearance of blood in his epidural catheter. The epidural catheter was removed, following which the patient developed motor and sensory loss. Rapid surgical decompression resulted in the recovery of the patient's lost neurologic function.

To minimize the risk of neurologic complications, a brief summary of the suggested guidelines pertinent to cardiac surgery should be followed:

1. New antiplatelet medication, such as ticlopidine and clopidogrel, should be discontinued 10 days before surgery. Aspirin should be stopped 7 days before surgery.
2. In the presence of coagulopathy from any cause, neuraxial blocks should not be performed.
3. Difficult or traumatic attempts may cause trauma to epidural vessels and, consequently, may increase the incidence of hemorrhage in the epidural space. Surgery should be delayed for 24 hours if a bloody tap occurs.
4. A minimum interval of 1 to 2 hours should be followed between the epidural placement and full or partial heparinization.
5. Preference should be given to the use of a midline approach for epidural placement because the lateral approach increases the risk of trauma to epidural veins.
6. Preference should be given to saline solution injection through the epidural needle to distend the epidural space before insertion of the catheter.
7. Removal of the epidural catheter should take place only after normal hemostasis has been restored postoperatively.
8. No anticoagulation or antiplatelet medication should be started while the epidural catheter is still *in situ*.
9. Close neurologic surveillance is mandatory.
10. Immediate availability of MRI and neurosurgical consult is mandatory.

Epidural Abscess and Spinal Cord Infarction

A large prospective database of studies has identified a frequency of 0.00% to 0.05% for epidural abscess in noncardiac surgery. Major risk factors for the development of epidural abscess associated with thoracic epidurals included insertion technique, duration of use, patient risk factors (e.g., immunocompromised, malignancy, diabetes, and chronic obstructive airways disease), and perioperative anticoagulant therapy.

The incidence of catheter-related infection and epidural abscess is likely to be similar in patients who have undergone cardiac surgery. However, a high rate of blood transfusions (potential for immunosuppressive effects), postoperative ventilation, and cardiovascular instability, which is pertinent to patients who have undergone cardiac surgery, may all contribute to the enhanced rate of catheter-related infections.

Although the denominator is unknown, there have been case reports of patients developing spinal cord infarction after cardiac surgery. The mechanism has been related to hypotension, relative anemia during cardiopulmonary bypass (CPB), dislodgment of atheromatous plaques from a calcified aorta, and the use of an intra-aortic balloon pump. It is possible that the incidence of spinal cord infarction may be increased in patients having an epidural catheter. The proposed mechanism may be related to a reduction in spinal cord perfusion pressure. The decreased perfusion pressure would occur during CPB when the perfusion pressure is routinely maintained in the range of 50 to 70 mm Hg and when the hematocrit levels are allowed to decrease to 20% or even lower. The perfusion pressure of the spinal cord may be compromised even further because of an increase in the tissue pressure caused by relatively large volumes of fluid infusion in the epidural space. However, the association of TEA and spinal cord infarction after cardiac surgery has not been reported.

TECHNICAL ASPECTS OF NEURAXIAL ANESTHESIA

Epidural Approach

Epidural anesthesia has been used successfully in patients undergoing coronary revascularization surgery as well as open heart surgery. An epidural catheter is sited either a day before the surgery or on the day of surgery. The level of insertion of the epidural catheter varies from C7/T1 to T2/T5. Establishing adequate neuraxial block is usually achieved by a bolus of ropivacaine 0.375% to 0.75%—5 to 8 mL, or bupivacaine 0.25% to 0.5%—5 to 12 mL, with or without opioid supplements (e.g., sufentanil 15 to 25 μg or fentanyl 20 μg). Maintenance of neuraxial anesthesia is managed by infusion of a local anesthetic supplemented by opioid or clonidine (e.g., ropivacaine 0.2% plus fentanyl 2 μg/mL at a rate of 5 to 14 mL/hour, or bupivacaine 0.5% with morphine 25 μg/mL 4 to 10 mL/hour, or bupivacaine 0.125% plus clonidine 0.0006% at a rate of 10 mL/hour). The average duration of epidural infusion is 3 ± 1.5 days.

Intrathecal Technique

Intrathecal analgesia in cardiac surgery has been used with great success since the 1980s. Although morphine is the most commonly used intrathecal opioid, the addition of intrathecal clonidine seems to augment the analgesic effects of morphine alone. The ideal or optimal dose of intrathecal morphine is not known. However, the effect of intrathecal anesthesia on duration of postoperative ventilation is expected to be dose dependent. Clearly, if the dose is too high, one would expect respiratory depression and prolonged ventilation time; conversely, if the dose is too low, the expected result would be poor analgesia. Utilizing intrathecal morphine dosage, we found a therapeutic window between the doses of 10 to 50 μg/kg (see Fig. 11-1). The optimal dose of intrathecal morphine with respect to the feasibility of early extubation, although providing adequate analgesia, appears to be in the range of 10 to 25 μg/kg.

Review: Regional anesthesia for cardiac surgery
Comparison: 08 Dose response for extubation time
Outcome: 01 Minutes to extubate

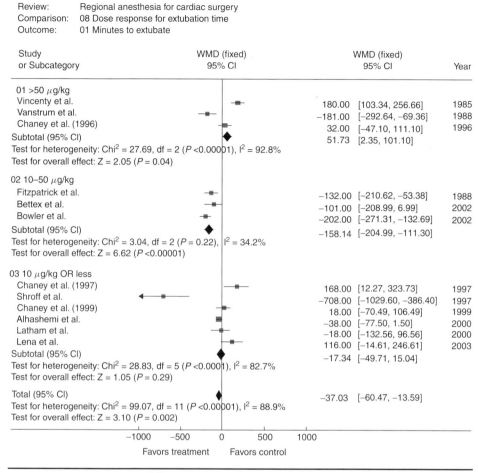

FIGURE 11-1. Dose-response difference in extubation time: Meta-analysis of intrathecal morphine in patients undergoing coronary revascularization surgery. Morphine dose of 10 to 50 μg/kg was most beneficial with respect to reduction of postoperative ventilation time. WMD, weighted mean difference.

High Spinal Anesthesia

Currently, there are two randomized controlled trials that have explored a feasibility of high spinal anesthesia in patients undergoing cardiac surgery. Lee et al. compared β-receptor desensitization and downregulation, as well as stress response between high spinal anesthesia and standard general anesthesia in patients undergoing coronary revascularization surgery. Patients in the spinal group received intrathecal hyperbaric bupivacaine, 0.75%—5 mL, before induction of anesthesia. The spinal group had significantly less atrial β-receptor dysfunction and lower serum concentrations of epinephrine, norepinephrine, and cortisol. In addition, patients in the spinal group had a higher cardiac index and a lower pulmonary vascular resistance index in the post-CPB period.

Another study randomized patients to receive intrathecal sufentanil 50 μg/morphine 0.5 mg, or intrathecal sufentanil 25 μg/morphine 0.5 mg/hyperbaric bupivacaine 9.75 mg as an adjunct to general anesthesia, or standard opioid-based general anesthesia with mock spinal anesthesia. Visual analog pain scores were significantly better in both spinal–general anesthesia groups when compared to the general anesthesia group. There was no difference in extubation times and length of stay between the three study groups.

Although the administration of high spinal anesthesia has been shown to be feasible in patients undergoing cardiac surgery, the requirements of vasoconstrictors during the pre-CPB period are increased.

Management of High Thoracic Epidural Anesthesia in an Awake Patient

The clinical experience of utilizing the high TEA as a sole anesthetic technique for coronary bypass surgery was introduced in the late 1990s. Clearly, this particular technique could only be utilized in off-pump beating heart coronary revascularization surgery. Although the early results were encouraging, the largest published case series to date is limited only to several hundred patients. The need for conversion to general anesthesia was reported in 5 out of 137 in the largest series and in 5 out of 71 patients in the remaining reports. The reasons for conversion included respiratory distress due to pneumothorax or phrenic nerve dysfunction and patient general distress. Although most patients undergoing awake off-pump coronary revascularization surgery required one or two coronary bypass grafts, multiple coronary bypass grafts have also been performed with this particular anesthetic technique. Excellent pain control, acceptable surgical conditions, and readiness to be discharged from the hospital within 1 to 3 days after surgery make it appealing to the enthusiasts of this technique. An epidural catheter is placed the day before the surgery in all patients. The level of epidural needle insertion varied from C7 to T3. The bolus to establish adequate neuraxial block and maintenance of anesthesia consisted of local anesthetic with or without opioids (e.g., bupivacaine 0.5%—5 mL plus bupivacaine 0.25%—5 to 16 mL with fentanyl 25 μg, or ropivacaine 0.5% and sufentanil 1.66 μg/mL at a rate of 20 to 30 mL/hour). Postoperative analgesia can usually be achieved with ropivacaine 0.16% plus sufentanil 1 μg/mL at a rate of 2 to 5 mL/hour.

CONCLUSION

Patients who were managed with the regional techniques benefited from superior postoperative analgesia, shorter postoperative ventilation, reduced incidence of supraventricular arrhythmia, and lower rates of perioperative myocardial infarction. The risk-to-benefit ratio therefore may be in favor of epidural and spinal anesthesia in patients undergoing coronary artery bypass graft surgery. However, meticulous adherence to guidelines for the use of regional techniques in cardiac surgery should be followed in order to avoid untoward neurologic events that are associated with this technique.

SUGGESTED READINGS

Djaiani G, Fedorko L, Beattie WS. Regional anesthesia in cardiac surgery: a friend or a foe? *Semin Cardiothorac Vasc Anesth.* 2005;9(1):87–104. Review.

Ho AM, Chung DC, Joynt GM. Neuraxial blockade and hematoma in cardiac surgery: estimating the risk of a rare adverse event that has not (yet) occurred. *Chest.* 2000;117:551–555.

Karagoz HY, Kurtoglu M, Bakkaloglu B, et al. Coronary artery bypass grafting in the awake patient: three years' experience in 137 patients. *J Thorac Cardiovasc Surg.* 2003;125:1401–1404.

Lee TW, Grocott HP, Schwinn D, et al. High spinal anesthesia for cardiac surgery: effects on beta-adrenergic receptor function, stress response, and hemodynamics. *Anesthesiology.* 2003; 98:499–510.

Liu SS, Block BM, Wu CL. Effects of perioperative central neuraxial analgesia on outcome after coronary artery bypass surgery: a meta-analysis. *Anesthesiology.* 2004;101:153–161.

Scott NB, Turfrey DJ, Ray DA, et al. A prospective randomized study of the potential benefits of thoracic epidural anesthesia and analgesia in patients undergoing coronary artery bypass grafting. *Anesth Analg.* 2001;93:528–535.

Chapter 12

Perioperative Monitoring in Cardiac Anesthesia

Daniel Bainbridge

Anesthesia is essentially a specialty of monitoring. Monitors such as pulse oximetry and end-tidal carbon dioxide were once novel experimental devices. Today, many additional monitors are available to aid in the management of patients undergoing cardiac operations. The purpose of this chapter is to review some commonly used cardiac, neurologic, and hemostatic monitors (see Table 12-1).

CARDIAC MONITORS

Pulmonary Artery Catheter

The pulmonary artery catheter is a standard monitor used for assessing cardiac output (CO) and preload through measurement of capillary wedge pressure. Its benefits are still controversial, with some advocating its routine use and others suggesting its selective use.

- Risks: Pulmonary hemorrhage, arrhythmia, and line infection.
- Indications for use: Ejection fraction (EF) <40%, severe heart failure.
  - Poor cardiovascular function.
  - Surgical: Aortic surgery, complex valve repair/replacement, minimal access surgery.
  - Postoperatively: Sepsis, refractory hypotension.
- Measurement: Proper measurement requires:
  - Appropriate position: West Zone 3.
  - Appropriate transducer height.
  - Avoid overwedging (see Table 12-2).

The pulmonary artery catheter allows accurate measurement of CO, central venous pressure (CVP), pulmonary artery (PA) pressure, and PA occlusion pressure (wedge). Systemic vascular resistance (SVR) and cardiac work are calculated measures. When used to measure preload, it is best to monitor trends or changes with interventions

▶ **TABLE 12-1** Standard Monitors

Cardiac monitors
Arterial line
Noninvasive blood pressure
Central venous line
V lead ECG (typically with continuous monitoring of leads II and V)
Other monitors
End-tidal carbon dioxide
Arterial saturations
Inspired oxygen
Ventilatory pressure

ECG, electrocardiograph.

(i.e., fluid boluses) because compliance alters the pressure–volume relation of the left ventricle (LV) and therefore affects the accurate measurement of preload.

Transesophageal Echocardiography

Transesophageal echocardiography (TEE) is used in the assessment of hemodynamics and cardiac anatomy during cardiac and aortic procedures.

- Risks: The most serious complication is esophageal perforation, which occurs in patients with esophageal pathology (i.e., esophageal stricture or esophageal carcinoma). More common complications include sore throat and difficulty with swallowing.
- Indications for use: Indications for use of TEE are listed in Table 12-3.
- Measurement: The TEE allows excellent anatomic and functional assessment of the heart. It is suggested that the complete American Society of Echocardiography/ Society of Cardiac Anesthesiologists (ASE/SCA) examination be performed intraoperatively to ensure interrogation of the all-important structures (i.e., myocardium, atria, valves, and aorta). In addition, a measure of diastolic and systolic heart function should also be performed. Diastolic function includes the E, A, S, and D waves. For systolic function, a regional and global estimate of LV function should be recorded. Additional measures should be performed based on cardiac pathology.

▶ **TABLE 12-2** Wedge Pressure

Wedge pressure overestimates preload	Mitral regurgitation
	Increased pulmonary vascular resistance
	Pulmonary vein compression
Wedge pressure underestimates preload	Mitral stenosis
	Artificial mitral valve
	Noncompliant LV
	Aortic insufficiency

LV, left ventricle.

▶ **TABLE 12-3** Indications for Use of Transesophageal Echocardiography

Class I indications	1. Evaluation of acute, persistent, and life-threatening hemodynamic disturbances
	2. Surgical repair of valvular lesions or hypertrophic obstructive cardiomyopathy or aortic dissection
	3. Evaluation of complex valve replacements requiring homografts or coronary reimplantation, such as the Ross procedure
	4. Surgical repair of most congenital heart lesions that require cardiopulmonary bypass
	5. Surgical intervention for endocarditis
	6. Placement of intracardiac devices during port-access surgery
	7. Evaluation of pericardial window procedures in patients with posterior or loculated effusions
Class IIa indications	1. Surgical procedures in patients at increased risk of myocardial ischemia, myocardial infarction, or hemodynamic disturbances
	2. Evaluation of valve replacement, aortic atheromatous disease, cardiac aneurysm, repair, and pulmonary embolectomy
	3. For the detection of air emboli

NEUROMONITORS

Bispectral Index

The bispectral index is a device that is used to measure the depth of anesthesia. This index is one of the number of devices that employs an electroencephalogram (EEG)-derived algorithm to generate a linear, dimensionless scale from 0 to 100, with 100 indicating fully awake and 0 indicating an isoelectric EEG.

■ Risks: Noninvasive device.
■ Indications for use:
   ● The device is indicated for all cases but may be selectively employed when awareness is of concern. This monitor is specifically used in young patients, emergency cases, and in patients with a prior history of awareness.
   ● The device may be beneficial in cases where an isoelectric EEG may be beneficial, for instance, during circulatory arrest.
■ Measurement: Two probes are placed on either side of the forehead. This provides a simple scale of 0 to 100. A value of 70 and lower is required to prevent awareness during anesthesia.

Near Infrared Spectroscopy

The near infrared spectroscopy measures cerebral brain oximetry relying on the relative tissue transparency to nearinfrared light (700 to 900 nm). It gives a measure of regional saturation of the capillary, arterial, and venous compartments.
■ Risks: Noninvasive device.
■ Indications for use:
   ● The device is used in patients at risk for stroke (i.e., elderly patients, patients with diabetes, and patients with previous stroke).

▶ **TABLE 12-4** **Measures of Thromboelastography**

Clotting time	R	Time until the initial fibrin formation. Analogous to an aPTT
Clot kinetics	K	A measure of the speed to reach a specific level of clot strength
Clot strength	MA	Represents the ultimate strength of the fibrin clot (measure of IIb/IIIa and platelet function)
Clot stability	LY 30	Measures the rate of amplitude reduction 30 minutes after

aPTT, activated partial thromboplastin time.

- The device is used in surgical cases that may interfere with cerebral perfusion (i.e., circulatory arrest, aortic arch repairs).
- Measurement: The near infrared spectroscopy provides information about cerebral saturation in both the left and right hemispheres. Normal saturation levels are between 60% and 75% (unlike pulse oximetry, cerebral oximetry measures arterial, capillary, and venous blood saturation). It does not require pulsatile flow to operate and is, therefore, useful during cardiopulmonary bypass. When cerebral saturations fall (in the setting of normal arterial saturations), certain measures may be used to increase saturations, such as increasing carbon dioxide CO_2), increasing blood pressure, ensuring that the head and neck are in neutral position, and checking the placement of the aortic cannula.

COAGULATION MONITORS

- Risks: Noninvasive assessment of coagulation.
- Indications for use: Used in patients at high risk for coagulopathy (i.e., emergency surgery, resternotomy, and pre-existing coagulopathy).

Many recent advances have been made in point-of-care testing to allow for shorter response times in the performance of coagulation testing. The following are some commonly used point-of-care tests employed during cardiac surgery.

Thromboelastograph

- Measures: The measures of thromboelastographs are listed in Table 12-4. The thromboelastograph has been demonstrated to be useful in reducing transfusion requirements following high-risk cardiac surgery.

Hepcon Heparin Management System

- Measures:
  - Activated clotting time (ACT): The time taken for whole blood to clot when activated usually with kaolin or celite.
  - Heparin dose response (HDR): Determines the amount of heparin that needs to be administered to achieve the target ACT specified by the user.
  - Heparin protamine titration (HPT): Determines the amount of protamine sulfate that needs to be given to neutralize circulating heparin.

SUGGESTED READINGS

Cheitlin MD, Armstrong WF, Aurigemma GP, et al. ACC/AHA/ASE 2003 guideline update for the clinical application of echocardiography: summary article: a report of the American College of Cardiology/American Heart Association Task Force on Practice Guidelines (ACC/AHA/ASE Committee to Update the 1997 Guidelines for the Clinical Application of Echocardiography). *Circulation.* 2003;108(9):1146–1162.

Raper R, Sibbald WJ. Misled by the wedge? The Swan-Ganz catheter and left ventricular preload. *Chest.* 1986;89(3):427–434.

Shanewise JS, Cheung AT, Aronson S, et al. ASE/SCA guidelines for performing a comprehensive intraoperative multiplane transesophageal echocardiography examination: recommendations of the American Society of Echocardiography Council for Intraoperative Echocardiography and the Society of Cardiovascular Anesthesiologists Task Force for Certification in Perioperative Transesophageal Echocardiography. *J Am Soc Echocardiogr.* 1999;12(10):884–900.

Shore-Lesserson L. Point-of-care coagulation monitoring for cardiovascular patients: past and present. *J Cardiothorac Vasc Anesth.* 2002;16(1):99–106.

Chapter 13

Perioperative Transesophageal Echocardiography

Annette Vegas

The role of intraoperative transesophageal echocardiography (TEE) has grown expo-nentially, and its use has become commonplace during cardiac surgeries. For patients who have undergone complex cardiac surgery and for those who are extremely ill, the surgeon requires a thorough understanding of individual patient cardiac structure and function to provide optimal patient care. The goal of an intraoperative TEE study is to conduct a complete but targeted examination on the basis of a specific indication. The echocardiographer provides timely information that may influence patient manage-ment. Depending on the institution, intraoperative TEE examinations are performed either by cardiologists or by anesthesiologists.

TECHNOLOGY

- Echocardiography was first used in the operating room (OR) in the early 1970s as heart surface (epicardial) scanning. The first publication of intraoperative m-mode TEE was in 1979, and the electronic phased array transducer was introduced in 1982. In the late 1980s, high-frequency biplane TEE probes and, subsequently, multiplane (omniplane) TEE probes provided high resolution, color mapping, and continuous wave Doppler assessment. New emerging technologies include three-dimensional im-aging, myocardial perfusion, and intraoperative dobutamine stress echocardiography.

- Medical ultrasound transducers emit sound in different ranges. The higher the ultrasound frequency, the less the tissue penetration and the better the image quality. Each transducer therefore trades off penetration for image quality.
  - The basic transthoracic (epicardial) transducer (2.5 MHz) requires greater tissue penetration through the chest wall to image the heart from the anterior to posterior position. The probe, in a sterile sheath, can be placed directly on the epicardial surface of the heart in patients who have a contraindication to TEE.
  - TEE uses a higher frequency 5-MHz probe positioned in the esophagus closer to the heart so that less tissue penetration is required. The heart is imaged from posterior to anterior.
  - An epiaortic scan places a 10- to 15-MHz probe directly on the aorta to image the aorta from anterior to posterior. This technique is sensitive for the detection of aortic atheroma.
  - Intravascular ultrasound uses a disposable 30-MHz ultrasound probe to image the heart from the inside. These catheters are used in the catheterization laboratory to assist with atrial septal defect (ASD) device closures.
- Technical limitations to the use of TEE in the OR include unfavorable OR lighting conditions, electrical cautery interference, and surgical manipulations of the heart. In addition, anesthesia also alters the loading conditions of the heart that affects interpretation of valvular regurgitation severity.

TRANSESOPHAGEAL ECHOCARDIOGRAPHY APPLICATIONS

- TEE permits a detailed examination of the heart structure and function. A specific echocardiographic mode interprets and displays the returning sound waves differently.
  - The two-dimensional mode shows normal or abnormal structural anatomy and allows quantification of size and assessment of myocardial and valvular function.
  - Color Doppler mode displays blood flow within the heart and great vessels using color. Normal flow is unidirectional and smooth (laminar). Regurgitant or stenotic valvular flow or flow through abnormal connections typically appears as turbulent flow. Quantification of flow by spatial mapping and vena contracta size determines lesion severity.
  - Pulsed or continuous wave Doppler mode displays information as a spectral trace of velocity versus time and demonstrates timing, direction, and amount of flow. Quantification of blood flow velocity permits calculation of pressure gradients and hemodynamic information.
  - TEE can be used in combination with special contrast agents to assess blood flow and myocardial viability.
- Current clinical applications for TEE (see Fig. 13-1) include the evaluation of native valve disease, prosthetic valve function, ventricular function, congenital heart disease, and risk of thromboembolism. TEE can also be used to diagnose aortic dissection, complications of endocarditis, and etiology of stroke. TEE is a valuable adjunct during percutaneous cardiac procedures, such as ASD device closures, and is used intraoperatively during cardiac surgical procedures.

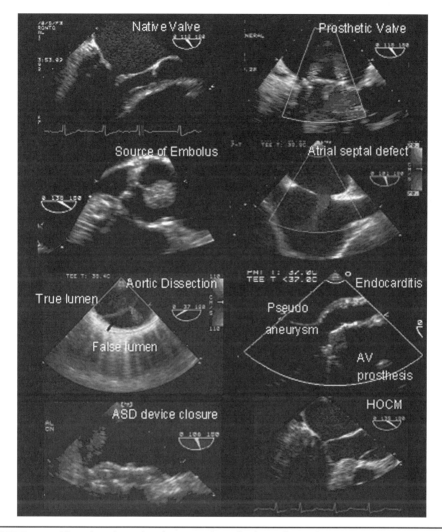

FIGURE 13-1. Clinical applications of transesophageal echocardiography (TEE).

■ Intraoperative TEE is used for a well-defined indication (see following text), addresses all clinically relevant issues, and provides immediate and definitive interpretation. By performing a complete examination and by looking at all cardiac structures and function, the echocardiographer confirms known pathology and identifies any new pathology. New unexpected findings can alter the course of the operation.

■ Intraoperative TEE is used for diagnosis to guide the surgical procedure, immediately assess surgical results, detect complications, and monitor ventricular function. The goal of the echocardiographer is to provide information based on which the surgeon and anesthesiologist can make informed decisions.

- TEE is a valuable diagnostic modality for perioperative patients who are hemodynamically unstable.

TRANSESOPHAGEAL ECHOCARDIOGRAPHY VIEWS

- Individuals interested in using TEE, whether cardiologists, surgeons, or anesthesiologists, must be fluent in the standardized nomenclature to describe and to communicate findings. The Society of Cardiovascular Anesthesiology (SCA) and the American Society of Echocardiography (ASE) jointly described the terminology in a landmark paper in 1999.
- The SCA recommends the examination of the heart using 20 different TEE views, which can conveniently be grouped together to image specific structures at different levels. As shown in Figure 13-2, the heart and great vessels can be imaged at three levels: the upper esophageal (UE), midesophageal (ME), and transgastric (TG) views.
  - These four UE views (and two ME views) examine the aorta (Fig. 13-2A) in different planes. They are crucial in determining the presence of aortic pathology such as aneurysms, dissections, or atheroma.

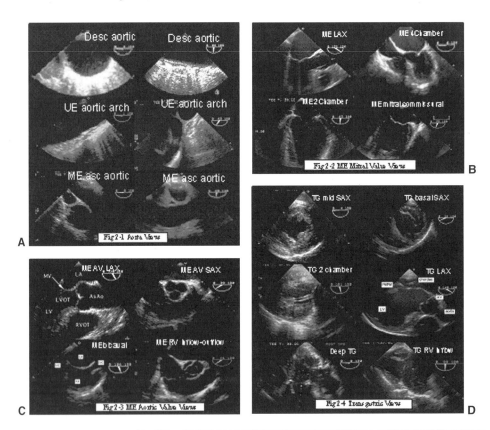

FIGURE 13-2. Society of Cardiovascular Anesthesiology (SCA) transesophageal echocardiography views.

- The eight ME views can be divided into two groups of four views. The four views in Figure 13-2B examine the left ventricle and mitral valve. The four views in Figure 13-2C look at the aortic, pulmonic, and tricuspid valves, as well as the intra-atrial septum.
- Finally, by advancing the probe into the stomach the six TG views (Fig. 13-2D) are attained. The classic doughnut view of the left ventricle is obtained at the base and the midportion of the heart and provides assessment of ventricular function. These views are also critical for Doppler alignment and assessing gradients across the aortic valve and left ventricular outflow tract (LVOT).

ROLE AND INDICATIONS

- The SCA and American Heart Association (AHA) have each produced guidelines for the use of echocardiography using three levels of recommendations. These guidelines are based on scientific evidence for clinical decision-making and on the effectiveness of echocardiography to influence patient outcome. The guidelines attempt to meet most patients' needs but consideration should be given to the individual patient, procedure, and setting. Table 13-1 summarizes the 1996 SCA guidelines for perioperative TEE.
- On the basis of these intraoperative TEE guidelines, not every patient undergoing cardiac surgery has a specific indication for TEE and would not benefit from an intraoperative TEE. However, in general, the new millennium elective cardiac surgery patient is older, has diabetes along with renal dysfunction and heart failure, and undergoes redo or complex surgery. End-organ reserve is low, therefore, improved accuracy and

▶ **TABLE 13-1** Society of Cardiovascular Anesthesiology Guidelines for Perioperative Transesophageal Echocardiography

Category 1	*Category 2*	*Category 3*
Strongest evidence, TEE useful	Weaker evidence, TEE may be useful	Little evidence, TEE infrequently useful
• Valve repairs	• Myocardial ischemia/infarct	• Myocardial perfusion, coronary artery anatomy
• Congenital heart	• Valve replacement	
• HOCM	• Cardiac aneurysms, thrombus	• Repair of cardiomyopathies
• Endocarditis	• Cardiac tumors, foreign bodies	• Repair thoracic aorta injuries
• Aortic Dissection+AI	• Pulmonary embolectomy	• Uncomplicated pericarditis
• Pericardial window	• Cardiac trauma	• Cardioplegia administration
• Hemodynamic instability	• Aortic dissections, no AI	• Placement of IABP, AICD, PAC
	• Aortic atheroma	
	• Assist devices	
	• Pericardiectomy	
	• Air emboli	

TEE, transesophageal echocardiography; HOCM, hypertrophic obstructive cardiomyopathy; AI, aortic insufficiency; IABP, intra-aortic balloon pump; AICD, automatic implantable cardioversion defibrillator; PAC, pulmonary artery catheter.

reliability in clinical decision-making may prevent an adverse outcome. In this setting, TEE is a reasonable choice as an intraoperative monitoring tool.

- Forty years after it was introduced into cardiac practice, the long-debated value of the Swan-Ganz catheter in cardiac surgery still remains unanswered. TEE is a superior monitor of myocardial ischemia, and both right and left ventricular myocardial function, and it is useful in determining relative volume status. TEE can make a new diagnosis that may alter clinical management. Unfortunately, it is an expensive program to start and requires special operator expertise. The Swan–Ganz catheter, while providing different information, comes at an economic price and requires less expertise. Neither technology has yet been proven to change patient outcome in any large studies.
- As a monitoring device, there is no compelling evidence that TEE changes clinical outcome. There is some evidence that TEE helps direct clinical management. TEE is invaluable in assessing valve function and in ensuring that correct operation is done. TEE is essential to confirm the adequacy of surgery and reduce the need for re-exploration. Post–cardiopulmonary bypass (CPB) TEE optimizes de-airing after open-heart procedures. Finally TEE has a limited role in detecting aortic atheroma and potentially identifying patients at risk for stroke.

CONTRAINDICATIONS AND COMPLICATIONS

- Contraindications to TEE include oropharyngeal, esophageal, and gastric pathology; lack of expertise; or lack of patient consent. Epicardial scanning using a standard transthoracic probe in a sterile sheath placed directly on the heart permits imaging if there is a contraindication to TEE or if there is a failure to insert the TEE probe.
- When used properly, TEE is safe without serious complications, as reported by Kallmeyer following 7,200 intraoperative TEEs. The most common complication is a sore throat, the most serious one being esophageal perforation in one patient. There is a low risk of infection; patients at risk for infective endocarditis do not require antibiotic prophylaxis for TEE.
- Echocardiography requires focused attention to acquire and to interpret the images. A TEE study during the vulnerable immediate post-CPB period can lead to distraction and reduction in patient care. It is controversial as to how a person can provide an adequate diagnostic study and anesthetic at the same time.
- Errors of interpretation can expose the patient to the additional risk of too much or not enough surgery or treatments. The SCA recognizes specific technical and cognitive skills required to be practiced by an advanced or basic echocardiographer.

SPECIFIC PERIOPERATIVE TRANSESOPHAGEAL ECHOCARDIOGRAPHY APPLICATIONS

Monitoring Myocardial Function

- The most important part of TEE for coronary artery bypass grafting (CABG) is the examination of the left ventricle (LV). The ASE and SCA recommend a *16-segment*

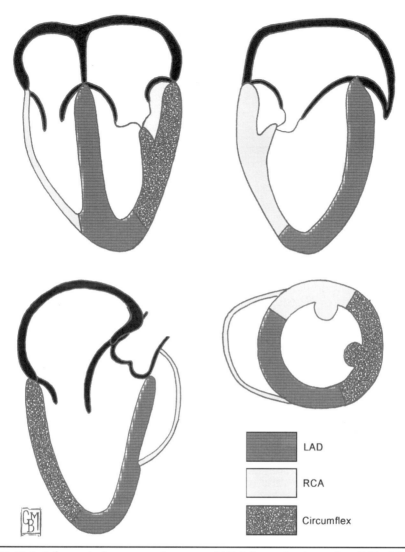

FIGURE 13-3. Left ventricular segmental anatomy. LAD, left anterior descending; RCA, right coronary artery.

model for examining the LV (see Fig. 13-3), dividing the basal and midventricular levels each into six segments and the apex into four segments. All 16 segments are examined by obtaining cross-sectional views of the LV, through the ME and TG windows, with assessment of size, global function, and regional wall motion. Either the right, left anterior descending, or circumflex coronary artery perfuses each segment.

■ In current clinical practice, analysis of LV segmental function is based on a qualitative visual assessment of the motion and/or thickening of a myocardial segment during systole. This qualitative grading scale (see Table 13-2) for wall motion has been used and is recommended: A hypokinetic segment thickens and moves inward, an

▶ **TABLE 13-2** Left Ventricular Segmental Function

		Wall Motion	Wall Thickening	Radius Change(%)
1	Normal	Inward	+++	>30
2	Mild hypokinetic	Inward	++	10–30
3	Severe hypokinetic	Inward	+	<10
4	Akinesis	None	0	None
5	Dyskinesis	Outward	0	None

akinetic segment does not thicken or move, and a dyskinetic segment fails to thicken and moves paradoxically outward during systole.

- TEE can assess quantitative ventricular function. Measurements of fractional area change (FAC), fractional shortening, and wall stress provide semiquantitative assessment of global ventricular function. Calculation of right and left ventricular cardiac output and ejection fraction is possible but requires time.

- Within seconds of the onset of myocardial ischemia, affected myocardial segments contract abnormally. TEE detects *new severe* segmental wall motion abnormalities (SWMA) in patients before ischemic ST—segment electrocardiogram (ECG) changes.

Valve Repairs and Replacement

TEE allows precise definition of valve anatomy, determines the mechanism of valve dysfunction, and quantifies the severity of the lesion. Substantial operator experience and thorough knowledge of anatomy and pathology are required for optimal results. Detailed anatomic information guides the surgeon's choice of surgical repair. Benefits to surgical valvular repair include reduced perioperative morbidity and mortality, preservation of the mitral apparatus with maintenance of ventricular function, no need for an anticoagulant, long-term durability, and freedom from reoperation.

Mitral Valve

- The mitral valve is a complex cardiac structure, better thought of as the mitral valve apparatus. It consists of two leaflets, annulus, chordae, papillary muscles, and LV wall. Abnormalities can occur at each level, so an accurate diagnosis guides the surgeon in the surgical options for mitral repair or replacement.

- The mechanism of mitral regurgitation (MR), as classified by Carpentier, is based on mitral leaflet motion:
  - Normal: dilated cardiomyopathy, perforated leaflet.
  - Excessive: prolapse, flail.
  - Restrictive: rheumatic, ischemic.

- Mitral valve prolapse (MVP) is a common pathology that is frequently repaired. The pre-CPB TEE determines the scallops involved (single, multiple), mitral annulus size, and direction and severity of the MR jet. The post-CPB TEE evaluates residual MR, presence of systolic anterior motion (SAM) of the anterior mitral valve leaflet (AMVL) and LV function under appropriate loading conditions.

Aortic Valve

- The aortic valve apparatus (root) is not a single anatomic structure but is comprised of the aortic annulus, valve cusps, sinuses of Valsalva, sino-tubular junction (STJ), and the proximal ascending aorta. The LVOT is the outflow portion of the LV just inferior to the aortic valve that supports the aortic valve annulus.
- The mechanism of aortic insufficiency (AI) can similarly be classified according to cusp mobility:
  - Normal: perforation, aortic root (aneurysm, dissection).
  - Excessive: prolapse.
  - Restricted: calcified, rheumatic.
    The severity of AI is difficult to quantify, particularly if an eccentric jet is present.
- The pre-CPB TEE evaluates aortic cusp number and mobility, measures the size of the aortic root, and measures the quantity and direction of AI. This information helps determine whether the aortic valve can be spared or needs replacement.

Valve Replacement

- Pre-CPB measurements of annulus size, presence, and location of calcification and involvement of multiple valves guides surgical management.
- TEE color Doppler has a high sensitivity for paravalvular leak post-CPB. Small leaks frequently improve after protamine administration. Immediately post-CPB, valve gradients may be high because of altered load conditions.
- Significant LVOT obstruction can occur with septal hypertrophy and hypovolemia postaortic valve replacement (AVR) for aortic stenosis. Preservation of mitral subvalvular structures and strut height may obstruct the LVOT post–mitral valve replacement (MVR).

Congenital Heart

- Practical constraints of TEE probe size limited the early introduction of intraoperative TEE in congenital cardiac surgery. New smaller TEE probes and epicardial scanning have become more frequent during pediatric congenital heart surgery.
- Echocardiography can define the congenital lesion and associated anomalies, assess ventricular function, and assess the adequacy of corrective or palliative procedures. Combined expertise in echocardiography and congenital heart disease is required to make an accurate assessment.
- Simple congenital lesions (ASD, ventricular septal defect [VSD], patent ductus arteriosus, and coarctation) can be easily imaged. Complex congential heart lesions (transposition of the great vessels, tetralogy of Fallot, and unichamber hearts) may be uncorrected, palliated, or completely corrected and difficult to image.
- Intraoperative TEE assesses lesion type, shunt direction, chamber size, right ventricular pressures and function, and associated anomalies. Post-CPB TEE determines the adequacy of repair of septal defects and identifies residual shunts, obstructions, and valvular insufficiency.

Hypertrophic Obstructive Cardiomyopathy

- Hypertrophic obstructive cardiomyopathy is an uncommon cardiac pathology worldwide. The surgical management of these patients involves a septal myectomy.

- The echo findings are complex and reveal a dynamic obstruction of the LVOT. The thickened septal ventricular muscle contracts, thereby causing anterior motion of the AMVL into the LVOT. Movement of the AMVL into the LVOT results in an eccentric posterior-directed jet of MR and turbulent flow in the LVOT.
- The pre-CPB TEE measures the maximal septal thickness, AMVL-septal contact point and the distance from the right coronary cusp, and peak LVOT gradient.
- Following myectomy, laminar flow is established through the LVOT and there is a reduction in the amount of MR. Post-CPB TEE establishes the absence of AMVL-septal contact, laminar LVOT flow, reduction in MR, provoked (post premature ventricular contraction) LVOT gradient >50 mm Hg, and absence of VSD.

Endocarditis

- It is now well established that echocardiography is the technology of choice for the diagnosis of endocarditis. According to the Duke criteria, the presence of vegetations, abscess, *new* partial dehiscence of a prosthetic valve, and *new* valvular regurgitation are major findings for the diagnosis of endocarditis. Echocardiography may also identify minor findings of new nodular valve thickening, valve perforations, and nonoscillating mass.
- TEE has proven to be sensitive and specific for detecting vegetations on native valves (100%), and less so on prosthetic valves (94%). Vegetations appear as irregular echodense, independently mobile masses. Echocardiography documents the location, number, and size of vegetations. All valves should be examined because multiple valves may be involved.
- TEE has proved to be more sensitive and specific compared to transthoracic echocardiography (TTE) for the diagnosis of endocarditis complications such as perivalvular extension (e.g., abscess, pseudoaneurysm, or fistula). Perivalvular abscess is particularly common in prosthetic valve endocarditis because the sewing ring is the primary site of infection. Prosthetic valve rocking occurs <40% circumferential ring dehiscence. Aortic abscesses (86%) are easier to detect than mitral abscesses (42%).
- Valve regurgitation may result from leaflet/cusp malcoaptation, leaflet perforation, torn chordae, flail cusp, or perivalvular leak. Intraoperative TEE defines the etiology of valve regurgitation and evaluates the adequacy of valvular repair or replacement.

Aortic Atheroma

- Stroke is one of the most devastating complications of cardiac surgery. Although the etiology of stroke in this setting is multifactorial, a major factor is thought to be a plaque at the site of aortic cannulation. TEE is useful in examining most of the aorta including the proximal ascending aorta, arch, and descending aorta. Atheroma can be detected in these regions.
- Although most of the thoracic aorta can be imaged by TEE, the trachea creates a blind spot in the distal ascending aorta where aortic cannulation commonly occurs.

This region is examined using an epiaortic probe in a sterile sheath placed directly on the ascending aorta. The aorta can be imaged in both short axis and long axis.

- Epiaortic scanning permits precise localization and characterization of plaque within the aorta. An epiaortic study is better than TEE and surgical palpation for identifying aortic plaque. The presence of aortic atheroma allows the surgeon to consider alternative strategies to aortic cannulation. Whether the identification of ascending aortic atheroma and altered surgical technique reduces stroke is yet to be proved.

Aortic Aneurysms and Dissection

- Aortic aneurysms are permanent, localized dilatation of the aorta, having a diameter of at least 1.5 times that of the expected normal diameter of a given segment.
- Aortic dissection involves a tear in the intima that allows blood to flow between the intimal and medial/adventitial layers, creating a false lumen. As blood separates these layers, the intima is compressed, creating a smaller true lumen. Aortic dissection usually occurs in the ascending aorta, within a few centimeters of the aortic valve, or in the descending thoracic aorta distal to the insertion of the ligamentum arteriosum. Risk factors for aortic dissection include bicuspid aortic valve, coarctation aorta, pre-existing aneurysm, Marfan syndrome, pregnancy, and hypertension.
- TEE has evolved to become the diagnostic modality of choice for aortic dissection. It is widely available and has the advantage of being performed at the patient's bedside with no interference in intensive monitoring or treatment. TEE is associated with a sensitivity rate of 98% and specificity rates of 77% to 98%.
- TEE evaluation of dissection includes assessment of the origin of the intimal tear, extent of the dissection, adequacy of perfusion in the lumens, LV function, and the presence of complications. Complications that may be detected using TEE include pericardial effusion, presence and severity of AI, and regional wall motion abnormalities from coronary dissection. The presence of a structurally normal aortic valve and AI may permit a valve sparing procedure. Post-CPB TEE documents residual AI.
- Identification of an intimal flap that separates the true and false lumens may be difficult. Multiple TEE views are required. The flap must first be distinguished from linear artifact and then the true and false lumens must be identified. The flap is usually mobile and flow appears in opposite directions on each side of the flap.

Hemodynamic Instability

- TEE provides invaluable information about patients who are hemodynamically stable in the intensive care unit (ICU), noncardiac OR, or recovery room. The patient who is hemodynamically unstable can be a challenge to manage. TEE permits assessment of cardiac function, diagnosis of valvular pathology, and pulmonary embolism.
- Qualitative TEE estimates ventricular filling and function and directs the administration of fluids, inotropes, and vasopressors. Echocardiography can differentiate severe ventricular dysfunction from other life-threatening causes of hypotension.

▶ **TABLE 13-3** **Echocardiographic Differential of Hypotension**

EDA	FAC	Etiology
↓↓	↑↑ >0.8	Hypovolemia
↑↑	↓↓ <0.2	LV failure
∅	↓↓ >0.8	↓ SVR, severe MR or AR, or VSD

EDA, LV end-diastolic cross-sectional area; FAC, LV fractional area change; LV, left ventricle; SVR, systemic vascular resistance; MR, mitral regurgitation; AR, aortic regurgitation; VSD, ventricular septal defect.

Severe hypovolemia is recognized as a marked decrease in end-diastolic area and as a marked increase in ejection fraction. Arterial vasodilatation, severe aortic regurgitation, MR, and VSD can manifest the same LV filling and ejection pattern in the TG midpapillary short-axis view. Using other TEE views and color Doppler, differentiating these etiologies of hypotension is facilitated.

- The echocardiographic characteristics of the most common causes of severe hypotension are summarized in Table 13-3.
- Cardiac tamponade can be a lethal complication in the postcardiac surgery patient and may result from a loculated compression of the heart. The result of an urgent TEE in the hemodynamically unstable postcardiac surgery patient is unpredictable. Clinical management is often modified as a result of the TEE finding.

SUGGESTED READINGS

Kallmeyer I, Collard C, Fox A, et al. The safety of intraoperative transesophageal echocardiography: a case series of 7200 cardiac surgical patients. *Anesth Analg.* 2001;92:1126–1130.

Quinones M, Otto C, Stoddard M, et al. Recommendations for quantification of doppler echocardiography: a report from the Doppler Quantification Task Force of the Nomenclature and Standards Committee of the American Society of Echocardiography. *J Am Soc Echocardiogr.* 2002;15:167–184.

Shanewise JS, Chueng AT, Aronson S, et al. ASE/SCA Guidelines for performing a comprehensive intraoperative multiplane transesophageal echocardiographic examination: recommendations of the American Society of Echocardiography Council on Intraoperative Echocardiography Board and the Society of Cardiovascular Anesthesiologists Task Force for Certification in Perioperative Transesophageal Echocardiography. *Anesth Analg.* 1999;89:870–884.

Thys D, Abel M, Bollen B, et al. Practice guidelines for perioperative transesophageal echocardiography: a report by the American Society of Anesthesiologists and the Society of Cardiovascular Anesthesiologists Task Force on Transesophageal Echocardiography. *Anesthesiology.* 1996;84:986–1006.

Wake PJ, Ali M, Carroll J, et al. Clinical and echocardiographic diagnoses disagree in patients with unexplained hemodynamic instability after cardiac surgery. *Can J Anaesth.* 2001;48:778–783.

Zoghbi W, Enriquez-Sarano M, Foster E, et al. Recommendations for evaluation of the severity of native valvular regurgitation with two-dimensional and doppler echocardiography. *J Am Soc Echocardiogr.* 2003;16:777–802.

Chapter 14

Essence of Cardiopulmonary Bypass Circuit and Intra-aortic Balloon Pump

Peter Allen

- With its introduction to clinical use in the 1950s, the heart–lung machine ushered in a revolution in the field of cardiac surgery. Today, >650,000 cardiac procedures are performed annually in the United States utilizing the heart–lung machine for cardiopulmonary bypass (CPB).
- The heart–lung machine is a series of electronically controlled pumps, which circulates blood through tubing diverted from the venous side of the heart. The blood then passes through an array of components and monitoring devices and returns oxygenated blood to the aorta. The heart–lung machine can perform the functions of systemic (occasionally regional) circulation, ventilation, and temperature regulation of the patient, thereby setting the stage to arrest the heart safely to provide a

motionless and bloodless field for the surgeon to perform many cardiac surgical procedures.

■ The heart–lung machine is used in the surgical setting for noncardiac cases such as thoracoabdominal aneurysms, neurologic procedures, rewarming of the accidental profound patients with hypothermia, and certain cancer treatments. The components of this technology can be utilized for extreme life-support measures outside the operating room to provide ventricular assistance or extracorporeal membrane oxygenation (ECMO) for cardiac or respiratory failure.

CARDIOPULMONARY BYPASS DESIGN AND COMPONENTS

■ Circuit design depends in part on the type of oxygenator used, either a bubble or membrane, and on the type of venous reservoir used. If the circuit employs a collapsible venous reservoir, blood-to-air exposure is reduced and the system is referred to as a closed circuit. The closed system requires a separate hard-shell cardiotomy reservoir to filter and return blood that is collected from the vent and pump suction to the circuit for autotransfusion back to the patient.

■ In contrast, open circuits incorporate the venous drainage, vent, and suction return in a single hard-shell reservoir. The suction blood passes through an integrated filter, whereas the venous drainage bypasses that filtering mechanism. This has eliminated the need for the collapsible venous reservoir bag; however, there is greater blood-to-air interface.

OXYGENATORS

■ Bubble oxygenators have a simple design, are inexpensive, and are open systems. Although they are no longer widely utilized in North America, bubble oxygenators are still utilized in other parts of the world. The mechanism of action is to have blood pass over a sparger plate, which allows a jet of oxygen to pass through a series of holes designed to make large bubbles. These bubbles transfer carbon dioxide (CO_2) and smaller size bubbles, which transfer oxygen (O_2) more readily. CO_2 regulation is controlled by the flow rate of 100% O_2 through the sparger plate. One hundred percent O_2 must be used to avoid nitrogen (N_2), which is relatively insoluble. This makes blood gas control somewhat imprecise because there is a poor control of the O_2.

■ Major disadvantages of the bubble oxygenator are handling of the formed elements (in particular of the red cell leading to hemolysis) and elimination of microembolism created by these bubbles. The design of the bubble oxygenator also has an inherent safety issue surrounding massive air embolism, which can easily occur if the reservoir inadvertently empties.

■ The membrane oxygenator has a mechanism of action much like a lung, in that the blood phase is separated from the gas phase by a semipermeable membrane. This membrane can be made of either polypropylene or a silicone rubber. The membrane material can be pleated, coiled, or made into hollow fibers. The basic principle remains the same, with oxygen and carbon dioxide diffusing across a semipermeable membrane. Because there is no direct blood-to-gas interface for oxygenation, this eliminates the concerns associated with N_2. This allows for the introduction of a combination of medical air and O_2 in the ventilating gas. Adjustments of the flow rate of the ventilating gas will control O_2, as is the case with the bubble oxygenator; however, perfusionists can now adjust the fraction of inspired oxygen (F_{IO}), giving them greater control over blood gases.

- Two added benefits of the membrane oxygenator are that the large volumes of freshly oxygenated blood need not be subjected to the defoaming step that is required with the bubble oxygenator. Therefore, silicone wash off is no longer a great concern. Suction blood in any circuit will still be subject to defoaming agents. However, the formed elements of blood are handled in a much gentler fashion with a membrane oxygenator, and this reduces the amount of hemolysis formed with the bubble oxygenator.

- Oxygenators used in routine bypass surgery tend to be concentric in design, routinely incorporating a heat exchanger for temperature control. The surface area of the patient and CPB circuit exposed to the ambient temperature of the operating room, surgeon preference (hypothermia or normothermia), and the surgical procedure all play a role in temperature regulation. Before passing through the oxygenator, blood passes over one side of the heat exchanger material, which is typically stainless steel, coated aluminum, or even plastic, whereas warm or cold water is circulated on the other side of the heat exchanger, thereby controlling the patient's temperature.

- At normothermia, the period of ischemic tolerance is approximately 5 to 6 minutes for tissues that receive a high distribution of blood flow such as the central nervous system, liver, and kidneys. Hypothermia reduces the oxygen consumption of these vital organs. As blood is cooled, there is both an increase of oxygen in plasma and a left shift in the oxyhemoglobin dissociation curve. The rule of seven doubles the ischemic tolerance time of tissues. Every 7°C reduction in temperature will double the ischemic tolerance, and, therefore, at 30°C, ischemic tolerance becomes 10 to 12 minutes, and at 23°C, the tolerance becomes 20 to 24 minutes.

- Hypothermia can be categorized from mild to profound (see Table 14-1). Mild-to-moderate hypothermia is generally used for straightforward routine open-heart procedures. Profound hypothermia with circulatory arrest is used for complex congenital heart repairs and for complicated adult situations such as those involving the arch vessels. The rates of cooling and rewarming must be closely controlled. In the adult, temperature gradients should not exceed 10°C to 12°C, and in the pediatric patient this gradient should not exceed 8°C.

TABLE 14-1 Categories of Hypothermia

Classification	Degrees	Safe Arrest Time (minutes)
Mild	32–37	4–5
Moderate	28–32	8–10
Deep	18–28	16–20
Profound	0–18	64–84

PUMPS

There are two main types of pumps routinely utilized on the heart lung machine.

1. The roller pump is a positive displacement pump. There is a direct relationship between the revolutions per minute (RPM) of the pump and the displacement of a fixed volume of fluid based on the size of tubing that is present in the raceway of the pump head. A roller pump can be used as an arterial pump to support circulation. It can be used as a sucker pump to clear blood from the operative field for autotransfusion after heparin has been administered, as a vent to decompress and de-air the heart, or as a cardioplegia pump to deliver the solutions to arrest the heart.
   - The roller pump is not load sensitive, and, therefore, if a clamp is placed across the tubing of the roller, the pump will continue to positively displace volume and potentially rupture the tubing or create a line separation at a connector. An improperly occluded pump head can also create hemolysis.
2. The centrifugal pump has a magnetically backed impeller coupled to an electric motor to create a constrained vortex. These types of pumps are load sensitive, and downstream loads such as a tubing clamp or the systemic vascular resistance (SVR) of the patient will affect the flow rates. Therefore, there is no direct RPM-to-flow rate relationship and, as such, a flow probe must be utilized to monitor actual flows. This translates into an element of circuit protection in that, if the downstream resistance is too high, no further forward flow will occur; therefore, the risk of tubing separation and rupture will become less of a potential issue.
   - The centrifugal pump has a couple of advantages for the patient. First, the flow of solution requires a fully primed pump head. Therefore, if the centrifugal pump looses its prime, gross air will not be pumped to the patient. The other touted benefit is gentle handling of the formed elements of blood, particularly the platelets. The inherent design of the centrifugal pump demands that it must be primed to produce flow. Therefore, the centrifugal pump must be used as an arterial or venous pump to circulate blood. It cannot be used in a vent or suction position.
   - Tubing ranges in diameter of 1/8" to 1/2" and is typically made of polyvinyl chloride (PVC). Tubing sizes are determined primarily by the flow that they are expected to deliver.

PRIMING SOLUTIONS

- The priming solution volume will cause a hemodilutional effect. Its constituents will have a great effect on the metabolic response of the patient, particularly if the patient is a child. Therefore, pump prime needs to take into consideration osmolarity (especially patients with renal failure), electrolytes, the patient's preoperative hematocrit value (Hct), and overall volume of the circuit.
- In most cases, the goal is to have a minimum Hct of 0.21 to discontinue CPB. In an effort to avoid excess hemodilution, the size of the oxygenator along with tubing sizes and lengths can be adjusted to a point to help offset this situation. In some situations, the addition of a hemoconcentrator into the circuit can also play a role in increasing the Hct by removing excess plasma water.

CARDIOPLEGIA DELIVERY SYSTEMS AND SOLUTIONS

■ Cardioplegia delivery systems range from straight crystalloid solutions resting on a bed of ice infused with a pressure bag, to more complex variable ratio blood cardioplegia delivery systems with their own heat exchangers, which cause less hemodilution to deliver the arresting solutions. With blood cardioplegia delivery systems, which have their own heat exchanger and slaved pumps to vary the ratio of blood, arresting solutions are delivered.

■ Although there are numerous variations of cardioplegia solutions used today, they all have potassium as the common denominator. Potassium concentrations in cardioplegia solutions can vary from 12 to 100 mEq/L depending on the type of delivery system utilized. The final concentration delivered to the myocardium should never exceed 40 mEq because a concentration more than this can possibly lead to endothelial damage due to calcium influx. The ideal solution should be slightly alkalotic to offset tissue acidosis from anaerobic metabolism during the arrest and should be slightly hyperosmotic to prevent cellular edema.

■ The temperature and methodology delivery of cardioplegia can vary from continuous normothermic cardioplegia to intermittent tepid or intermittent cold cardioplegia. The simple act of arresting the heart can reduce myocardial oxygen consumption (Mvo_2) by up to 97%. The low viscosity of cold crystalloid cardioplegia can easily reach the subendocardial layers, and this rapidly cools the myocardium and results in a sustained arrest. Blood cardioplegia may require more frequent doses to maintain the arrest; however, it is a more physiologic solution that carries oxygen more readily and avoids the hemodilution effect that is associated with straight crystalloid solutions.

■ A warm induction cardioplegia arrest will improve oxygen uptake by the myocardium, resulting in improved postischemic myocardial performance. A warm, or "hot shot," of cardioplegia before cross clamp removal will increase myocardial metabolic recovery.

■ Cardioplegia is commonly delivered in an antegrade fashion to the myocardium through a cannula in the aortic root. Retrograde delivery is frequently utilized if there is severe proximal stenosis of the coronary arteries, aortic insufficiency, or valve surgery. Care must be taken to monitor and maintain coronary sinus pressures between 35 and 50 mm Hg. Higher pressures can result in a rupture of the coronary sinus; lower pressures indicate that the cannula is no longer seated properly.

ANCILLARY EQUIPMENT AND MONITORS

A variety of filters are utilized by the heart–lung machine. These range from prebypass filters to arterial line filters to remove unwanted items such as microdebris and gaseous emboli.

Some of the commonly found ancillary equipment and monitors on the heart–lung machine include:

■ Temperature probes to monitor arterial, venous, and cardioplegia temperatures.
■ Transducers with high-pressure alarms with pump shut off interfaces, to monitor various line pressures.
■ Venous saturation monitors.
■ Arterial Po_2 probes.

- Online or continuous blood gas/electrolyte/Hct monitors.
- Sampling manifolds.
- Ultrasonic bubble detectors.
- Level sensors.
- Timers.
- Emergency hand cranks.
- Computer interfaces to trend flows, monitored parameters, blood work results, cardiac indexes, and to provide pulsatile flow if desired.
- Anesthetic vaporizers (i.e., Forane).

CONTRAINDICATIONS FOR CARDIOPULMONARY BYPASS

- Intracerebral hemorrhage.
- Epidural hematoma.
- Subdural hematoma.
- Massive trauma.

Figure 14-1 describes the cardiopulmonary bypass circuit.

CONDUCT OF BYPASS

- Communication between the surgeon, perfusionist, and anesthesiologist is the cornerstone to patient safety during the conduct of cardiopulmonary bypass.
- Heparin must be administered before cannulation. Activated clotting time (ACT) is routinely monitored throughout the case to monitor the anticoagulation effect of heparin.
- Maintenance of circulation is no longer dependent on "homeostatic" mechanisms but depends on "cardiac output" (CO). In normothermic adults, generally accepted pump flows are in the range of 2.2 to 2.5 L/minute/m². In patients with hypothermia, lower flow rates of 1.8 L/minute/m² may be acceptable. In pediatrics, two methods of flow rates have been reported utilizing either a body surface area (BSA) calculation of 1.8 to 3.5 L/minute/m² or a weight calculation of 70 to 150 mL/kg/minute. It must always be kept in mind that the "set" blood flow may be considerably less to the patient due to losses from physiologic shunts (bronchial blood flow), purge lines, and vent suction.
- Although acceptable flow rates are fairly well established, there is considerable controversy about acceptable arterial pressures during CPB. At any given flow rate there is marked variability in arterial pressure from patient to patient. The overriding concern with low arterial pressures is adequacy of organ perfusion, which depends on O_2 consumption, blood flow distribution, and intrinsic autoregulatory capability of various vascular beds. Perfusion pressure is determined by the interaction of blood flow and overall arterial impedance, which is primarily a function of vasomotor tone and blood viscosity.
- Regulation of pressure on bypass is interplay between pump flow rates and/or pharmacology to manipulate the patient's SVR. Mean arterial blood pressures in the adult patient are generally maintained between 50 and 70 mm Hg. Pressures below

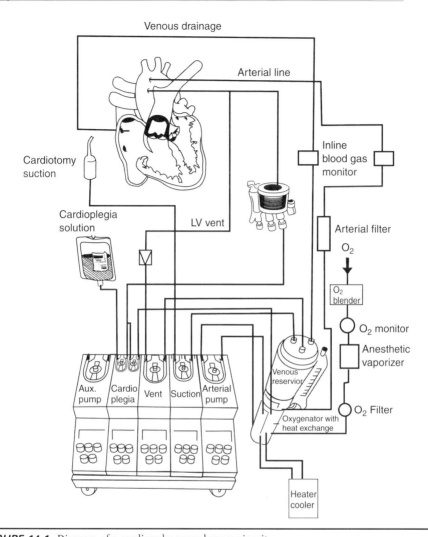

FIGURE 14-1. Diagram of a cardiopulmonary bypass circuit.

50 mm Hg are associated with electroencephalogram (EEG) changes. Risks of high mean arterial pressure (MAP) include rapid rewarming of the ischemic myocardium through noncoronary collateral flow, cerebral hemorrhages, and pump-tubing separation. Hypertensive states are usually an indication that anesthetic agents may need to be addressed and, therefore, cannot be treated by simply reducing the pump flow alone. The surgeon, because of flooding of the surgical field, may request reduction of pump flows. These times are monitored by the perfusionist and announced to the surgeon on a minute-to-minute basis.

- Initiation of bypass usually results in a drop in MAP at adequate pump flows, which is a result of lowered SVR (phenomenon A) related to the resultant hemodilution, which causes a decrease in blood viscosity and a loss of vascular tone because of the dilution of circulating catecholamines. This can be dealt with through increases in pump flows, administration of vasopressors, or through a combination of both. (Phenomenon A is less likely to occur if a blood prime is used.) This situation will generally settle down after 5 to 10 minutes. Phenomenon A can be followed by an increase of SVR known as *phenomenon B*, a resultant episode of hypertension caused by a closure of microvasculature, generation of C3a, C4a, and changes in blood viscosity as caused by third spacing and hypothermia.

Drugs commonly used to raise SVR and MAP

1. Phenylephrine 100 to 200 μg bolus.
2. Norepinephrine 4 mg/250 mL 5% dextrose solution (D5W) as infusion.

Drugs commonly used to lower SVR and MAP

1. Anesthetic agents: propofol, inhalational agent, narcotics, benzodiazepines.
2. Direct agents: sodium nitroprusside, 50 mg/250 mL D5W as infusion.

PULSATILE VERSUS NONPULSATILE FLOW

- Nonpulsatile flow is a common standard because it is easy to use and it is compatible with patient survival. Some evidence suggests that pulsatile flow during CPB provides a more physiologic milieu and probably better tissue perfusion.
- There are conflicting studies on the subject, likely because of the difficulty of isolating pulse contour from many other operant factors during CPB. There are problems associated with pulsatile bypass. The arterial inflow cannula has a cross-sectional area that is 8 to 10 times smaller than the aorta. During the pressure pulse, the transcannula pressure gradient across the cannula must be sharply increased to at least 400 mm Hg over the pressure that is seen during nonpulsatile perfusion if the same total flow is to be maintained to benefit renal function. This is difficult to obtain with either the roller or the centrifugal pump heads without increasing the likelihood of various jet-related effects including hemolysis, shearing of aortic atherosclerotic plaques, aortic dissections, cannula site leaks, and dislocations.
- Despite the lack of outcome studies, pulsatile flow may be advantageous in patients with coronary artery disease at risk for ischemia/infarct, chronic arterial hypertension, or chronic end organ insufficiency (renal, hepatic).

ALPHA-STAT VERSUS pH-STAT BLOOD GAS MANAGEMENT

- The major goal of blood gas management is to provide optimal perfusion to the vital organs. Alpha-stat and pH-stat are the two currently used methods during extracorporeal circulation. Alpha-stat measures the blood gas sample at 37°C irrespective of patient temperature. Hypothermia increases the CO_2 plasma solubility. The pH strategy measures the blood gas sample at 37°C and then makes adjustments on the basis of patient temperature. Proponents to pH-stat suggest that the increased CO_2 prevents the shifting of the oxyhemoglobin curve to the left, thereby enhancing oxygen delivery to the tissues.

- Alpha-stat management has demonstrated the preservation of autoregulation of cerebral blood flow (CBF), thereby maintaining a constant flow despite changes in pressure during CPB and despite a nonpulsatile flow pattern, hemodilution, and hypothermia. Studies on CBF and acid–base balance have demonstrated a correlation between CBF and cerebral oxygen consumption during hypothermia, with cerebral perfusion pressures ranging from 20 to 100 mm Hg. Alpha-stat management at temperatures of 28°C has also demonstrated considerable elevation of coronary blood flow, preserved left ventricular function, and increased left ventricular oxygen consumption and lactate utilization.

- With pH-stat, the additional presence of CO_2, a known potent vasodilator, can cause a luxury perfusion to the brain with higher pump-flow rates. This may be a benefit to neurologic protection in preparing a patient for a period of profound hypothermia with circulatory arrest. It must be kept in mind that CBF varies widely with perfusion pressure; this is associated with increased concentration of CO_2, which is a potent vasodilator. This can paradoxically increase regional ischemia by diverting blood away from maximally dilated collateral vessels and can reduce the driving pressure to areas supplied by critically stenosed vessels. Higher CBF might also increase the amount of microaggregates and air delivered into the microcirculation.

- The debate continues over the kind of management strategy that is the best. The answer most likely rests on the type of case being performed. Current recommendations are to use alpha-stat for adults undergoing moderate hypothermia CPB and pH-stat during cooling in profound hypothermia pediatric patients.

COMPLICATIONS OF CARDIOPULMONARY BYPASS AND AVAILABLE COUNTER MEASURES

- As blood is circulated through the CPB circuit, it is exposed to a comparatively large foreign surface area. This artificial environment has been associated with damaging effects such as hemolysis, platelet aggregation, and activation of complements C3a and C5a, leading to leukocyte activation and free-radical production. The collective adverse reactions have been implicated as the cause of systemic inflammatory response syndrome (SIRS). Surface-modifying agents create a biocompatible surface. These coating agents have been proven to reduce SIRS and preserve platelet function and are currently finding their way in the various components of extracorporeal circuit.

- The combination of the inflammatory process, reperfusion injury, deflated lungs, changes in blood flow patterns while on CPB, and drop of colloid osmotic pressure (COP) that causes capillary leaking in the lungs can set up a form of adult respiratory distress syndrome in the postoperative phase known as "pump lungs." Sometimes referred to as postperfusion lung, patients with a history of poor pulmonary function preoperatively, smokers, and obese patients are the most susceptible to this condition.

- The use of membrane oxygenators, along with arterial line filters, to remove platelet aggregates, leukocyte clumps, and other debris is a standard practice in most institutions today. Vigilance to maintain COP by volume expanders such as albumin, or hydroxyethyl starch to the pump prime, and avoidance of high pulmonary artery pressures to prevent over distending the heart and pulmonary vasculature should be practiced. Biocompatible circuits are also effective in preventing this condition.

RENAL COMPLICATIONS

■ Extracellular, interstitial fluid shifts, and renal blood flow are affected by the composition of the pump prime, COP, endocrine changes related to dilution, and temperature changes, along with reduced pressures and pump flows.

■ Acute renal failure requiring hemodialysis has been reported in 2% of patients. Patients with poor preoperative renal function, multiple exposures to angiographic dyes, and multiple homologous blood transfusions are at the highest risk.

■ The potential of renal failure increases with bypass time, infection, and with low cardiac output states. Patients who have undergone valve surgery are twice as likely to develop renal failure. Excessive shear stresses can cause hemolysis. Hemoglobinuria may develop in those cases where the resulting free hemoglobin load exceeds the ability of the proximal tubules to reabsorb the load.

■ Maintenance of COP with the addition of either albumin (which also helps to coat non-surface modifying agent [SMA] circuits), hydroxyethyl starch, or Pentaspan in the pump prime will help prevent fluid shifts. Mannitol, renal dose dopamine, and furosemide can be used to promote diuresis. Proper occlusion of the pump heads, avoiding excess suction, and proper cannula selection will decrease hemolysis related to shear stress.

NEUROLOGIC COMPLICATIONS

■ Neurologic deficits post-CPB of a variable degree are common. These complications are usually transient and often so subtle that they can only be detected with careful pre- and postoperative examination. The incidence of stroke has been reported to be as high as 5%. The nature of the insult tends to be the result of an embolic event. These emboli can be air, thrombus, fat, calcific debris, or circuit debris.

■ Manipulation of a diseased ascending aorta during cannulation and application of the cross clamp is thought to cause the most cerebral emboli. The use of epiaortic scanning can help the surgeon determine the best location for cannulation and cross clamping the aorta. Newer arterial cannula designs such as a softer flow pattern to prevent shearing of plaque or a filter to trap plaque from the aorta are beginning to gain popularity.

■ Hyperglycemia can exacerbate ischemic brain injury. The stresses of CPB and rewarming can increase glucose levels even in the patient without diabetes. Hypothermia also suppresses the insulin response, causing glucose levels to rise. Insulin may be required in an effort to limit blood glucose levels to <200 mg/dL.

■ Pericardial-shed blood has been associated with lipid microembolization, and there is some evidence that shed blood can be highly thrombogenic. Pericardial- or mediastinal-shed blood can be filtered or processed in a cell saver to eliminate these harmful effects.

■ To prevent massive air embolism during the pump run, vigilance is required to maintain safe operating levels in the venous reservoir. It is interesting to note that although massive air embolism is a real potential issue, microair embolism can be a greater one. Preventing microair being generated from any source, from or into the circuit, must be practiced. For example, air entrained into the venous line will generate microgaseous air emboli on the side of the circuit. For management of blood gases, alpha-stat pH management has been shown to be the optimal strategy for neurologic protection during moderate hypothermic bypass.

- To prevent air coming out of solution, warming and cooling gradients must not exceed 10°C for adults and 8°C for pediatric patients. Careful attention must also be given when rewarming because hyperthermic perfusion of the brain can exacerbate ischemic events.
- Before the removal of the cross clamp, especially with open-heart cases, the operating room table should be placed in Trendelenburg position. Proper venting of the aortic root should also be ensured at this time to remove any gaseous emboli from the heart. Transesophageal echo is one of the latest additions to cardiac surgery, and it is a wonderful tool to assess whether there is any air remaining in the heart.
- Postbypass, especially with valve procedures, small bubbles of air from the heart or air entrained from and around the aortic purse strings can be noted in the aortic cannula. For this reason, it is important to confirm that the arterial line is clear before any transfusion of volume from the pump once the patient is off bypass.

HEMATOLOGIC EFFECTS OF CARDIOPULMONARY BYPASS

- CPB causes a number of alterations to the coagulation system. There is a dilutional effect on all of the coagulation factors, especially on factor V that tends to follow the dilutional effect of the decrease in Hct. These levels tend to return to normal levels within 48 hours.
- Plasma proteins will adhere to a foreign surface within seconds of contact, and this occurrence will be closely followed by cellular elements and fibrinogen. Platelet adhesion by platelet fibrinogen receptors is then stimulated, which results in a loss of platelet membrane glycoprotein IIb/IIIa fibrinogen receptors. This stimulation of platelet adhesion to the foreign surface area of the CPB circuit after the initiation of CPB will last a few minutes and will stop because fibrinogen is covered by platelet fragments.
- After this activation, there is a recovery of platelet morphology that occurs on bypass; however, with a prolonged or strong stimulation these reversible aggregates can transform into secondary aggregates, which secrete thromboxane from dense granules. Activated platelets, with loss of surface proteins and/or granules, are no longer able to function. Postbypass, there is a recovery of platelet function and volume, which would indicate the recruitment of younger and larger platelets into circulation.
- Primary fibrinolysis is stimulated by the release of thromboplastic tissue substances from disrupted endothelium, which is rich in plasmin activator substances and has contact with the foreign surface of the CPB circuit. Prekallikrein activation occurs from surface contact and hypothermia. Activation of the fibrinolytic system by the intrinsic pathways seems to be limited to the onset of bypass, whereas the extrinsic system seems to be affected later on CPB. However, there can be an imbalance between the ability to form a clot and the strength of the lytic process.

- Although there are alterations to the coagulation system from CPB, this occurrence does not inevitably predict post-CPB bleeding. Diagnosis of excessive bleeding in the postbypass stage needs to be assessed after the administration of protamine and careful examination of the surgical field. Bleeding falls into either surgical bleeding, which is controlled by surgical techniques, or nonsurgical bleeding, which is the generalized ooze from multiple sites and exposed raw surfaces such as the sternum and skin edges (see Chapter 18 for detail on antifibrinolytic agents).
- The modification of CPB circuits is currently coming on the scene with the aim of decreasing priming volumes to reduce the dilutional effects of both the coagulation system and hemoglobin. This will also decrease the foreign surface area of the CPB circuit. Creating a biocompatible surface using SMA coated on the circuits will preserve platelet function. Albumin added to the pump prime will lay down a protein coat on non-SMA circuits.
- If the patient's initial hemoglobin count and size of the patient permit, intraoperative autologous blood sequestration from the venous line, upon initiation of bypass of 15% of the patient's circulating volume, can provide a rich source of fresh clotting factors for intraoperative post-CPB transfusion.

FAILURE TO WEAN FROM BYPASS

Occasionally, despite maximal inotropic support, some patients cannot be weaned from CPB (see Chapter 15). This is often the result of a stunned myocardium, which requires a tincture of time and additional mechanical support to recover. Patients with a grade III-IV ventricle are at greatest risk. The support of an intra-aortic balloon pump (IABP) may be required to wean the patient from CPB and provide the myocardium to recover postoperatively in the intensive care unit.

INTRA-AORTIC BALLOON PUMP

Mechanism of Action and Role

- The IABP is the most common mechanical ventricular assist device in use today. The IABP has the potential of increasing cardiac output by 10% to 15% without an increase in myocardial oxygen demand. The role of the IABP is temporary mechanical support for a reversibly failing myocardium. The intra-aortic balloon (IAB) is a long narrow balloon fixed on to a catheter tube, which is inserted into the thoracic aorta, generally percutaneously, using the Seldinger technique through the femoral artery.
- The primary goal of IABP therapy is to increase myocardial oxygen supply and to decrease myocardial oxygen demand. This is achieved with three simple principles: counter-pulsation, diastolic augmentation, and afterload reduction. To meet the first mechanism of action, the IABP must be able to counterpulse against some element of ventricular ejection.
- The IABP console shuttles helium via through an electronic-controlled pneumatic system to inflate and deflate the IAB in synchronization with the cardiac cycle.
- Rapid inflation of the balloon with the onset of diastole after the aortic valve has closed (dicrotic notch on the arterial waveform) increases the volume in the aorta.

This will result in a higher diastolic pressure and will counter pulse blood toward the coronary arteries, thereby increasing the oxygen supply to the myocardium.

■ Deflation of the IAB will, in effect, reduce the volume in the aorta and thereby decrease the afterload, which the left ventricle has to pump against to open the aortic valve. The result is a decrease in oxygen demand.

■ As a result of the afterload reduction, the time spent in the isovolumetric phase of the cardiac cycle is shortened and the left ventricle can then spend more time in the ventricular ejection phase. This translates into a higher stroke volume and thus sets the stage for a higher cardiac output.

Indications

■ Refractory ventricular failure.
■ Cardiogenic shock.
■ Refractory unstable angina.
■ Impending infarction.
■ Mechanical complications related to infarction, that is, decrease of shunt across ventricular septal defects (VSDs) or mitral regurgitation.
■ Ischemia related to intractable ventricular arrhythmia.
■ Cardiac support for anesthetic induction of general surgical cases.
■ Cardiac support high-risk angiograph or angioplasty patients.
■ Septic shock.
■ Failure to wean from cardiopulmonary bypass.
■ Intraoperative pulse flow generation.
■ Support for failed angioplasty and failed valvuloplasty.
■ First line of ventricular assist for bridge to transplant.

Contraindications

■ Severe aortic regurgitation.
■ Abdominal or thoracic aortic aneurysm (femoral approach).
■ Severe calcific aortoiliac disease.
■ Severe peripheral vascular disease (with cardiac surgery, consider transthoracic approach).
■ Aortic dissection.
■ End-stage heart disease not awaiting transplant.

Balloon Operation

Commonly Found Controls on an Intra-aortic Balloon Pump Console

■ On/Off switch: turns console on or off.
■ Zero button: uses to zero the arterial line.
■ Autofill button: fills empty balloon.
■ Triggers: chooses electrocardiogram (ECG), pacing, pressure or internal rate.
■ ECG: select different leads and adjust size (look for largest R wave).
■ IABP balloon frequency: 1:1, 1:2, or 1:3.

- Augmentation: minimum to maximum inflation of balloon.
- Inflation/Deflation slide controls: for setting optimal beginning and end of balloon inflation.
- Standby: temporarily stops balloon from inflating (i.e., to flush balloon, deal with artifact) or starts the balloon.
- Reference line: moves to help set timing and compare pressures.
  Three parameters can be adjusted during operation of the IABP: trigger, timing, and augmentation.
  - Trigger modes: Trigger is the signal that the system uses to identify the beginning of the cardiac cycle and starts IAB inflation. Triggers that can be used include the ECG, which is the gold standard for triggering; arterial pressure; and internal rates on the IABP console.
  - Timing: Timing is the relation between inflation and deflation of the IAB in concert with systole and diastole. Inflation must occur just after the closure of the aortic valve for proper diastolic augmentation, which is represented by the dicrotic notch on an arterial pressure waveform. Deflation must be complete just as the aortic valve opens for proper afterload reduction. Reference to the aortic pressure waveform and adjustments to the inflation and deflation-timing controls will determine optimal timing.
  - Augmentation: Augmentation can be varied by the ratio of heart rate to inflation frequency (1:2, 1:1) and the degree to which the balloon is inflated each time (percent augment).

Conventional Timing versus Real Timing

- Conventional timing: The computer of the IABP console memorizes the R-to-R interval of the ECG, or the peak-to-peak pressures of the arterial waveform to establish a logarithm to determine the inflation interval of the IAB during diastole. This method of timing is best established with R-to-R intervals that are equal. In the event of irregular intervals found with arrhythmias, IABPs that are in use today are sophisticated enough to deflate the balloon if an R wave is sensed. Occasionally, some arrhythmias such as those found with atrial fibrillation can be difficult to track.
- Real timing: can be of assistance with some of these situations. Real timing deflates the IABP in relation to systole. Despite the arrhythmia, the delay between the QRS complex and the opening of the aortic valve, which is known as the pre-ejection period (PEP), remains relatively constant, as does the ejection time, and, therefore, the remaining time of the cycle is diastole. Hence, changes in diastolic times caused by arrhythmias will not have a great effect on augmentation.

Primary Effects of Intra-aortic Balloon Pump Therapy

Inflation

- Rapid inflation of the balloon just after the aortic valve has closed (dicrotic notch) markedly elevates and augments diastolic pressure and displaces blood volume.

The further into diastole that inflation begins, the lower the diastolic augmentation pressure and the less the hemodynamic advantage.
- Its effects:
  - ▲ Increase coronary blood flow.
  - ▲ Augment perfusion to the aortic arch and distal systemic circulation.
  - ▲ Increase coronary collateral circulation.

Deflation

- Balloon deflation occurs just before the aortic valve opens or during isovolumetric contraction. This reduces aortic end diastolic pressure (AoEDP), thereby lowering the resistance which the left ventricle must eject against in systole.

Deflation has two rules:
1. Balloon AoEDP should be lower than the AoEDP of the patient.
2. Balloon-assisted systole should be lower than the systole of the patient.
   - Its effects:
     - ▲ Reduction of AoEDP achieved by the balloon's deflation just before the next systole enables the left ventricle to eject against a lower resistance (afterload reduction); aim for 8 to 10 mm Hg (maximum 15 mm Hg).
     - ▲ The systole following balloon inflation should be lower than unassisted systole. This decreases afterload and reduces the maximum tension required in systole.
     - ▲ MvO_2 is decreased because cardiac work during isovolumetric contraction is reduced.
     - ▲ Cardiac output is increased.
     - ▲ Reduction in peak left-ventricular pressure generated during systole reduces left-to-right shunting secondary to VSD and reduces the amount of regurgitation in mitral insufficiency.

Monitoring

- Following insertion of an IABP, a chest x-ray (CXR) should be obtained to ensure optimal placement. The tip of the balloon should be in the descending aorta below the origin of the left subclavian artery and above the renal arteries. On CXR, the balloon marker is roughly at the left second intercostal space. If the balloon tip is not visualized on CXR, try shooting an x-ray with IABP on standby.
- Urine output is monitored on an hourly basis. IAB placement can migrate and potentially block the renal artery.
- The balloon is always put as a standby before flushing the arterial line. Sampling blood through the arterial port is avoided. The IABP *in situ* should *never* be turned off except for removal.
- Vigilance is required to avoid the IABP complications listed in Table 14-2. Distal leg perfusion, urine output, and daily platelet counts are closely monitored. Prompt removal of the IAB catheter should occur with ipsilateral limb ischemia, visceral ischemia, or balloon rupture.

▶ **TABLE 14-2   Potential Complications and Side Effects of Intra-aortic Balloon Pump Therapy**

Bleeding at insertion site
Infection at insertion site
Coagulopathies such as thrombocytopenia
Vascular injuries, that is, aortic tear or dissection
Limb ischemia
Air embolism from pressure monitoring line; always remember the monitoring tip of the balloon is pointing at the arch vessels; blood samples should only be drawn from this line as a last resort; fiber optic technology is currently available for pressure monitoring on some IAB catheters
Balloon rupture, potential gas embolus; blood seen in the gas drive line is evidence of a balloon rupture; there will also be a loss of augmention seen on the arterial waveform; most IABP consoles will have an alarm status for this event and will stop pumping
Never let a balloon stay immobile in the patient for a period of >30 min; clot formation can occur related to stagnant blood flow on the balloon
Compartment syndrome

IAB, intra-aortic balloon; IABP intra-aortic balloon pump.

- It might be difficult to diagnose cardiac arrest in a patient who is paced and has an IABP. The IABP is turned off and, if the arterial or pulmonary artery trace is flat, chances are that the patient has no CO. Chest compression is started and the IABP is put on pressure setting until establishment of effective cardiac output; then 1:1 rate with ECG trigger is resumed.
- The balloon inflates with helium and has a nonthrombogenic surface and hence does not require systemic heparinization. Follow institutional protocols with regards to heparinization.
- Proper IABP timing is shown in Figure 14-2.

Weaning and Removal

- The decision to wean the patient from the IABP is usually made when the patient's hemodynamics are stable with a cardiac output of >2.2 L/minute/m^2. There are two different approaches to weaning: frequency reduction and volume reduction.
- Frequency reduction is the most common form of weaning. The IABP frequency is turned back from 1:1 to 1:2 to 1:3 over a period of hours. During this time, appropriate hemodynamic parameters (e.g., blood pressure [BP], CO, urine output) are checked. If the patient remains stable, the IABP may be discontinued.
- In volume reduction, the patient is monitored in the same way as in frequency reduction. With this method, the volume of the IAB is reduced by 20% increments without decreasing the frequency. This method tends to be a more physiologic approach to weaning in that it does not cause as rapid a change to afterload reduction. Caution must be used to avoid decreasing the IAB to <20% of its original volume, as there is the potential to create stagnant flow areas across the IAB and promote thrombus formation on the catheter.
- In either process, stable patients may be extubated before IABP removal. The manufacturer's recommendations for weaning are always considered. The IAB is removed once pumping has been discontinued.

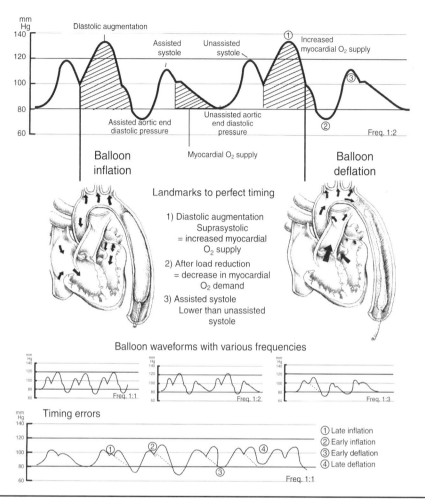

FIGURE 14-2. Diagram of arterial waveform variations during intra-aortic balloon pump (IABP) therapy.

Intra-aortic Balloon Pump Removal Techniques

1. The insertion site is inspected to ensure a routine percutaneous insertion. Some femoral cut-down balloon catheters and all transthoracic balloon catheters require operative surgical removal.
2. The coagulation status should always be checked and corrected before removal of the IAB.
3. Uncontrolled hypertension should be avoided during the removal by sedating the patient or using vasodilators (nitroglycerin) to prevent excessive bleeding.
4. The insertion site is cleaned with Betadine and the stay sutures are removed. The console should be turned off and it should be ensured that the balloon is deflated. The site of the percutaneous insertion point should be determined, and pressure should be applied just cephalad and directly over the artery. The tip should be pulled

smoothly and it should be ensured that the tip is intact and back bleeding occurs to remove any clot. The site should be compressed manually with sterile gauze for 20 to 30 minutes. Compression should be forceful enough to prevent bleeding, but not to occlude the vessel entirely.

5. After removal, patients are on bed rest for 4 hours with a sandbag over the removal site.

SUGGESTED READINGS

Bert AA, Stearns GT, Feng W, et al. Normothermic cardiopulmonary bypass. *J Cardiothorac Vasc Anesth*. 1997;11:91–99.

Brodie J, Johnson R. *The manual of clinical perfusion*. Augusta, GA: Glendale Medical Corporation; 1997.

Consensus statement: an evidence based approach to improving cardiovascular perfusion practice. Available at: www.outcomeskeywest.com/forum. Accessed 2004.

Gravalee GP, Davis RF, Utley JR, eds. Cardiopulmonary bypass. *Principles and practice*. Baltimore, MD: Williams & Wilkins; 1992.

Hornick P, Taylor K. Pulsatile and nonpulsatile perfusion: the continuing controversy. *J Cardiothorac Vasc Anesth*. 1997;11:310–315.

Murkin JM. Con: blood gases should be corrected for temperature during hypothermic cardiopulmonary bypass. *J Cardiothorac Vasc Anesth*. 1988;2:701–707.

Quaal S. *Comprehensive intra-aortic balloon pumping*. St Louis, MO: Mosby; 1984.

Chapter 15

Weaning from Cardiopulmonary Bypass and Low Output Syndrome

Annette Vegas

Successful weaning from cardiopulmonary bypass (CPB) requires a team approach with the surgeon, anesthetist, and perfusionist. Anticipating which patient might be difficult to wean is at best inaccurate, but experience supports age, preoperative cardiac function and length of CPB, and aortic cross-clamp as major risk factors. In anticipating a difficult wean, the choice of prophylactic pharmacologic agents is variable. The early and timely introduction of mechanical support is preferred to preserve end-organ function and allow the heart time to recover.

PREPARATION FOR WEANING FROM CARDIOPULMONARY BYPASS

- Weaning from CPB describes the smooth transition from 100% mechanical support of CPB to 100% physiologic support of the patient in the face of myocardial dysfunction and abnormal systemic vascular resistance (SVR). Attention is paid to the details outlined in Table 15-1 to ensure safe and successful weaning from CPB.
- The patient is warmed to a core temperature of $>36.5°C$. Temperature is measured in the nasopharynx because Swan-Ganz temperature is inaccurate with no flow through the lungs.

▶ **TABLE 15-1 Checklist before Weaning from Cardiopulmonary Bypass**

Surgery complete
Core temperature >36.5°C
Reperfusion time adequate (>8 min)
Metabolic milieu: HCT >20, K^+ <6.0 meq/L, HCO_3^- >20 mmol
Stable HR/rhythm (sinus rhythm 70–100 bpm)
Ventilator on: 100% FIO_2, adequate minute ventilation (PCO_2 <40 mm Hg)
Monitors rezeroed: check for arterial line discrepancy
Additional volume (PRBC, blood products, colloid, crystalloids)
Drugs prepared and mechanical support available

HCT, hematocrit; K^+, potassium; HCO_3^2, bicarbonate; HR, heart rate; FIO_2, fraction of inspired oxygen; PRBC, packed red blood cells.

- The reperfusion time is at least 8 minutes to replenish myocardial adenosine triphosphate (ATP) stores and wash out metabolites from the coronary circulation.
- An adequate metabolic milieu (hematocrit >20, serum potassium $[K^+]$ <6.0 mmol and bicarbonate $[HCO_3^+]$ >20 mmol) is essential before CPB weaning. These values are assessed from the warm arterial blood gas (ABG) sent by the perfusionist.
- The patient requires a heart rate (HR) of 70 to 100 beats per minute (bpm), preferably sinus rhythm, for adequate cardiac output to compensate for a lower stroke volume that is associated with myocardial dysfunction. For many patients, this is the most crucial factor to successful CPB weaning.
  - If the HR is slow, the heart can be atrial, A-V sequential, or ventricular paced using temporary epicardial pacer wires. Failure to pace may result from elevated serum potassium levels or from technical problems with the leads, cables, or pacer box.
  - A fast HR will typically slow down with atrial filling. Reducing or eliminating exogenous catecholamines, administering β-blockers, or cardioverting a supraventricular tachycardia may improve the HR.
  - Persistent ventricular irritability (tachycardia or fibrillation) may reflect inadequate myocardial perfusion or persisting ischemia. Management options include defibrillating (5 to 20 J), raising mean perfusion pressure, correcting the metabolic milieu, and/or administering antiarrhythmics such as magnesium sulfate (1 to 2 g), lidocaine (1 to 1.5 mg/kg), or amiodarone (150 mg).
- The lungs are re-expanded with two to three breaths to a peak pressure of 30 to 40 cm H_2O, with visual confirmation of bilateral lung expansion. In addition to recruiting atelectatic areas, this maneuver helps remove trapped air in the pulmonary veins. The fraction of inspired oxygen (FIO_2) is 100%, and the minute ventilation is adjusted to maintain a PCO_2 of 40 mm Hg.
- Monitors connected to the patient are reset and rezeroed. There may be a discrepancy between peripherally monitored arterial blood pressure (BP) and central aortic pressure, which gradually resolves over the post-CPB period. More accurate pressure monitoring may be obtained from a noninvasive BP cuff, an aortic root line, or a femoral arterial line.

- A discussion with the perfusionist helps determine whether there is enough volume in the pump to come off CPB. In the absence of sufficient volume, the perfusionist or anesthesiologist may administer additional colloids or crystalloids. It is preferred to administer blood and blood products through a peripheral line to avoid trauma to transfused cells associated with the pump.
- Low cardiac output, low mean arterial pressure (MAP), high preload, and poor myocardial oxygen delivery accompanies the crucial period of myocardial dysfunction at the end of CPB. Routinely administered drugs, which vary with institutional practice, as well as additional inotropes, vasopressors, vasodilators (including nitric oxide [NO]), and mechanical support (intra-aortic balloon pump [IABP]), should be available to treat the patient as needed.

WEANING FROM CARDIOPULMONARY BYPASS

- Over a short time, the perfusionist leaves blood in the patient by reducing venous return from the patient with a partial clamp on the venous line. The right side of the heart begins to fill and the central venous pressure (CVP) and pulmonary artery trace become pulsatile. The aortic cannula flow is reduced, and, gradually, the patient's native circulation begins to function. CPB is discontinued provided the heart is able to generate an adequate systolic blood pressure (SBP) with a reasonable preload. The venous line is completely clamped and the aortic pump head is turned off.
- If needed, additional volume in increments of 50 to 100 mL may be transfused through the aortic root line to optimize preload. Overfilling the heart has to be avoided, even if the SBP appears low because overdistention impairs ventricular contractility.
- Following CPB, an optimal SBP of 90 to 120 mm Hg needs to be maintained. Most patients can tolerate a relatively low SBP 60 to 80 mm Hg for 3 to 5 minutes, and often it is a short time before the patient's heart begins to function well without support. Adequacy of systemic perfusion by observing patient color, urine output, and absence of acidosis has to be monitored. The measured cardiac output and calculated SVR give further information on whether to manipulate afterload or contractility if the SBP is low and the filling pressures are adequate.

FAILURE TO WEAN FROM CARDIOPULMONARY BYPASS

- If the patient is doing poorly, the simplest and fastest solution is to go back on CPB. The reasons for failure to wean from CPB may include:
  - Incomplete repair (e.g., graft failure, prosthetic valve dysfunction, and failed native repair).
  - Inadequate myocardial protection (e.g., left ventricular distention, inadequate cooling, inadequate cardioplegia, ventriculotomy, prolonged ventricular fibrillation, air or debris in coronaries, surgical trauma, and prolonged CPB >120 minutes).
  - Reperfusion injury to the myocardium.
  - Inadequate preload or overload (ventricular distention).
  - Unstable cardiac rhythm.
  - Low SVR.

▶ **TABLE 15-2** Options for Weaning from Cardiopulmonary Bypass

Right Ventricular Failure	*Left Ventricular Failure*	*Biventricular Failure*
Milrinone	Dopamine	Dopamine
Norepinephrine ± NTG	Epinephrine	Epinephrine
Nitric oxide	Dobutamine	Dobutamine
Isoproterenol	Milrinone ± norepinephrine	Milrinone
PGE$_1$	IABP	Norepinephrine
Epinephrine	Ventricular assist device	IABP
Avoid N$_2$O, acidosis, low PO_2		Mechanical assist
Ventricular assist device		

NTG, nitroglycerin; IABP, intra-aortic balloon pump; PGE$_1$, prostaglandin E$_1$.

- The consequences of failure to wean from CPB include (a) myocardial damage, (b) prolonged CBP time, (c) potential systemic hypotension/organ damage, (d) need for multiple inotropes, and (e) use of mechanical assistance. There is a potential for a coagulopathy and an increased need for blood products in the post-CPB period.
- Successful weaning from CPB may require further (a) reperfusion on CPB, (b) hemodynamic manipulation with pharmacotherapy, and/or (c) improved preload or pacing. In addition, the patient may benefit from investigations such as repeat arterial blood gas (ABG), transesophageal echocardiography (TEE) (cardiac assessment), or Doppler of coronary graft patency. This helps determine whether ventricular support (i.e., pharmacologic or mechanical) or more surgical manipulation (e.g., redoing graft, replace rather than repair valve) is needed. There is no simple recipe of drugs or single formula to memorize; instead, the management options for patients are individualized as outlined in Table 15-2.

PROPHYLACTIC PHARMACOTHERAPY

- Myocardial dysfunction after coronary artery bypass graft (CABG) is a common problem, with predictable recovery patterns during the first 24 hours of postoperation. Myocardial function initially improves during the first few minutes post-CPB but then begins to deteriorate until 4 to 6 hours after surgery, when gradual improvement in function begins and complete recovery occurs within 24 hours. Worse preoperative myocardial dysfunction may require a longer recovery time.
- In everyday clinical practice, hemodynamic data available during separation from CPB is limited; filling pressures and visual evaluation of contractility are to be relied upon to guide therapy. Despite pre-existing myocardial dysfunction, some patients will not require support to separate from CPB. The short-term need for inotropic drug support appears to be an indicator of postoperative ventricular dysfunction only, and the use of inotropes *per se* does not influence long-term outcome in the surgical population.
- Various intraoperative and preoperative predictive factors associated with the perioperative use of inotropes were studied in different surgical populations (see Table 15-3). Rao et al. analyzed risk factors for low cardiac output in 4,558 post-CABG patients at the Toronto General Hospital (TGH). They reported the use of inotropes in

▌ **TABLE 15-3   Predictive Factors for Postoperative Inotropic Support in Cardiac Surgery**

Rao			Butterworth		
Variable	*%*	*Odds*	*Variable*	*P*	*Odds*
Low EF	27	5.7	Old age (>60 y)	0.0003	4.3
Emergency surgery	27	3.7	CHF	0.04	2.4
Repeat surgery	25	4.4	LVEF <0.40	0.02	1.43
Female sex	16	2.5	Anesthetist	0.002	3.5—0.19
Recent MI	16	1.4			
Older age (>70 y)	13	1.5			
Diabetes	13	1.5			
LM disease	12	1.4			
Three vessel disease	10	1.3			

EF, ejection fraction; CHF, congestive heart failure; LVEF, left ventricular ejection fraction; MI, myocardial infarction; LM, left main.

9.1% (412/4,558) of patients and a higher mortality rate (16.9%) for patients requiring inotropes. Butterworth reported on 149 patients undergoing valve repair and found a 52% (78/149) incidence of inotropic use.

■ Vasodilatory shock occurs during CPB and may be defined as MAP <60 mm Hg, cardiac index (CI) >2.5 L/minute, and/or norepinephrine dependence. Argenziano, in 1998, reported an 8% (11/145) incidence of vasodilatory shock in cardiac surgery patients. Through the multivariate analysis, low ejection fraction and the preoperative use of angiotensin-converting enzyme inhibitors (ACEI) were found to be positive predictive factors for vasodilatory shock. Christakis et al., in 1994, prospectively looked at phenylephrine requirements as a measure of vasodilatory shock in 555 patients undergoing CABG. They found that normothermic CPB and longer reperfusion time tend to be positive predictive factors, but left ventricular ejection fraction (LVEF) <0.40, advanced age, and peripheral vascular disease tend to be negative predictors of pressor use. Patients who had low SVR intraoperatively continued to have low SVR in the early postoperative period. They reported no difference in morbidity (stroke, left internal mammary artery [LIMA] spasm) and mortality in the highest requiring pressor group.

■ Choice and dosing of inotropic agent depends on the pathophysiology of the patient's pre-existing heart disease and reperfusion injury.

 ● Patients with chronic congestive heart failure (CHF) have higher circulating catecholamines and an activated renin-angiotensin system, which have the following effects:

  ▲ Deplete myocardial norepinephrine stores; therefore, indirect acting agents are less effective.

  ▲ Decreases β_1 receptor density; therefore, normal $\beta_1:\beta_2$ (80:20), in failing heart $\beta_1:\beta_2$ (60:40).

  ▲ β_1 desensitization; therefore, the effectiveness of β_1 receptor agonists that are used alone may have a plateau effect.

- "Stunned myocardium" can be defined as failure of myocardial function in normal or ischemic areas to return to baseline after periods of hypoxic injury or reperfusion.
- Inotropes will not reverse actively the ischemic dysfunctional myocardium. Stunned myocardium will respond to inotropes, indicating that ATP stores can be recruited to restore proper ventricular function. The ideal inotropic drug would increase contractility and ventricular ejection without elevations in HR, SVR, and myocardial oxygen consumption (Mvo_2). There is *no* ideal inotrope at present.

INDIVIDUAL AGENTS

Calcium Chloride

- Severe ionized hypocalcemia (Ca_i) reduces myocardial contractility and SVR. Mild hypocalcemia ($Ca_i > 0.80$ mmol/L) produces little detrimental effects on patients who are critically ill. Ionized calcium concentrations have been reported to decrease, increase, or remain unchanged during CPB. Intraoperative ionized calcium levels are not routinely measured.
- Clinical studies demonstrate the ability of calcium chloride ($CaCl_2$) to increase myocardial contractility, MAP, and SVR during separation from CPB. $CaCl_2$ in 5 mg/kg to 10 mg/kg doses considerably increases MAP and ionized calcium concentration in the blood but has no effect on cardiac index. Laboratory and clinical evidence suggests that in the absence of ionized hypocalcemia or volatile anesthetics the administration of calcium does not improve contractility but increases SVR.
- At some institutions, 1 g $CaCl_2$ is given routinely by the perfusionist into the pump when separating from CPB. In patients who have ventricular hypertrophy, high MAP or short CPB runs, $CaCl_2$ may be omitted.

Adrenergic Agonists

- Sympathomimetics include naturally occurring (endogenous) catecholamines, synthetic catecholamines, and synthetic noncatecholamines. These drugs act directly or indirectly on specific adrenergic receptors: β_1 (increases HR and inotropy), β_2 (smooth muscle relaxation), α_1 (postsynaptic vasoconstriction), and α_2 (presynaptic vasoconstriction) (see Table 15-4).
- Endogenous epinephrine mediates the stress response. Exogenous epinephrine is frequently used to support stunned reperfused myocardium. Most clinical studies have shown minimal hemodynamic differences between exogenous catecholamines in patients undergoing cardiac surgery. Epinephrine, dopamine, and dobutamine increase stroke volume at equivalent doses at the expense of increased HR and Mvo_2.
- There is little evidence that β adrenergic receptor antagonists (esmolol) can be administered to selectively inhibit tachycardia without also inhibiting the ability of an adrenergic agonist to increase stroke volume.
- At the TGH, dopamine is frequently run as a background infusion (1 to 5 μg/kg/minute) on CPB to (a) maintain MAP sufficient to run propofol, (b) increase or decrease renal effects, and (c) facilitate weaning from CPB. Low-dose epinephrine

▶ **TABLE 15-4 Action of Drugs on Adrenergic Receptors**

Agent	Action	α_1	α_2	β_1	β_2	Dopamine
Epinephrine	Direct	+++	+++	++	++	Ø
Norepinephrine	Direct	+++	+++	+	Ø	Ø
Dopamine	Direct	++	+	+	+	+++
Dobutamine	Direct	Ø	Ø	+++	++	Ø
Isoproterenol	Direct	Ø	Ø	+++	+++	Ø
Phenylephrine	Indirect	+++	+++	Ø	Ø	Ø

is a reasonable second choice, though patients who develop high dose requirements for early mechanical support (IABP) or additional pharmacologic therapy (milrinone/norepinephrine) are considered. It should be remembered that epinephrine also squeezes the venous system; thus, filling pressures may increase and require the addition of a small venodilating dose of nitroglycerin. Dobutamine is a popular intraoperative inotrope at some institutions.

Phosphodiesterase Inhibitors

■ These are synthetic noncatecholamine, nonadrenergic inotropes that act to inhibit phosphodiesterase (PDE) III resulting in elevated intracellular cyclic adenosine monophosphate (cAMP). These drugs have the advantage of increasing contractility and cardiac output while decreasing pulmonary capillary wedge pressure (PCWP), SVR, and pulmonary vascular resistance (PVR). There is no effect on HR or Mvo_2.

■ Because these drugs do not act on β_1 adrenergic receptors, they are synergistic with β_1 agonists and can have an added benefit when both classes of agents are used. These agents may prevent myocardial ischemia by dilating arterial conduits and inhibiting platelet thrombus formation. The drugs may be difficult to titrate and may cause considerable systemic hypotension, necessitating the addition of a vasopressor.

■ **Amrinone** was the initial prototypical PDE inhibitor. When compared with epinephrine, amrinone appeared to be as effective as epinephrine, but more prone to produce vasodilatation. Owing to problems with thrombocytopenia, amrinone has been replaced with later generation PDE inhibitors.

■ **Milrinone** is a second-generation PDE. The European Multi-center Trial Group evaluated its efficacy post-CPB. This study showed improved cardiac output at doses of 50 μg/kg IV bolus + infusion 0.50 μg/kg/minute (half-life; 50 minutes). Higher doses further reduced BP and were associated with more arrhythmias.

■ **Enoximone** is an imidazolam PDE inhibitor that is widely available in Europe.

■ Milrinone has gained favor as the first-line drug of choice for patients with right ventricular (RV) failure or high pulmonary artery (PA) pressures. A loading dose of 50 μg/kg is given by the perfusionist into the pump before separation and, if necessary, an infusion is started. Low-dose norepinephrine is the vasopressor of choice to maintain an adequate MAP.

Nitric Oxide

- NO is an endogenous endothelial-derived relaxing factor. Vascular endothelial cells contain the isoenzyme NO synthetase, which is responsible for the production of NO from L-arginine. NO traverses to vascular smooth muscle cells, resulting in smooth muscle relaxation and vasodilation. Inhaled NO has the advantage of being delivered directly to the pulmonary alveoli and the pulmonary circulation; it acts locally on the pulmonary circulation before inactivation locally by hemoglobin (half-life; 1 minute). Therefore, NO improves ventilation-perfusion (V/Q) matching as it is delivered to areas with ventilation and will improve perfusion to those areas.
- Exogenous NO is toxic, producing methemoglobin and nitrogen dioxide. Routine monitoring for these toxins is recommended.
- PVR following cardiac surgery may cause RV failure, decreased cardiac output, and systemic hypotension. Attempts to use intravenous vasodilators to decrease PVR in this setting may also decrease SVR and exacerbate systemic hypotension. Several studies have convincingly demonstrated that inhaled NO may selectively decrease PVR following cardiac surgery.
- Treatment is started at 20 to 80 parts per million (ppm), and commonly 40 ppm is tried. The effect of NO is relatively rapid and the following parameters are monitored:
  - PVR = (mean pulmonary artery pressure [PAP] – PCWP/cardiac output) $\times$ 80 (normal PVR = 50 – to 150 dynes/second/cm^5) .
  - RV function: PAP, cardiac output/CI, MAP, CVP, PCWP, mixed venous O_2.
  - Oxygenation: oxygen saturation (Sao_2), arterial oxygen (Pao_2), alveolar-arterial gradient (A-a gradient).

Vasopressin

- Arginine vasopressin (AVP) has long been recognized as a potent hormonal regulator of blood volume and BP through antidiuresis and its release either in response to osmotic changes or as a baroreflex-mediated response.
- Hypotension, post-CPB, is typically associated with a measured increase in AVP levels to concentrations of 100 to 200 pg/mL. In most cases of vasodilatory shock, AVP levels on weaning from CPB were inappropriately low for the degree of arterial hypotension, in contrast to the previously reported elevated levels.
- In certain states (e.g., septic shock, post-CPB) with low measured AVP, hypotension has been reversed with exogenous AVP infusion. For patients receiving left ventricular assist devices (LVADs), up to 42% may have profound vasodilatory shock requiring high-dose vasopressors and inotropes. The addition of a small dose of AVP (0.9 units/minute) raised MAP and permitted a reduction in norepinephrine use.
- Vasopressin is used in the setting of low SVR (i.e., warm shock) with high norepinephrine requirements in the perioperative cardiac surgery patient. An infusion of vasopressin 40 units/100 mL D5W is started at 0.05 to 0.1 unit/minute (3 to 6 units/hour). For patients with normal renal function, AVP is weaned rapidly over 2 to 3 hours once catecholamine requirements normalize. If the patient has impaired renal function, AVP is weaned slowly over 12 hours when renal function improves.

Thyroid Hormone, Glucose Insulin Potassium, Steroids

- In a euthyroid cold patient, measured, free T3 increases with heparin and falls to the lower limit of normal on CPB, and then continues to fall for up to 24 hours postoperatively. Thyroid hormone in animals has been shown to increase myocardial contractility by consuming less energy substrate than normal. Preliminary studies in humans used a dose of 0.8 μg/kg IV at release of aortic x-clamp, followed by 0.8 μg/kg over 6 hours, and then tapered. Despite the theoretical benefit of T3 on myocardial contractility, thyroid hormone is not used in patients who are warm, euthyroid, and unable to wean from CPB.
- The metabolic cocktail of glucose (D50W 1 g/kg) + insulin 1.5 units/kg + KCl 10 mmol has positive inotropic effects, although the cellular mechanisms are not clear. Human studies suggest some benefit for the management of low cardiac output in septic shock, and it is not used in weaning patients from CPB.
- Steroids were briefly advocated in the management of septic shock, but lost favor when they failed to document any improved outcome in two multicenter trials.

Mechanical Support

- In addition to inotropic support regimens, early use of mechanical support can preserve end-organ function while allowing the heart time for recovery. Currently available mechanical support options include (a) IABP, (b) portable cardiopulmonary pump systems, and (c) ventricular assist devices (VAD). The criteria for the institution of more aggressive support from ventricular assist devices include poor patient hemodynamics of low cardiac output, elevated PAP, elevated CVP, and tachycardia with arrhythmias on at least two high-dose inotropes.
- An IABP reduces afterload and augments coronary perfusion, but provides only a modest 15% to 20% increase in cardiac output. The balloon catheter is easily inserted percutaneously at the bedside through the femoral artery.
- Portable cardiac pump systems consist of a centrifugal pump, heat exchanger, and membrane oxygenator. The simplest device is extracorporeal membrane oxygenation (ECMO), a CPB system with venoarterial cannulation placed through either the femoral or intrathoracic vessels. In the postcardiac surgery patient, this remains a salvage technique with poor survival outcomes.
- There are currently two paracorporeal ventricular assist devices available for short-term mechanical circulatory assist; the Abiomed BVS 5000 (Abiomed Inc., Denver, Colorado) and Thoratec (Thoratec Corp., Berkeley, California). The mean time for ventricular support is hours to days, and survival from post-CPB myocardial failure is 25% to 46%.

SUMMARY

Keys to successful weaning include adequate communication with the patient, a little patience, checking and rechecking the parameters summarized in Figure 15-1, and choosing the best drug.

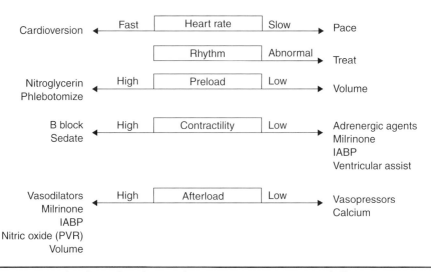

FIGURE 15-1. Outline for cardiopulmonary bypass wean. IABP, intra-aortic balloon pump; PVR, pulmonary vascular resistance.

SUGGESTED READINGS

Argenziano M, Chen JM, Choudhri AF, et al. Management of vasodilatory shock after cardiac surgery: identification of predisposing factors and use of novel pressor agent. *J Thorac Cardiovasc Surg.* 1998;116:973–980.

Butterworth JF, Legault C, Royster RL, et al. Factors that predict the use of positive inotropic drug support after cardiac valvular surgery. *Anesth Analg* 1998;86: 461–467.

Christakis GT, Fremes SE, Koch JP, et al. Determinants of low systemic vascular resistance during cardiopulmonary bypass. *Ann Thorac Surg* 1994;58:1040–1049.

Goldstein DJ, Oz MC. Mechanical support for postcardiotomy cardiogenic shock. *Semin Thorac Cardiovasc Surg.* 2000;12(3):220–228.

Griffin M, Hines R. Management of perioperative ventricular dysfunction. *J Cardiothorac Vasc Anesth.* 2001;15(1):90–106.

Rao V, Ivanov J, Weisel RD, et al. Predictors of low cardiac output syndrome after coronary artery bypass. *J Thorac Cardiovasc Surg.* 1996;112(1):38–51.

Royster R. Myocardial dysfunction following CPB: recovery patterns, predictors of inotropic need, theoretical concepts of inotropic administration. *J Cardiothorac Vasc Anesth.* 1993;7(4 Suppl. 2): 19–25.

Chapter 16

Pulmonary Hypertension and Right Ventricular Dysfunction Postcardiopulmonary Bypass

Achal K. Dhir and Fiona E. Ralley

Pulmonary hypertension, defined as mean pulmonary arterial pressure (PAP) >25 mm Hg, is a common postoperative finding after heart surgery. Cardiopulmonary bypass (CPB), an extreme form of physiologic derangement, commonly results in injury to the pulmonary vascular structures. CPB-induced endothelial damage causes an elevation in pulmonary vascular tone, leading to pulmonary hypertension. Pulmonary vascular resistance (PVR) is the primary clinical determinant of right ventricular afterload. It is unusual for the right ventricle (RV), which actively contributes to the loading of the left ventricle, to be able to generate a mean pressure >40 mm Hg. Any rise in PVR compromises RV performance and cardiac output. Acute pulmonary hypertension reduces stroke volume of the RV by suddenly increasing its afterload, increasing its end-diastolic volume, and reducing its ejection fraction. Chronic pulmonary hypertension, on the other hand, causes right ventricular hypertrophy and dilation because of progressive systolic pressure overload, resulting in gradual RV dysfunction. Performance of the RV is also affected directly by ischemia and CPB. RV dysfunction, coupled with abrupt rises in PVR and associated pulmonary hypertension can result in perioperative right ventricular failure (RVF).

PATHOPHYSIOLOGY

With abrupt increases in PVR, the left ventricular filling is limited by reduced RV stroke volume. The left ventricle (LV) is also compressed as the interventricular septum (IVS) moves paradoxically to the left during systole. Bowing of the IVS reduces left ventricular volume in early diastole and impairs left ventricular filling. These mechanisms lead to low cardiac output and reduced systemic arterial pressure. With elevated right

145

ventricular wall stress, coronary blood flow to the RV, which normally occurs during both phases of the cardiac cycle, is reduced. Systemic hypotension caused by any reason worsens RV failure due to myocardial ischemia. Increased RV end-diastolic pressure is reflected back as increased right atrial and central venous pressures (CVP). An acutely dilated and dysfunctional RV may also stretch the tricuspid ring with the development of tricuspid regurgitation. Hypoxemia in RV dysfunction occurs because of reduced cardiac output, reduced pulmonary blood flow, and right-to-left intracardiac shunting (in the presence of patent foramen ovale or atrial septal defect). Because the right coronary artery supplies the atrioventricular (AV) node in approximately 85% of individuals and the sinoartrial (SA) node in approximately 60% of individuals, any disturbance in the right coronary arterial blood supply may precipitate atrial arrhythmias.

MECHANISM OF POSTCARDIOPULMONARY BYPASS RIGHT VENTRICULAR DYSFUNCTION

Severity of post-CPB pulmonary vasoconstriction appears to correlate with CPB-induced endothelial injury, leading to an imbalance of coexisting vasodilator and vasoconstrictor functions. There is CPB-induced reduction in prostacyclin (PGI_2) and nitric oxide (NO) levels, and an elevation in thromboxane A_2, catecholamine, adhesion molecule, and endothelin levels. The exact mechanism of CPB-induced endothelial injury and of alteration and imbalance of vasoactive substances is still not fully understood. The most important mechanism responsible for endothelial dysfunction during cardiac surgery appears to be related to ischemia-reperfusion injury and an exaggerated inflammatory response. Administration of protamine may cause a complement-mediated reaction. A true protamine reaction is infrequent, but once it occurs, it leads to catastrophic pulmonary hypertension and subsequent RV failure.

CAUSES OF RIGHT VENTRICULAR DYSFUNCTION

A passive increase in pulmonary artery pressure, as seen in left ventricular failure, is the most common cause of RV dysfunction. Overall impaired performance of the RV may be associated with:

- RV ischemia/infarction.
- Acute or chronic pressure overload.
- Acute or chronic volume overload.
- Nonischemic contractile dysfunction.

DIAGNOSIS OF RIGHT VENTRICULAR DYSFUNCTION

Early diagnosis and prompt institution of therapy is required to prevent RVF and a poor outcome. The diagnosis of RV dysfunction can be based on the following:

- Awareness of existing preoperative and intraoperative risk factors such as mitral valve disease, chronic LV dysfunction, some congenital cardiac lesions, chronic parenchymal lung disease, pulmonary embolism, and prolonged CPB.
- Clinical signs:
  - Systemic hypotension and features of low cardiac output.
  - Distended neck veins (raised CVP).

- Tricuspid regurgitation.
- Hypoxemia.
- Increased airway pressure (sometimes wheezing).
■ Pulmonary artery catheter findings of:
  - Elevated right atrial, RV end-diastolic, and PAP.
  - Normal or low pulmonary wedge pressure (unless RV dysfunction is secondary to left ventricular failure).
  - Elevated PVR.
  - Reduced RV stroke work index, RV ejection fraction, and cardiac output.
■ Transesophageal echography (TEE) is one of the most important tools for diagnosing pulmonary hypertension and RV dysfunction; it can show:
  - Increased RV/LV size ratio.
  - Volume and pressure overloaded RV with reduced function.
  - Paradoxical septal bulging.
  - Tricuspid and pulmonary regurgitation.
  Three-dimensional echocardiography and pulsed tissue Doppler should make accurate volumetric analysis possible in the near future.

MANAGEMENT STRATEGIES

Management of pulmonary hypertension and associated RV dysfunction can be classified as follows:

■ Prevention of pulmonary hypertension.
  - Off-pump surgery when possible.
  - Avoidance of factors that increase PVR (see Table 16-1).
  - Following strategies to reduce PVR (see Table 16-2).
  - Following general measures to reduce CPB-induced endothelial dysfunction and systemic inflammatory response (aprotinin, ultrafiltration, high dose steroids, etc.).

▌ **TABLE 16-1** Factors Increasing Pulmonary Vascular Resistance

1. Sympathetic stimulation
• Light anesthesia
• Pain
2. Acidemia
3. Hypoxemia
4. Hypercarbia
5. Hypothermia
6. Increased intrathoracic pressure
• Controlled ventilation
• Positive end expiratory pressure
• Atelectasis

Reprinted with permission from Lovell AT. Anaesthetic implications of grown-up congenital heart disease. *Br J Anaesth.* 2004;93(1):129–139.

▌ TABLE 16-2 Factors Reducing Pulmonary Vascular Resistance

1. Increasing Pao_2
2. Hypocarbia
3. Alkalemia
4. Minimizing intrathoracic pressure
• Spontaneous ventilation (if possible)
• Normal lung volumes
• High frequency and jet ventilation
5. Avoidance of sympathetic stimulation
• Deep anesthesia
6. Pharmacologic methods
• Vasodilators

Reprinted with permission from Lovell AT. Anaesthetic implications of grown-up congenital heart disease. *Br J Anaesth.* 2004;93(1):129–139.

- Therapy for RV dysfunction/failure (see Table 16-3):
  - Preload optimization.
  - Inotropic support (contractility).
  - Vasodilators (afterload reduction).
  - Vasoconstrictors (maintaining perfusion pressure).
  - Mechanical assist devices.

TREATMENT

- Preload optimization: Volume loading was traditionally used for RV infarction. However, in the presence of a raised PVR, volume loading of the RV is ineffective, and with a high RV end-diastolic pressure, further loading of the RV may in fact reduce LV preload. In general, preload should be augmented only if the CVP is <10 mm Hg.
- Inotropic support: This is the cornerstone of current therapy for pulmonary hypertension and RV dysfunction and includes improving contractile performance of the RV and reducing its afterload by pulmonary vasodilation.
  - β-adrenergic agonists: Dopamine and epinephrine have been shown to improve biventricular performance even with a raised PVR.
  - Inodilators: These improve contractility and reduce afterload (vasodilation), thereby improving cardiac output and reducing PAP. Drugs in this category are isoproterenol, dobutamine, and phosphodieterase (PDE)-III inhibitors (amrinone, milrinone, enoximone, etc.).
  - Digoxin is useful in improving contractility and controlling atrial arrhythmias.
- Vasodilators:
  - Nonselective vasodilators: The systemic hypotension that is produced by nonselective vasodilators sometimes limits their use. Commonly used drugs are nitroprusside, nitroglycerin, hydralazine, and α-adrenergic blocking drugs (phentolamine, tolazoline, phenoxybenzamine).

▌ **TABLE 16-3** Therapeutic Interventions in Pulmonary
                 Hypertension and Right Ventricle Dysfunction

General measures	
• Hyperventilation, Alkalosis	Maintain $Paco_2$ at 25–30 and pH 7.5
• Oxygen	Prevents hypoxic vasoconstriction
• Sedation and muscle relaxation	Prevents rise in PVR
Inotropes/inodilators	Improve contractility, reduce afterload
β-adrenergic agonists	
• Dobutamine	2–20 μg/kg/min
• Dopamine	Up to 5 μg/kg/min
• Epinephrine	0.05–0.2 μg/kg/min
• Isoproterenol	0.02–20 μg/kg/min
PDE-III Inhibitors	
• Inamrinone	5–20 μg/kg/min (maintenance)
• Milrinone	Bolus 50 μg/kg then 0.5–0.75 μg/kg/min
• Enoximone	Bolus 0.5 mg/kg then 5–10 μg/kg/min
Vasopressors	Maintain coronary perfusion
• Norepinephrine	0.05–0.2 μg/kg/min
• Vasopressin	1–5 units/h
Vasodilators	
Nonselective	
• Diltiazem	Effective orally
• Nitroprusside	0.1–4 μg/kg/min
• Nitroglycerin	0.1–7 μg/kg/min
• Phentolamine	1–20 μg/kg/min
• Tolazoline	Bolus 0.5–2 mg/kg, then 0.5–10 mg/kg/h
Semi-selective	
• Prostacyclin (epoprostenol)	2.5–20 ng/kg/min
• PGE_1 (iloprost)	0.05–0.4 μg/kg/min
Selective	
• Inhaled nitric oxide	0.05–80 ppm
• Inhaled prostacyclin	20,000 ng/mL (8 mL/h via nebulizer)
Miscellaneous (PDE-V inhibitors)	
• Dipyridamole	0.2 mg/kg slow IV
• Sildenafil	50 mg PO q8h
Mechanical support	
• IABP	Unload left heart, improve coronary perfusion to left and right heart
• PABC	Unload right heart
• RVAD	Rest right heart

PVR, pulmonary vascular resistance; PDE, phosphodieterase; IABP, intra-aortic balloon
    pump; PABC, pulmonary artery counter pulsation balloon; RVAD, right ventricular as-
    sist devicoc.
Modified from Balser JR, Butterworth J. Cardiovascular drugs. In: Hensley FA, Martin
    DE, Gravlee GP, eds. *A practical approach to cardiac anesthesia.* 3rd ed. Philadelphia, PA:
    Lippincott Williams & Wilkins; 2003:46.

- Semiselective vasodilators: Prostaglandins such as PGE_1 and PGI_2 (prostacy-clin, epoprostenol) have more specific vasodilatory effects on the pulmonary circulation because a substantial proportion gets metabolized in the lungs in a single pass. However, they too can cause systemic hypotension if given through the intravenous route.

- Specific pulmonary vasodilators: NO, if given through the inhaled route, immediately dilates the pulmonary vessels, binds to hemoglobin, and gets inactivated. It has no systemic vasodilatory effects, and it has been used successfully in different types of pulmonary hypertension (valve/transplant/congenital cardiac surgery and primary pulmonary hypertension). Inhaled in doses of 0.55 to 80 parts per million (ppm), it reduces PVR immediately and improves oxygenation and shunt fraction, and it easily combines with oxygen and forms nitrogen dioxide (NO_2), which is potentially toxic. Inhaled NO requires a special delivery system along with monitoring of both NO and NO_2 fractions; it also causes formation of methemoglobin and, if stopped abruptly, can cause dangerous rebound pulmonary hypertension. Broad heterogeneity of response to inhaled NO in adult patients who have undergone cardiac surgery is well known. Approximately 30% of patients may not respond to inhaled NO.

  Inhaled aerosolized prostacyclin appears promising, with little systemic hypotensive effects. It has a stable, nontoxic metabolite, not requiring any specific monitor. It has been shown to be superior to conventional vasodilators in treating pulmonary hypertension in children and has been used successfully after heart transplant in adults.

- Miscellaneous: PDE inhibitors—These agents increase intracellular cyclic adenosine monophosphate (AMP) levels in the myocardium, thereby causing positive inotropy, and increase cyclic guanosine monophosphate (GMP) levels in the vasculature, causing vasodilation. Isoform-III of PDE is specific to the myocardium, and inhibitors of this enzyme are used as inodilators. Aerosolized milrinone has been used in the inhaled form for its pulmonary vasodilatory properties alone or to enhance the effects of inhaled prostacyclin with no systemic vasodilation. Inhibitors of isoform-V of PDE specifically increase cyclic GMP concentration in the pulmonary circuit. These agents have been used to treat pulmonary hypertension, especially in patients who are nonresponders to inhaled NO therapy. Two available drugs, dipyridamole and sildenafil, have been used separately and successfully in treating post-CPB pulmonary hypertension.

■ Vasoconstrictors: These drugs are essential to maintain systemic blood pressure and coronary perfusion, especially when using nonspecific vasodilators. Norepinephrine improves cardiac function and maintains coronary perfusion by raising blood pressure in the failing heart. There have been case reports of the successful use of infusions of norepinephrine through an intra-aortic or left atrial line (to maintain systemic blood pressure [BP]) and of PGE_1 or prostacyclin through the right atrial or PA line (to reduce pulmonary hypertension).

■ Mechanical support:
  - Intra-aortic balloon counterpulsation or pump (IABP) improves RV function by improving LV function.

- Pulmonary artery counter pulsation balloon (PACB) has been used successfully in treating resistant RV failure despite IABP and full pharmacologic support.
- RV assist devices (RVAD) are useful as a bridge to recovery or to transplantation. RVAD flow should be carefully monitored so as not to overwhelm the left ventricle (if it has not been bypassed). These devices may be extra- or intracorporeal and could be used univentricularly or biventricularly. Drawbacks include the inability to generate pulsatile flow, difficulty in chest closure, and requirement of invasive monitoring and systemic heparinization. The ABIOMED biventricular support (BVS) 5000 is a pneumatic device, which is relatively safe, simple to maintain, and is ideal for short-term support (average 7 days).

SUGGESTED READINGS

Balser JR, Butterworth J. Cardiovascular drugs. In: Hensley FA, Martin DE, Gravlee GP, eds. *A practical approach to cardiac anesthesia*. 3rd ed. Philadelphia, PA: Lippincott Williams & Wilkins; 2003:46.

De Wet CJ, Affleck DG, Jacobsohn E, et al. Inhaled prostacyclin is safe, effective, and affordable in patients with pulmonary hypertension, right heart dysfunction, and refractory hypoxemia after cardiothoracic surgery. *J Thorac Cardiovasc Surg*. 2004;127:1058–1067.

Haraldsson A, Kieler-Jensen N, Ricksten SE. The additive pulmonary vasodilatory effects of inhaled prostacyclin and inhaled milrinone in postcardiac surgical patients with pulmonary hypertension. *Anesth Analg*. 2001;93:1439–1445.

Lovell AT. Anaesthetic implications of grown-up congenital heart disease. *Br J Anaesth*. 2004;93(1): 129–139.

Riedel B. The pathophysiology and management of perioperative pulmonary hypertension with specific emphasis on the period following cardiac surgery. *Int Anesthesiol Clin*. 1999;37(2):55–79.

Solina AR, Ginsberg SH, Papp D, et al. Dose response to Nitric oxide in adult cardiac surgery patients. *J Clin Anesth*. 2001;13:281–286.

Chapter 17

Perioperative Blood Conservation in Cardiac Surgery

Bruce D. Spiess

Cardiac surgery has historically accounted for approximately 20% of the blood product consumption in the United States. There are changes in this percentage as new surgical techniques have come into vogue.

Red blood cell transfusions are utilized approximately 14 million times per year in the United States for more than 4 million patients. The demand continues to grow and supplies of available allogeneic banked blood are not keeping pace with the demand.

The nation's blood supply hit its lowest nadir, as well as the lowest demand rate, in 1997 (Fig. 17-1). It was at that time that the blood banking industry managed to essentially defeat human immunodeficiency virus (HIV). Throughout the 1990s, the blood banking industry developed more screening systems, voluntary withdrawals, look backs, surrogate testing, and, eventually, nucleic acid testing (NAT) for viral deoxyribonucleic acid (DNA).

In late 1999, the risk of contracting HIV was somewhere between 1:1.4 to 2.4 million units transfused. The risk for contracting hepatitis C was closing in on 1:1 million units transfused. It should be noted, however, that hepatitis B is still a relatively possible threat, with its risk running between 1:50,000 to 100,000 units transfused. Other viruses are far more common. One need look no further than the recent brush with West Nile virus that had the risk of contraction by blood transfusion during the summer of 2001 at 1:400 to 4,000 units. Transfusion transmitted virus (TTV), a cricovirus (like severe acute respiratory syndrome [SARS] and avian flu) is present in 52% of all blood transfused, and 1% of patients who receive a blood transfusion seroconvert. Prions are

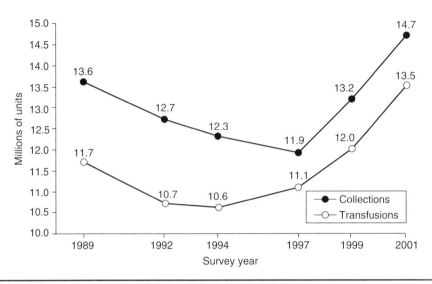

FIGURE 17-1. Allogeneic and red cell collections and transfusions.

now a worry in the blood supply as the first and now a second case of prion transmission through blood have been just announced. That might or might not be of concern to patients with cardiac disease because the time from infection to disease is variably long (years to decades). So, the major focus of blood banking has now shifted from viral transmission to other complications of transfusion and the ever-present anxiety of supply.

RISKS OF TRANSFUSION

Adverse Events

Today the most common causes of adverse events after transfusion are:
- ABO-Rh incompatibility.
- Transfusion related acute lung injury (TRALI).
- Immunosuppression secondary to transfusion.

Immunosuppression is, in this author's opinion, the number one risk factor in blood transfusion. For this reason alone, it is well worth instituting a blood transfusion reduction program in cardiac surgery. Allogeneic blood carries cytokines, white cells, and other humeral agents that contribute to a down regulation of the recipient's ability to fight infection. If nonleukoreduced blood is infused, the white cells from the donor implant in the recipient's bone marrow and actually reproduce. Donor DNA has been isolated from recipients for up to 1 year after transfusion. The donor white cells acutely depress helper T-cell function. It is unclear how long this effect lasts, but it is clearly evident for the first 24 to 36 hours after a single unit transfusion. Cytokines are present in allogeneic blood, and the infusion of 1 unit of blood after cardiac surgery has been shown to increase circulating cytokines in the recipient by as much as 15-fold. The effect of this inflammatory insult is as yet unstudied. It may play roles in endothelial cell dysfunction and attachment of platelets and white cells to areas of inflammation, but it may also contribute to secondary feedback down regulation of white cell activity 12 to 24 hours after infusion. Other growth factors and inhibitors do seem to be present in banked blood even if it has been white cell reduced. Therefore, one cannot simply say that the solution to all the immunologic and inflammatory problems is to leukoreduce the blood.

Approximately 1% of patients are seroconvert positive after transfusion. No one has ever done a definitive study to implicate transfusion as a major cause of non-Hodgkin lymphoma, but some associations and links are present. In orthopedic surgery, the risk of perioperative infections increases substantially with transfusion. Odds ratios increase between 1.3- and 3.5-fold if patients are transfused allogeneic as opposed to autologous blood. It should be noted that autologous blood by itself is immunosuppressive, and even euvolemic hemodilution blood has some increased levels of cytokines and other agents that are mild immunosuppressives.

Interestingly, the latest work examining the use of leukoreduced versus non-leukoreduced blood in randomized trials has shown that patients had a minimal (0.5-day) difference in length of stay if they were transfused leukoreduced blood after cardiac surgery. However, for those patients receiving no blood as compared to either group that did receive blood, the difference in length of stay was more than 4 days. The definitive prospective randomized trial of transfusion or no transfusion for heart surgery is yet to be performed and needs to be done to establish whether decreased extent of transfusion in patients could lead to the reduction of infection (e.g., pneumonia).

COST OF RED CELLS TRANSFUSION

Today, a unit of red cells for purchase from the American Red Cross or a community-based blood center costs somewhere between $150 to $350. It is projected that by 2007 the cost will increase to more than $500. The rate of rise in cost per unit is increasing ever more steeply each year, and shortages will drive the costs even higher. Each new NAT test adds from $7 to $15 per unit. Leukoreduction adds about $35 per unit and autologous donation almost doubles the cost.

TECHNIQUES TO ACCOMPLISH REDUCTION IN TRANSFUSION

Table 17-1 lists a large number of potential strategies to decrease dependency upon banked blood. The remainder of this chapter discusses a number of these options but does not exhaustively search the literature on each one. Much of the literature has used a single technique in cardiac surgery and then compared that prospectively or retrospectively to patients wherein the technique has not been employed. Each institution should practice a multimodule approach in anesthesia and surgical techniques, and pharmacologies in reducing blood products transfusion.

Transfusion Trigger/Permissive Anemia

By allowing more permissive anemia, the demand for blood will decrease in a given cardiac surgical unit. Most cardiac teams have a predetermined trigger for transfusion.

▶ **TABLE 17-1   Techniques to Accomplish Blood Transfusion Reduction in Cardiac Surgery**

Permissive anemia (changed transfusion trigger)
Meticulous hemostasis
Intraoperative cell salvage
Postoperative cell salvage (mediastinal reinfusion)
Erythropoietin utilization
Anesthetic techniques (postoperative epidural/intrathecal narcotics)
Euvolemic hemodilution (intraoperative autologous donations)
Autologous predonation
Enhanced coagulation testing
Coagulation treatment algorithm
Aprotinin
Lysin analogs
DDAVP
Critical care limitation of blood draws
Small bypass circuits
Heparin coated/bonded circuits
New anticoagulants
RAP
Factor VIIIa/rescue therapies

DDAVP, des amino-D-arginine-vasopressin; RAP, retrograde autologous prime.

In several recent surveys of transfusion utilization, the range of red cell transfusion was huge. Some centers transfuse up to approximately 85% of patients, whereas others have reported as low as 2% transfusion rates. The mortality rates from centers transfusing less blood are very acceptable.

There is extensive literature examining the effects of hematocrit (Hct) on the outcome after heart surgery. One study looked at intensive care unit (ICU) entry Hct, the sum total of everything that happened in the operating rooms, and found that patients with the lowest Hct had the fewest myocardial infarctions (MIs) and congestive heart failure (CHF). In some high-risk subgroups they also had the lowest death rate. This study did control for transfusion and had extensive controls for confounders. In a study of renal failure, lowest Hct on bypass was found to relate to increased mortality. But, when transfusions were taken into account, the mortality rates increased with transfusion, giving the take-home message that although anemia is bad, trying to treat the anemia may be worse.

Using an arbitrary way of transfusing, triggered by a preconceived Hct number, at any time during the operation is not physiologic. Oxygen-carrying capacity deficits are to be treated with red cell transfusion and not with arbitrary laboratory values. Finding one or many different ways to assess oxygen supply and demand for a patient with cardiac disease is probably more physiologic than transfusing based upon an arbitrary, although heartfelt, Hct transfusion trigger. We have adopted such a strategy in our institution and have therefore routinely accepted Hct levels both on bypass and in the ICU that heretofore were not tolerated. This is certainly not to say that transfusion is not utilized at our institution, but the basic paradigm has considerably changed. As a result, the utilization of transfusion within our institution has also changed. Today, approximately 20% of all patients who undergo heart surgery receive any red cells during their entire hospital stay. At its lowest nadir, only 8% of patients were transfused, simply because there is no absolute lowest Hct on bypass or on entry to the ICU. It depends upon the clinical picture the patient presents, as well as the aforementioned measures of oxygen supply and demand. Therefore, each institution is left to designing their transfusion trigger. We firmly believe that using an oxygen deficit definition will conserve blood, and the data so far support that patients do as well or better with this paradigm change.

Meticulous Surgical Hemostasis

If a center is genuinely particular about blood transfusion reduction, then certain politically hard questions have to be addressed. This may mean that the chief of surgery should get metrics on his or her surgeons' length of surgery, as well as their utilization of blood products, chest tube bleeding, reoperation rates, and, ultimately, the length of hospital stay and morbidity and mortality. For each institution, there will clearly be a right and a wrong way of collecting the metrics and dealing with the results.

Cell Salvage

Banked blood does not supply adequate oxygen delivery. Only fresh blood or native red cells can do that. Therefore, conserving red cell mass by salvage is one very valuable technique. There are arguments raging in the anesthesia and surgical literature right now about the use of mediastinal direct harvest to the pump, cardiotomy suction versus suction to a cell salvage device. It appears that fat emboli and thrombin generation are increased when direct mediastinal harvest to the cardiopulmonary bypass (CPB) machine is routinely carried out.

Cell salvage machines can be set up with a reservoir on suction and anticoagulation of the captured blood. Cell savers in use today concentrate the cells to between a 55% to 70% Hct and resuspend them in normal saline. They require at least 500 mL of suction fluid to be able to cycle, but more importantly, they are usually preprogrammed to fill, centrifuge, and empty only when the bowl has finished cycling and has a volume at the correct concentration of cells. There is a widespread misconception that cell-saver blood has residual heparin or other anticoagulants after processing. There is absolutely no need to administer protamine to cover any blood from the cell saver. There is also essentially no coagulation protein presence or any platelets left. There may well be activated white cells, some level of cytokines created merely from the cell processing, and some bradykinins generated from contact. But once the wash cycle has been performed, these should be greatly reduced and are certainly less than those present in the mediastinum or from the bypass system alone.

One question that is often asked is whether it is better to wash blood from the bypass machine at the end of the case through the cell saver or directly reinfuse it to the patient. It seems that there is no right answer to this, and this author is not aware of any well-performed study to tell us which is better. If one wants to increase the Hct of the patient, cell saver processing of the blood might well help boost the Hgb by a gram per liter or so after surgery. The loss of platelets and coagulation proteins will be the result, and one has to wonder how much is gained by a slight increase in oxygen carrying capacity/concentration of red cells. Very often, with a patient who has normal renal function, the kidneys will concentrate the red cells within several hours and the Hct will increase.

Every red cell is precious and it should be the standard in the operating room that all lap sponges and other sources of red cells be harvested. Soaking these in saline, which is then processed through the cell saver, shows meticulous attention to harvesting every native red cell. Once again, this one technique alone may not be enough to decrease transfusion needs, but it should be considered as part of an overall program.

The cost of cell saver hardware can be an added part of the surgical budget. Today, cell saver inserts are roughly the same cost as 1 unit of red cells. The cost of the sterile reservoir, saline, and some anticoagulant is approximately 20% of the cost of a unit of red cells and is well worth setting up for every cardiac case. The only real contraindications to utilization of cell salvage are overwhelming sepsis and direct tumor resection. Both of these have been debated in the literature and may actually be relative contraindications. Cell savers have been utilized in sickle disease without worsening of outcomes although it is unclear whether some sickling will occur in the cell saver machine.

Autologous Predonation

Preoperative autologous donation has been in and out of vogue. In heart surgery in the United States, it is utilized <1% of the time. However, this is different in other countries. In Western Europe, where heart surgery often has prolonged waiting periods, there are centers wherein autologous predonation is utilized in >50% of patients.

For patients with stable angina undergoing coronary artery bypass grafting (CABG) surgery, it does seem reasonable to consider delaying surgery for 1 to 3 weeks while 1 to 3 units of autologous blood is harvested. It can be done safely in a monitored environment with some fluid reinfused. Autologous blood has all the same dysfunctional oxygen carrying capacity as does allogeneic blood aged the same way in the blood bank. Therefore, the use of autologous blood will not necessarily improve the recipient's oxygen delivery any better than allogeneic blood. There are still some mild, inflammatory, and downregulating effects even of autologous predonated blood. Autologous blood harvest may well decrease the patient's entry Hct such that his or her hemodilution during surgery brings him or her closer to a transfusion trigger. The efficacy of autologous predonation can certainly be increased by effective iron therapy and/or the combination of a shot or two of erythropoietin. Erythropoietin is expensive and is not recommended for patients who have their own normal erythroblastic capabilities.

Erythropoietin Therapy

Erythropoietin therapy has been approved for use in increasing red cell mass for patients with renal disease and for those who are anemic before surgery. High-dose erythropoietin can be administered with a major iron boost at the same time, and a reactive erythrocytosis is present within 5 to 7 days. Maybe more importantly, the patient's own marrow is activated and, postoperatively, the time for rebound of red cell mass can be reduced. Once again, there are no large studies to guide the interested anesthesia and surgery groups about using erythropoietin for cardiac surgery. Carefully predetermined groups of patients at particularly high risk for transfusion might well benefit. What can be said for epo therapy can also be said for high-dose iron therapy. There does exist some literature that the use of some iron preparations may well help boost erythropoiesis, especially in the groups of patients who are debilitated and otherwise with little iron store. Again, as a group comes together to plan, it seems that such therapy should be discussed as an option even if surgery needs to be postponed.

Euvolemic Hemodilution

Euvolemic hemodilution is very easy to accomplish and is quite inexpensive. The cost of preloaded blood storage bags with citrate preservative is only a few dollars. The cost of volume infusions to replete the circulating volume taken out with the phlebotomy may be in the range of $30 to $60, and then one should have a mechanical rotating platelet shaker available in the operating room to keep the euvolemic autologous blood stirred so that platelets do not clump. Euvolemic intraoperative hemodilution has been carried out in many surgeries. It has proven to be very cost effective in prostate and orthopedic surgery. In heart surgery, it has not independently been proven widely to be effective alone.

Euvolemic hemodilution, if utilized, will provide a ready volume of high Hct autologous blood for reinfusion at the end of surgery. Platelet function within the bags should be as close to normal as actually possible. The red cells will have near normal functioning 2,3-diphosphoglycerate (DPG) and, therefore, transport oxygen as well as the patient's cells that have been in the body all along. Also, the use of euvolemic blood will decrease circulating Hct and therefore decrease the Hct on bypass, as well as in the early few minutes of postweaning from the bypass machine. If that causes a patient to reach a transfusion trigger it may then be counterproductive, but the blood would be available in the operating room to be reinfused immediately.

In patients with relatively normal body size and red cell concentration, it is easy to take 1 to 3 units of red cells before going onto bypass for a CABG surgery. This can be done while the internal mammary artery is being taken down (usually about 30 to 60 minutes).

Circuit Priming, Size, Retrograde Autologous Prime

In CPB, the risk for transfusion is determined by gender, body size, and relative anemia of patients being operated on. A normal CPB circuit will require 1,500 to 2,000 mL of either crystalloid or colloid to prime. It is hemodilution that is the largest driver for transfusion in cardiac surgery. Newer circuits and indeed entirely new bypass machines have circuit volumes of approximately 500 mL. Even if one is using the full-sized circuits, then cutting tubing or eliminating dead space as much as possible is worthwhile (see Chapter 14).

Retrograde autologous prime (RAP) is a technique performed by the perfusionist just as the team is ready to switch onto bypass circulation. The venous, arterial, or both limbs of the bypass circuit are slowly drained back, removing their colloid or crystalloid prime. It is quite possible to get as much as 800 mL or more back out of the circuit by using this technique. It therefore becomes possible to cut the single largest cause of transfusion, hemodilution, by 50%. In our institution, it is utilized now in approximately 50% of cases and does make a difference in our level of hemodilution. The team needs to assess how often the perfusionists then have to give fluid during the case to be able to maintain circulating volume. RAP techniques are not independently going to reduce blood transfusion requirements substantially but can be part of an overall program. In one study, it only accounted for a 4% drop in blood transfusion rate.

Postoperative Mediastinal Cell Salvage

The postoperative mediastinal cell salvage technique uses the standard sterile chest tube drainage system, filters the collected fluid, and simply rehangs that fluid to be run in through the intravenous line. Studies using this technique have had mixed results in decreasing blood utilization. The red cells collected, unfortunately, come with a high price in biochemical contaminants. Chest tube drainage is, at best, a fluid with Hct equal to that of the circulating blood. At the end of surgery, intravascular blood is already hemodiluted. As time goes by, the chest tube drainage contains more lymph or other cellular leakage products and less pure blood. Although what appears in the chest tube is red, it does not mean that there are a majority of red cells. Few studies have ever tested chest tube output Hct before reinfusion. What is collected may well have undergone clot formation and secondary degradation due to fibrinolysis. Therefore, the D-dimer, fibrinopeptides, cytokines, white cells, thrombin, and platelet activating substance concentrations are larger. In one study of more than 2,000 patients, it was shown that reinfusion of mediastinal blood may actually worsen the outcome. Therefore, reinfusion is not recommended by this author as part of an overall realistic blood transfusion reduction strategy; however, in rare catastrophic bleeding, wherein blood products are not readily available, its use could be lifesaving. In such a case, it is most likely that blood accumulating in the chest tubes is closer in composition to that of the circulating blood, and the most probable cause of bleeding might be surgical bleeding.

Aprotinin, Synthetic Antifibrinolytics, and Des-Amino-D-Arginine-Vasopressin

Today, prophylactic use of antifibrinolytics has become almost universal for on-pump heart surgery. Aprotinin, a 56 amino acid nonspecific serine protease inhibitor, is very effective both in decreasing the postoperative chest tube drainage as well as in transfusion utilization. The lysine analogue drugs, tranexamic acid and ε-amino caproic acid (Amicar), are competitive antagonists for lysine attachment to plasminogen. They block the conversion of plasminogen to active plasmin. Aprotinin does so at a very low dose, but it also inhibits a wide range of inflammatory reactions. Both the lysine analogues and aprotinin decrease bleeding. Des-amino-D-arginine-vasopressin (DDAVP) is an analog of vasopressin without any vasoconstrictive properties. If anything, it is a moderate vasodilator. DDAVP increases the release of von Willebrand factor (VWF) from platelets and endothelial cells in some patients. VWF is important in the adherence and aggregation of platelets to areas of endothelial damage. The dosages and coagulation management of these medications are detailed in Chapter 18.

Enhanced Coagulation Management

Profound coagulation changes occur during heart surgery. The administration of large dosages of unfractionated heparin sets up a series of adverse events that leads to partial platelet activation, partial fibrinolysis, depression of the body's own antithrombotic buffering capacity, and other far-ranging effects. The administration of protamine to reverse heparin further creates side effects that can portend moderate to severe coagulopathic bleeding. Hemodilution, protein consumption, and the production of a number of coagulation inhibitors also contribute to the complexity of coagulation abnormalities. Monitoring heparin and protamine anticoagulation and reversal has been historically performed by the use of activated clotting times (ACT). Other variations of the basic ACT technology using different concentrations of activators has led to the ability to do an in-operating room bioassay for heparin concentration as well as dose response curves.

Monitoring platelet number and some coagulation parameters would seem reasonable in an effort to direct therapy. The therapies for the patient with coagulopathy and cardiac disease are really quite few. Platelet infusion, cryoprecipitate, fresh frozen plasma (FFP), DDAVP, aprotinin, and now activated factor VIIa are all that is available. The standard coagulation tests (prothrombin time [PT], activated partial thromboplastin time [aPTT], fibrinogen [Fib], and platelet count [PC]) either individually or collectively are very inaccurate in predicting severe or adverse bleeding after cardiac surgery (15% to 50% predictive accuracy).

Thromboelastography (TEG) is an old technology that gained rebound popularity with the advent of liver transplantation. TEG examines clot strength over time, and the key factors creating clot strength are platelet number, function (particularly GPIIB/IIIa binding sites), fibrinogen, and factor XIII cross-linking. The TEG has been shown in approximately 20 publications to be the best predictor of perioperative severe coagulopathic bleeding for heart surgery. It is particularly effective at predicting a surgical bleed. If the TEG is normal and the patient has abnormal chest tube output, then with >95% confidence it can be said that surgical bleeding is responsible. Algorithms using the TEG-guided (along with PT, Fib, and PC) utilization of coagulation products has shown tremendous decreases in the demand for such products with no difference in overall chest tube outputs for the patients. New techniques with the TEG look promising to be able to ferret out adenosine diphosphate (ADP) and aspiring inhibited platelet dysfunctions. TEG has reduced the use of platelets and FFP by more than one third in some series.

MISCELLANEOUS AND EMERGING TECHNOLOGIES

Heparin-bound or -coated circuits in some hands have been shown to be beneficial. It is, however, most beneficial when the overall heparin dosage can be decreased; many centers have not grown comfortable with doing that as well as using these circuits. Unfortunately, manufacturing companies have been unwilling to invest the money to do a large and definitive properly controlled study.

Both the use of platelet concentrates harvested during the operation and autologous platelet gel have some literature showing efficacy in decreasing bleeding. The platelet gels may also improve wound healing.

New anticoagulants are being tested. These include the direct thrombin inhibitors bivalirudin and argatroban. It is too early to comment upon data about bleeding from prospective randomized studies with bivalirudin, but in angioplasty patients, bleeding has been less than with heparin/protamine, with and without antiplatelet agents, and outcome has been improved. Both bivalirudin and argatroban have been used for patients with heparin-induced thrombocytopenia.

Human recombinant factor VIIa has been utilized as a rescue therapy for severe coagulopathic bleeding after heart surgery. It will shortly undergo prospective testing in heart surgery. From the published case reports, it does sometimes appear to work miracles but all should be forewarned that it is expensive and so far not attempted for widespread usage. It cannot be recommended at this time as part of an overall transfusion reduction schema.

SUGGESTED READINGS

Defoe GR, Ross CS, Olmstead EM, et al. Northern New England Cardiovascular Disease Study Group. Lowest hematocrit on bypass and adverse outcomes associated with coronary artery bypass grafting. *Ann Thorac Surg.* 2001;71:769–776.

Fang WC, Helm RE, Krieger KH, et al. Impact of minimum hematocrit during cardiopulmonary bypass on mortality in patients undergoing coronary artery surgery. *Circulation.* 1997;96: II194–II199.

Hardy JF, Harel F, Belisle S. Transfusions in patients undergoing cardiac surgery with autologous blood. *Can J Anaesth.* 2000;47:705–711.

Hardy JK, Martineau R, Couturier A, et al. Influence of haemoglobin concentration after extracorporeal circulation on mortality and morbidity in patients undergoing cardiac surgery. *Br J Anaesth.* 1998;1:38–45.

McGill N, O'Shaughnessy D, Pickering R, et al. Mechanical methods of reducing blood transfusion in cardiac surgery: randomized controlled trial. *BMJ.* 2002;324:1299.

Moskowitz DM, Klein JJ, Shander A, et al. Predictors of transfusion requirements for cardiac surgical procedures at a blood conservation center. *Ann Thorac Surg.* 2004;77:626–634.

Shore-Lesserson L, Manspeizer HE, De Perio M, et al. Thromboelastography-guided transfusion algorithm reduces transfusions in complex cardiac surgery. *Anesth Analg.* 1999;88:312–319.

Spiess BD. Establishing a blood-conservation program: a pharmacologic approach. *J Cardiothorac Vasc Anesth.* 2004;18(Suppl.):1S–42S.

Spiess BD, Ley C, Body SC, et al. Hematocrit value on intensive care unit entry influences the frequency of Q-wave myocardial infarction after coronary artery bypass grafting. *J Thorac Cardiovasc Surg*. 1998;116:460–467.

Spiess BD, Royston D, Levy JH, et al. Platelet transfusions during coronary artery bypass graft surgery are associated with serious adverse outcomes. *Transfusion*. 2004;44:1143–1148.

Vamvakas EC, Carven JH. RBC transfusion and postoperative length of stay in the hospital of the intensive care unit among patients undergoing coronary artery bypass graft surgery: the effect of confounding factors. *Transfusion*. 2000;40:832–839.

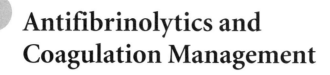

Chapter 18

Antifibrinolytics and Coagulation Management

Jacek M. Karski and Keyvan Karkouti

Usually, a small proportion of patients bleed excessively and require re-exploration of the mediastinum after cardiac surgery depending on surgical techniques, length of cardiopulmonary bypass (CPB), and pre-existing diseases. Approximately one half of these patients have coagulopathies and the other half have surgically correctable bleeding.

POSTCARDIOPULMONARY BYPASS COAGULOPATHY

Postoperative coagulopathy results from an activation of fibrinolysis and platelet dysfunction. Fibrinolysis is due to thrombin generation, fibrin production, and activation of factor XII. Platelet dysfunction is due to fibrinolysis and plasmin formation, with redistribution of platelet receptors.

Although there is no consensus about the nature of damage inflicted on platelets by CPB, the end point remains the same. Platelet damage causes excessive blood loss after surgery performed under CPB.

Recent use of powerful antiplatelet agents in patients with acute coronary syndrome increased the risk of bleeding in these patients.

PREDICTORS OF POSTOPERATIVE BLEEDING

Predictors of patients with excessive bleeding (>750 mL in 6 hours) are indicated in Table 18-1. Preoperative coagulation results do not predict patients at high risk for bleeding.

▶ **TABLE 18-1** Predictors of Excessive Bleeding

Patients with sepsis
Preoperative liver dysfunction
CHF acute aortic dissection
Complicated reoperations for congenital surgery
Coagulopathies (preoperative)
Prolonged CPB time (>120 min)
Renal failure
Aspirin and antiplatelet therapy

CHF, congestive heart failure; CPB, cardiopulmonary bypass.

The results of abnormal postoperative coagulation confirm the presence of ongoing coagulopathy from fibrinolysis and platelet dysfunction. These changes in the coagulation system start immediately after sternotomy and persist for up to 24 hours after surgery.

Coagulopathy can occur in patients with routine operations and normal preoperative coagulation profiles.

PREVENTION OF POSTOPERATIVE BLOOD LOSS

There are mechanical and pharmacologic ways to reduce blood loss after cardiac surgery. Some methods have been proven to be effective, whereas others are of questionable value.

Mechanical Methods to Reduce Blood Loss

- Suctioning of blood back to CPB circuit from the operating field, which requires early heparinization.
- Hemodilution with whole blood collection and retransfusion of all blood from CPB after surgery.
- Autotransfusion after cardiac surgery: The effectiveness of autotransfusion in reducing the need for blood transfusion is well documented (the procedure is used less in patients receiving antifibrinolytics before surgery).
- Presurgical blood donation with or without erythropoietin is effective. There is limited application in cardiac surgery because of the urgency of the surgery, degree of illness, and cost of the autologous predonation program.
- Use of a cell saver during the pre-CPB period is unpopular because it is expensive. Its popularity increased with off-pump surgery.
- Platelet plasmapheresis followed by reinfusion of autologous platelet concentrate is not a very popular method.

Pharmacologic Methods

- Pretreatment with antifibrinolytic agents before surgery is the most effective method for reducing bleeding and transfusion requirements after CPB.

- Use of antifibrinolytics after surgery is controversial but is popular when patients receive tranexamic acid.
- Postoperative use of desmopressin (des amino-D-arginine-vasopressin [DDAVP]) in patients with suspected platelet dysfunction.
- Use of synthetic factor VII after surgery in patients with intractable bleeding.
- Preoperative treatment of anemia by increasing the hemoglobin level through intake of iron and erythropoietin is used only in selected nonurgent cases.

ANTIFIBRINOLYTICS

Antifibrinolytic drugs reduce blood loss and blood transfusion requirements after cardiac surgery when given to the patient before surgery. The role of antifibrinolytics in the treatment of postoperative bleeding is less defined.

Synthetic antifibrinolytic agents (e.g., ε-aminocaproic acid and tranexamic acid) bind to lysine sites on plasminogen. They prevent the interaction of plasminogen with fibrin and inhibit its activation to the active protease form, plasmin. They also bind to plasmin and prevent its binding to fibrin, thereby leading to its destruction. Tranexamic acid (TA) blocks plasmin-induced platelet activation during CPB, thereby preserving platelet function and promoting hemostasis after surgery.

Aprotinin, a serine proteinase inhibitor, inhibits plasmin, complement activation, plasma, and tissue kallikreins. Laboratory studies and *in vitro* experiments show that aprotinin can protect platelet function during CPB. Preservation of platelet receptors in patients receiving aprotinin correlates to a reduction of postoperative bleeding and blood transfusion requirements.

Aprotinin (Trasylol)

Aprotinin is a single-chain polypeptide isolated from cow lung, which expresses activity in kallikrein inhibitor units (KIU). It is a potent antifibrinolytic that inhibits kallikrein and also modifies complement activation.

A number of clinical studies prove the effectiveness of giving aprotinin before and during CPB to reduce blood loss (by 36%) and blood transfusion requirements (by 50%).

The high dose of aprotinin used in these studies was calculated on the basis of the need for complete inhibition of kallikrein *in vivo*, at a blood level of 200 KIU/mL. The effectiveness of a low-dose aprotinin infusion (half-dose regime) has not been proven to reduce bleeding or to decrease the need for postoperative transfusion. A different regimen of aprotinin dose, based on its pharmacokinetics in patients undergoing cardiac surgery, is outlined in Table 18-2.

Tranexamic Acid (Cyklokapron)

The tranexamic acid has an antifibrinolytic effect through the following mechanisms:
- Formation of a reversible complex with a modified plasminogen.
- Competitive inhibition of the activation of enterokinase and noncompetitive inhibition of its proteolytic activity.
- Having a weak effect on thrombin and an even weaker inhibitive effect on plasmin.

▶ TABLE 18-2 Dose Regimen of Aprotinin (Kallikrein Inhibitor Units)

Type of Regimen	Loading Dose	CPB Dose	Maintenance Dose	Blood Level
High	2×10^6	2×10^6	0.5×10^6/h	200 KIU/mL
Half-high	2×10^6	2×10^6	0.25×10^6/h	50 KIU/mL
(Levy) high	52,000/min $\times$ 30 min	26,000/min $\times$ 60 min 500,000 in CPB	10,400/min	200 KIU/mL
(Levy) low	Divide the levy dose by a factor of 5	—	—	50 KIU/mL

CPB, cardiopulmonary bypass.

The elimination half-life of TA is 80 minutes, and approximately 90% of the dose is recovered from the urine after 24 hours. Direct comparison of potencies indicates that TA is six to ten times more potent than ε-aminocaproic acid and sustains greater antifibrinolytic activity in rat tissue.

Data from our earlier studies indicate that a single IV dose (10 g or 125 mg/kg) of TA given to patients before sternotomy:

■ Reduces the number of patients who bleed excessively (>750 mL in 6 hours) from 18% to 2%.
■ Reduces blood loss by 50% over the first 6 hours in the postoperative period and by 35% over the first 24 hours following surgery when compared to placebo.
■ Reduces the need for packed red blood cell (PRBC) transfusion in patients who are excessively bleeding when compared with patients who are not bleeding.

We currently recommend 100 mg/kg of TA (given as a single IV bolus before sternotomy) for surgical patients under moderate to deep hypothermia (<29°C) and/or for those at high risk or bleeding. Surgical patients with a low risk for bleeding under mild hypothermia (>33°C) will need only 50 mg/kg of TA before surgical incision. Our pharmacokinetic study indicated that alternatively, a loading dose of 30 mg/kg (12.5 mg/kg in the low-dose group) followed by an infusion of 16 mg/kg/hour (6.5 mg/kg/hour in the low-dose group) for the duration of surgery will provide comparable levels of TA in patients with cardiac disorders put on CPB.

ε-Aminocaproic Acid (Amicar)

Pretreatment with ε-aminocaproic acid reduces blood loss by 30% and blood transfusion requirements in the postoperative period.

The range of dose varies from 5 g to 9 g given IV before surgery followed by a continuous IV infusion of 1 g/hour for 6 hours to a dose of 15 g given as a single bolus before surgery.

In our retrospective comparison of the effectiveness of ε-aminocaproic acid (15 g) to TA (10 g), there was no considerable difference in reduction of blood loss. However, TA (10 g) was more effective in reducing the occurrence of excessive bleeders and in reducing the blood transfusion requirement. In the recent, yet unpublished study on

311 patients, we have proven that only 19 (14%) patients in TA group versus 37 (25%) in placebo group needed red blood cell transfusion in routine coronary artery bypass graft (CABG) surgery.

Comparison of Effectiveness of Aprotinin Versus Tranexamic Acid

Direct comparison of the effectiveness of aprotinin versus TA suggests that either drug given preoperatively reduces blood loss to the same extent in low-risk patients.

Meta-analysis does not show any considerable differences in the reduction of blood loss between patients pretreated with either aprotinin or synthetic antifibrinolytics. Patients receiving aprotinin had a considerably reduced postoperative blood transfusion requirement when compared to placebo.

There has been no study to date that compares the effectiveness of these drugs on blood loss and transfusion requirements in high-risk patients. Our recent (yet unpublished) case-controlled study on more than 1,000 patients failed to prove the superiority of aprotinin over TA in reducing bleeding or the need for blood transfusion in high-risk patients with bleeding and with cardiac disease.

Antifibrinolytics and Risk of Thrombosis

There is a possible risk of an increased thrombotic tendency during treatment with any fibrinolytic inhibitor. To date there is no published report of thrombotic complications in patients with cardiac disorders receiving antifibrinolytics perioperatively.

Recent studies addressed the issue of early graft occlusion in patients receiving preoperative aprotinin therapy and showed no difference in graft patency among treatment groups. Our study, which was recently accepted for publication, done on 311 patients showed no difference in early saphenous graft closure (up to 30 days) between placebo and TA group.

Desmopressin (Des Amino-D-Arginine-Vasopressin)

Desmopressin increases the level of the von Willebrand factor and improves platelet function. In only 4 of 13 trials, there was a significant reduction in blood loss when DDAVP was given to prevent postoperative bleeding in cardiac surgery. The role of DDAVP in reducing blood loss during cardiac surgery is limited to its postoperative use in patients with bleeding and with uremia or in patients who are on preoperative acetylsalicylic acid (ASA) therapy.

Factor VII Administration

Massive blood loss, defined as the loss of one blood volume or the transfusion of >5 units of red cells, occurs in approximately 10% of patients who undergo cardiac surgery with CPB.

In about one fifth of these cases, or 2% of the overall cardiac surgery population, blood loss becomes refractory to standard hemostatic interventions. Surgical outcome in patients with massive refractory blood loss is generally dismal—risk of death, for example, is increased by more than ten-fold.

As a consequence, there has been a great deal of interest in the use of recombinant factor VIIa (rF-VIIa)—a novel hemostatic agent that is currently approved only for hemophiliac patients—as salvage therapy for patients with massive, intractable hemorrhage after cardiac surgery, although its safety and efficacy for this indication have not been examined by any randomized controlled clinical trials.

In cardiac surgery, a single dose of 35 to 70 μg/kg, given as an intravenous bolus, seems to be effective in most cases. A second dose may be required in some patients.

Given that rF-VIIa is supplied in 2.4 and 4.8 mg vials, we have adopted the following dosage schedule: 4.8 mg (approximately 70 μg/kg) intravenous bolus for patients with severe, uncontrolled blood loss and 2.4 mg (approximately 35 μg/kg) intravenous bolus for patients with less severe, controlled blood loss.

Until such time that the risks of rF-VIIa in cardiac surgery are quantified, its use should be limited to cases where standard hemostatic interventions have already been tried and failed. It is only in these cases where the risks of ongoing hemorrhage far outweigh the potential risks of rF-VIIa therapy.

BLOOD PRODUCT ADMINISTRATION

Blood and blood products should be transfused only with a strict medical indication. The prophylactic use of blood products is not indicated in modern cardiac surgery. Our algorithm for management of microvascular bleeding is presented in the subsequent text.

PRBCs are given only to maintain hematocrit levels to be not <24% during and after CPB (whereas in older, high-risk, and chronically ill patients hematocrit levels are to be maintained at >28%). This new indication of maintaining higher levels of hematocrit than the previously recommended levels came from a yet unpublished study from our institution performed on 6,000 patients. The study indicated that hematocrit <24% during CPB is associated with increased risk of neurologic and renal complication in patients undergoing cardiac surgery.

Treatment of Bleeding

- Platelets (5 units) are transfused if the platelet count is <50 × 1091-1.
- Fresh frozen plasma (2 units) is transfused if international normalized ratio (INR) is >1.5 times the normal value.
- Ten units of cryoprecipitate is given if fibrinogen is below 1 g/L.
- Protamine sulfate (50 to 100 mg) diluted in 50 mL of normal saline and infused over 30 minutes is given in the cardiovascular intensive care unit (CVICU) if the activated clotting time (ACT) exceeds the baseline value by >10%.
- Patients who bleed >200 mL/hour for 2 consecutive hours or >400 mL in 1 hour are treated with repeated primary doses of TA given over 30 minutes.
- Desmopressin (16 to 20 μg) diluted in 50 mL of normal saline and infused intravenously over 30 minutes is given to patients with bleeding and with renal failure and to patients on ASA.
- Factor VII—2.4 mg IV is repeated in 30 minutes if bleeding continues.

▶ **TABLE 18-3 Blood Transfusion Prevention in Cardiac Surgery**

- Patient hemoglobin preoperatively >120 g/L (iron supplement)
- TA 100 mg/kg IV before sternotomy for high-risk patients
- TA 50 mg/kg IV for all routine patients
- Reinfusion of pump blood at the end of the procedure
- TA (repeat primary dose over 30 min) for patients bleeding >400 mL in the first hour or 200 mL for 2 consecutive hours
- Desmopressin 16–20 μg IV for patients with bleeding and with renal failure or recent ASA intake
- Postpone surgery (if possible) after antiplatelet agents for a minimum of 72 h
- Factor VII—2.4 mg IV repeated in 30 min if bleeding continues
- Strict adherence to blood and blood product transfusion protocol

TA, tranexamic acid.

SUMMARY

The combination of both mechanical and pharmacologic means of reducing blood loss and transfusion requirements in cardiac surgery seems to be the most logical way of preventing the need for blood transfusion.

Table 18-3 summarizes the pharmacologic strategies to minimize the risk of blood and blood product transfusion in cardiac surgery.

SUGGESTED READINGS

Dowd N, Karski J, Cheng D, et al. Pharmacokinetics of tranexamic acid during cardiopulmonary bypass. *Anesthesiology.* 2002;97:390–399.

Karkouti K, Beattie WS, Wijeysundera DN, et al. A propensity-score matched case-control analysis. *Transfusion.* 2005.

Karkouti K, Beattie WS, Wijeysundera DN, et al. Recombinant factor VIIa (rF-VIIa) for intractable blood loss after cardiac surgery. *Annals of Thoracic Surgery.* 2005.

Karski J, Djaiani G, Carroll J, et al. Tranexamic acid and early saphenous vein graft patency in conventional coronary artery bypass graft surgery: A prospective randomized controlled clinical trial. *J Thorac Cardiovasc Surg.* 2005;130(2):309–314.

Karski JM, Teasdale SJ, Norman P, et al. Prevention of post bypass bleeding with tranexamic acid and ε-aminocaproic acid. *J Cardiothorac Vasc Anesth.* 1993;7:431–435.

Karski JM, Teasdale SJ, Norman P, et al. Prevention of post cardiopulmonary bypass bleeding with high dose tranexamic acid. Double blinded, randomized clinical trial. *J Thorac Cardiovasc Surg.* 1995;110:835–842.

Lupacis A, Fergusson D. Drugs to minimize peri-operative blood loss in cardiac surgery. *Anesth Analg.* 1997;85:1258–1267.

Chapter 19

Heparin-Induced Thrombocytopenia and Alternatives to Heparin

Fiona E. Ralley

Thrombocytopenia postcardiac surgery is not uncommon, but in a small proportion of patients it may herald the development of a rare but serious complication of heparin therapy. There are two distinct forms of heparin-induced thrombocytopenia (HIT), with different clinical profiles (see Table 19-1). HIT-1 is associated with a mild-to-moderate reduction in platelet count within the first 1 to 4 days of treatment, which usually returns to normal values once heparin is stopped. HIT-2 occurs due to the production of an antibody against a heparin-platelet factor 4 complex, leading to a paradoxical procoagulant state. Once this procoagulant state has been produced, its effects can last from days to weeks even after the discontinuation of all sources of heparin. Patients undergoing cardiac surgery are at particularly great risk for the development of this syndrome. Although the prevalence of antibodies to heparin-platelet factor 4 complex by enzyme-linked immunosorbent assay (ELISA) may be as high as 61% at 5 days postcardiac surgery, the incidence of actual clinical HIT-2 is estimated to be between 1% and 3%, with a complication rate of 51% and mortality rate of 37%. Studies have shown that the morbidity and mortality of HIT-2 are consequences of the venous and arterial thrombi that characterize the disorder. Usually, venous thrombotic events

▶ **TABLE 19-1 Characteristics of Heparin-Induced Thrombocytopenia HIT-1 and HIT-2**

Characteristic	HIT-1	HIT-2
Etiology	Nonimmune mediated	Immune mediated
Onset time	1–4 d	5–10 d
Prognosis	Resolves when heparin stopped	May have serious consequences
Platelet count	Mild thrombocytopenia (usually $>100 \times 10^9$/L)	30%–50% reduction from baseline (often $<<100 \times 10^9$/L)
Complications	May be associated with thrombosis	Thromboembolism, myocardial ischemia, pulmonary embolus, limb amputation, stroke
Diagnosis	Exclusion of other causes	Detection of antibodies
Length of treatment	6–14 d	Minimum of 6 mo

HIT, heparin-induced thrombocytopenia.

predominate, but in postcardiac surgical patients arterial thrombi are more common, often affecting large lower-limb arteries, but may also involve mesenteric, renal, cerebral, and pulmonary arteries. In addition, there is an occasional need to perform urgent cardiac surgery on patients with a recent diagnosis of HIT-2, which presents a unique challenge in choosing an alternative anticoagulant regimen to heparin (see Table 19-2).

PATHOPHYSIOLOGY OF HEPARIN-INDUCED THROMBOCYTOPENIA

Heparin-Induced Thrombocytopenia-1

- HIT-1 causes only mild-to-moderate thrombocytopenia ($>10,000\times10^9$).
- Its mechanism of action is thought to be due to heparin-induced platelet clumping but is not immunologic.
- The alternative name for this condition is nonimmune heparin-associated thrombocytopenia.

▶ **TABLE 19-2 Anticoagulation Alternatives for Cardiac Surgery in Patients with Heparin-Induced Thrombocytopenia-2**

1. Standard heparin protocol (only for surgery) once antibody titers are absent
2. Ancrod (*Arvin*)
3. Danaparoid sodium (*Orgaran*)
4. Argatroban (*Novastan*)
5. r-Hirudin (*Lepirudin*)
6. Hirulog (*Angiomax*)
7. Factor Xa inhibitor (*Arixtra*)
8. Initial treatment with antiplatelet agent (ileoprost, epoprostenol, tirofiban) then standard heparin protocol for surgery

HIT, heparin-induced thrombocytopenia.

Heparin-Induced Thrombocytopenia-2

- HIT-2 is an immune-mediated disorder, caused by heparin-dependent immunoglobulin G (IgG) antibodies (HIT-IgG) binding to a confirmationally modified epitope on platelet factor 4 (PF4). The binding of heparin and other glycosamino-glygans to PF4 alters its shape, rendering it immunogenic. The IgG–PF4–heparin immune complexes bind to platelets through the platelet Fc receptors. The occupancy of these platelet Fc receptors activates intracellular protein kinases, thereby initiating platelet activation and aggregation, with the generation of platelet-derived microparticles. These microparticles are procoagulant and probably trigger the HIT-2 thrombotic complications.
- The triggered prothrombotic risk remains from days to weeks.
- Heparin obtained from bovine lung is more likely to produce HIT than the heparin from porcine intestine.
- Unfractionated heparin is more likely to cause HIT-2 than low-molecular weight heparin because heparin chains bind to PF4 in relation to their chain length.

DIAGNOSIS OF HEPARIN-INDUCED THROMBOCYTOPENIA

The diagnosis of HIT can only be made after the other sources of thrombocytopenia have been excluded. Reduced platelet count directly after cardiac surgery is common because of hemodilution and platelet consumption. However, the lowest platelet count is usually seen by the second or third postoperative day and it is followed by a subsequent thrombocytosis. Therefore, thrombocytopenia during the first 4 days after cardiac surgery is rarely due to HIT. Other causes of thrombocytopenia to be considered in this group of patients are septicemia, multiorgan failure, and rarely post-transfusion purpura.

Diagnosis of HIT-2 is confirmed by:

- The detection of HIT-IgG antibodies, as determined by ELISA for heparin–PF4 complex using goat antihuman antibody or
- By a heparin-induced platelet aggregation study (HIPAA).

As reference laboratories often are required to do these assays, there may be a delay in obtaining confirmation of the diagnosis. Due to the high sensitivity of these tests, a negative result usually rules out HIT-2. However, a positive test does not necessarily confirm the diagnosis of HIT-2 (see preceding text).

MANAGEMENT OF HEPARIN-INDUCED THROMBOCYTOPENIA

Clinical suspicion of HIT (thrombocytopenia, resistance to heparin anticoagulation, or thrombosis during heparin therapy) still remains the first criteria for stopping heparin therapy. Early recognition and treatment of HIT leads to a marked reduction in morbidity and mortality.

- Stop all forms of heparin (including low-molecular weight heparin [LMWH], flush solutions, heparin-bonded catheters) and start a rapidly acting, nonheparin anticoagulant (Table 19-3).

- Avoid prophylactic platelet transfusions.
- Start warfarin only once thrombocytopenia has resolved to avoid venous limb gangrene, a condition that arises from warfarin, causing an initial reduction in protein C and factor VII, which lead to a prothrombotic state that may require surgical thromboembolectomy.
- Surgery is to be delayed if possible until HIT-IgG antibodies are not detectable (up to 100 days). An "off-pump" technique may be considered because only one third to one half the dose of anticoagulant would be required (see following text).

Recent guidelines recommend that an alternative anticoagulant to heparin (see Table 19-3) be started in patients with both HIT-1 and with HIT-2. Initially, this was not thought to be necessary for patients with HIT-1; however, this new suggestion is based on the evidence that, if left untreated, the patients with HIT-1 are at an equally high risk for developing a thrombotic event in the ensuing days. Currently, there are three anticoagulants that have been approved for the treatment of HIT, argatroban (*Novastan*, United States, Canada), lepirudin (*Refludan*, United States, Canada), and danaparoid sodium (*Orgaran*, Canada, Europe). However, none of these anticoagulants have been approved for use in patients for cardiopulmonary bypass (CPB).

❱ **TABLE 19-3 Alternative Anticoagulants to Heparin**

Drug	Source	Chemical Structure	Mechanism of Action	Cross-Reactivity with Heparin Antibodies
Ancrod	Malayan pit viper venom extract	Thrombinlike enzyme	Proteolysis of fibrinogen	No
Danaparoid	Porcine mucosa extract	Mixture of heparan, dermatan, and chondroitin sulfates	Inhibits factor Xa >thrombin	Yes:10%
Argatroban	Synthetic peptide	Arginine analog 66-amino acid	Directly inhibits thrombin	No
Hirudin	Leech salivary gland extract	Polypeptide	Directly inhibits thrombin	No
Lepirudin	Cloning and expression in yeast cells	Recombinant form of hirudin	Directly inhibits thrombin	No
Bivalirudin	Synthetic peptide	Hirudin-derived peptide	Directly inhibits thrombin	No
Arixtra	Synthetic ultra-LMWH	Pentasaccharide	Direct factor Xa inhibitor	No

LMWH, low-molecular weight heparin.
Modified with permission from McNama P, Vegas A. Heparin associated thrombocytopenia and alternatives to heparin. In: Cheng DCH, David TE, eds. *Perioperative care in cardiac anesthesia and surgery.* Texas: Landes Bioscience; 1999;71–77.

ALTERNATIVES TO HEPARIN FOR CARDIOPULMONARY BYPASS

Ancrod (*Arvin*)

- Ancrod is derived from the venom of the Malayan pit viper.
- It is a proteinase enzyme that is composed of 17 amino acids (MW 37,000 Da).
- The anticoagulant effect of this drug is produced by selectively depleting the plasma of fibrinogen by splitting the fibrinogen molecule enzymatically to produce fibrinopeptide A, which is an unstable form of fibrinogen that is rapidly removed from the circulation without affecting the activity of any other clotting factors.
- Defibrinogenation with 1 to 2 U/kg body weight should not be carried out within a period of <6 hours to avoid overwhelming the capacity of the liver and reticuloendothelial system (RES) to harvest the fibrin and to prevent a hyperviscosity syndrome.
- The patient's plasma fibrinogen must be decreased to 0.5 g/L before starting CPB, thereby requiring up to 12 hours for defibrinogenation.
- Its rate of metabolism continues to change, with an initial half-life of 3 to 5 hours that can extend to 9 to 12 days.

Dosage Regimen for Cardiopulmonary Bypass

- The initial infusion of the anticoagulant at 8.4 U/hour must be started at least 12 hours before surgery.
- Fibrinogen concentrations should be measured every 4 hours after initial infusion.
- The infusion rate should be increased to aim for a fibrinogen concentration of 0.4 to 0.8 g/L.
- The infusion should be discontinued once this target level has been reached.
- Fibrinogen levels should be remeasured at regular intervals, and if the level is found to be >0.8 g/L, the infusion should be restarted at 2.1 U/hour.

In a study of 20 patients who received ancrod for anticoagulation for undergoing CPB, the patients had uneventful surgery, but the requirement for perioperative blood products was significantly higher as compared to a control group that received heparin. In addition, there have been other reports of the pump clotting off, even with adequate defibrinogenation.

Danaparoid Sodium (*Organ*)

- Danaparoid sodium is a low-molecular-weight (6,000 Da) heparinoid, which is derived from the porcine intestinal mucosa.
- It consists of a mixture of polysulfated glycosaminoglycans (heparan sulfate 84%, dermatan sulfate 12%, and chondroitin sulfate 4%).
- Its mode of action is by accelerating the activity of antithrombin III (ATIII) against factor Xa and factor IIa, which is similar to that of heparin but with much greater effect on anti-Xa. It is a potent thrombin inhibitor that binds to PF4 and in high doses inhibits platelet activation by the HIT-IgG.

- Cross-reactivity of HIT-IgG for danaparoid, leading to an exacerbation of HIT, has occurred in rare situations (up to 10%) and, therefore, necessitates a screening test before its use.
- It has a long half-life of 25 hours (anti-Xa activity), with no effect on international normalized ratio (INR) and partial thromboplastin time (PTT).
- There is no specific antidote to danaparoid.
- It is now no longer available in the United States.

Dosage Regimen for Cardiopulmonary Bypass

- Administer an initial intravenous(IV) bolus of 125 U/kg after sternotomy.
- The priming dose is 3 U/mL.
- Maintain a continuous infusion of 7 U/kg, which should be stopped 30 minutes prior to the end of CPB.
- An additional bolus of 1,250 U should be given if clots are seen.

Dosage Regimen for Off-Pump Coronary Artery Bypass (OPCAB)

- Administration of an initial bolus of 2,250 U is followed by an infusion of 150 U/hour.
- A target level of anticoagulation of 0.6 U/mL must be achieved.

The first use of danaparoid sodium during CPB was in 1990 by Doherty et al. Although effective as an anticoagulant, its use is associated with a considerable increase in postoperative blood loss. A review of 47 patients who received danaparoid as anticoagulation for CPB found that 36% of them had re-exploration for bleeding and 43% received >13 units of blood products.

Argatroban (*Novastan*)

- Argatroban is a small synthetic peptide (MW 527 Da) derived from L-arginine that has a half-life of 54 minutes.
- It exerts its anticoagulant effects by competitively and reversibly inhibiting thrombin, independent of ATIII.
- Argatroban is cleared primarily by the liver, with minimal renal clearance.
- It does not have any cross-reaction with heparin antibodies.
- Anticoagulant dosage is 2 μg/kg/minute (not to exceed 10 μg/kg/minute) by IV infusion to achieve a therapeutic level of 1.5 to 3 times the baseline activated partial thromboplastin time (aPTT), reaching a steady state within 1 to 3 hours.
- No antidote is available.
- No formation of antibodies on administering of repeated doses has been reported to date.

Dosage Regimen for Cardiopulmonary Bypass

- Initial bolus of 0.1 mg/kg should be administered before CPB.
- There is no requirement of additional drug in the pump prime.

- Continuous infusion of 5 to 10 μg/kg/minute during CPB is to be adjusted to maintain an activated clotting time (ACT) of 300 to 400 seconds.
- Infusion of the drug is discontinued at the end of CPB.

Dosage Regimen for Off-Pump Coronary Artery Bypass

- A continuous infusion of argatroban at the rate of 2.5 μg/kg/minute should be started after induction for 1 hour before off-pump coronary artery bypass (OPCAB) surgery.
- Discontinue infusion after revascularization has been completed.

Only limited experience has been reported on the use of argatroban in patients with acute HIT who underwent cardiac surgery. Several case reports describe the successful use of argatroban as an anticoagulant for OPCAB.

Hirudin (*Lepirudin* and *Desirudin*)

- Hirudin is produced from the salivary gland of the medicinal leech.
- It is a single-chain-65-amino-acid polypeptide (MW 7,000 Da).
- It is immunicologically distinct from heparin and does not cause thrombocytopenia.
- Hirudin completely inhibits all the procoagulant actions of thrombin by interacting with both the fibrinogen-binding and catalytic sites of thrombin, independent of ATIII.
- Its duration of action ranges from 80 minutes (normal renal function) to 200 hours (with renal insufficiency).
- There is no known antidote for this anticoagulant.
- Recombinant forms that are now manufactured are lepirudin (*Refludan*) and desirudin (*Revasc*).

Lepirudin

- Lepirudin is a recombinant form of hirudin, which has been derived from cloning and expression in yeast cells.
- Its elimination half-life is 0.8 to 2 hours in patients with normal renal function.
- To avoid the formation of clots, a hirudin level that is >2 μg/mL is required; therefore, a level of 4 μg/mL is the aim during CPB.

Dosing Regimen for Lepirudin for Cardiopulmonary Bypass

- An initial bolus dose of 0.25 mg/kg should be given 10 minutes before CPB.
- A bolus of 0.20 mg/kg should be added to the pump prime.
- A continuous infusion of 0.5 mg/minute should be maintained until 15 to 30 minutes before termination of CPB.
- Supplemental bolus doses (5 to 25 mg) are to be given to ensure a plasma level of 3.5 μg/mL (as determined by ecarin clotting time [ECT]).
- After the termination of CPB, 5 mg of lepirudin is added to the pump circuit volume to prevent clotting.

■ Post-CPB, a cell saver should wash out the drug from the pump blood prior to retransfusion.

The first reported use of lepirudin during CPB was in 1994 by Pötzsch et al.; it requires individualized dosing that is adjusted by frequent plasma drug level for use in patients undergoing CPB. At high concentrations used during CPB, the aPTT is unreliable because of a flattening effect at these concentrations. In the United States and Canada, there is a point-of-care commercial ECT method available, which can be requested on humanitarian grounds for the specific situation of CPB for a patient with acute HIT (Rapidpoint Coag, Bayer Diagnostics, Toronto, Ontario, Canada, and Tarrytown, NY, USA). The ECT should be maintained between 200 and 300 seconds during CPB. Unfortunately, major bleeding has, to date, been frequently associated when hirudin or r-hirudin has been used for anticoagulation in patients with HIT-2 who require CPB.

Formation of antibodies to r-hirudin has been reported in 56% to 74% of treated patients, but they do not appear to cause an allergic reaction. This antibody formation may, however, delay renal elimination of these active hirudin–antihirudin complexes, leading to excessive anticoagulation.

Bivalirudin (*Angiomax*)

■ Bivalirudin is a short-acting synthetic peptide (20 amino acids) with a lower MW than hirudin.
■ It directly inhibits thrombin with a minimal immunologic activity and with a half-life of 25 minutes.
■ It has two small peptide sequences that bind directly to the fibrinogen-binding site and the catalytic site of thrombin.
■ Binding to thrombin is reversible by plasma enzymes that cleave the binding of bivalirudin to thrombin.
■ It can be used in patients with hepatic or renal impairment.
■ The intraoperative monitoring of anticoagulation requires the ECT to be determined.

Dosage Regimen for Cardiopulmonary Bypass

■ An initial IV bolus dose of 1.5 mg/kg should be administered followed by a continuous infusion at the rate of 2.5 mg/kg/hour during CPB.
■ A bolus of 50 mg should be added to the priming solution.
■ ECT should be maintained between 400 and 500 seconds.
■ Maintain a core temperature of 37°C after CPB.
■ A bolus of 50 mg should be added to the residual pump volume followed by a continuous infusion at 50 mg/hour.

Dosage Regimen for Off-Pump Coronary Artery Bypass

■ An initial bolus of 0.75 mg/kg should be followed by a continuous infusion at the rate of 1.75 mg/kg/hour until the end of revascularization.

In a study of 20 patients undergoing primary coronary artery bypass grafting in whom bivalirudin was used as the anticoagulant for CPB, all the patients underwent successful surgery and there was no requirement for surgical re-exploration. The mean chest-tube drainage in the first 12 hours postoperatively was 700 mL. Anticoagulation was monitored by ECT in these cases. Bivalirudin is now suggested as the drug of choice in patients with HIT-2 and renal impairment. Several case reports also describe the successful use of bivalirudin for the "off-pump" cardiac surgery in patients with HIT-2 where ACT coagulation monitoring was used due to the lower drug concentration required during "off-pump" surgery (see preceding text).

FACTOR Xa INHIBITORS

Fondaparinux (Arixtra)

- Fondaparinux is a synthetic pentasaccharide, which mimics the site where heparin binds to ATIII.
- It acts as a selective inhibitor of activated factor X, with AT as a cofactor.
- It does not have any effect on aPTT and PT and does not bind to PF4.
- The plasma anti-Xa activity peaks at 2 hours and corresponds directly to fondaparinux levels.
- There is no cross-reactivity with antibodies associated with HIT.
- A dosage of 2.5 mg/day is the standardized prophylactic dose with a long half-life of 17 hours.
- There is no specific antidote and it is not neutralized by protamine.
- It is a new agent for the treatment of HIT, and so far there are no reports of its use for CPB.

MODIFICATION OF HEPARIN EFFECT

Pretreatment with an agent that blocks the activation of platelets when exposed to heparin has been given prior to standard heparinization protocols without adverse effects. Classes of drugs that have been used for this pretreatment include prostaglandins and the short-acting platelet antiglycoprotein IIb/IIIa receptor antagonists.

ANTIPLATELET AGENTS

Epoprostenol (Flolan)

- Epoprostenol is a naturally occurring prostaglandin I_2 that is not metabolized during the passage through the pulmonary circulation.
- It inhibits platelet activation by stimulating adenylate cyclase and by increasing cyclic adenosine monophosphate (cAMP).
- Its administration is by continuous infusion because of its short half-life of 6 minutes.
- It inhibits HIT antibodies with doses ranging from 15 to 30 ng/kg/minute.
- Standard heparin doses can be utilized once there is complete platelet inhibition.
- Infusion is to be continued until 15 minutes post protamine administration.

■ Its main side effect is vasodilation leading to profound hypotension, needing vasopressors.

Dosage Regimen for Cardiopulmonary Bypass

■ Infusion of the drug at the dosage of 5 ng/kg/minute is started after induction and increased by stages of 5 ng/kg every 5 minutes until the dose of 30 ng/kg/minute is reached.
■ Standard heparin dose is to be given at this time for an ACT >480 seconds.
■ Fifteen minutes after protamine reversal, the infusion is decreased by 5 ng/kg every 5 minutes until the infusion is stopped.
■ Norepinephrine infusion (0.05 to 0.1 μg/kg/minute) as required to keep the mean arterial pressure (MAP) >75 mm Hg.

In a recent case report, epoprostenol was given to three patients before systemic heparinization for CPB. Platelet inhibition was monitored with a hemoSTATUS II assay. No patient returned for re-exploration and there was no increased need for transfusion of blood products.

Tirofiban (*Aggrastat*)

■ Tirofiban is an antiglycoprotein IIb/IIIa agent that competitively inhibits the platelet fibrinogen receptor.
■ It is short acting, with a half-life of 2 hours and with predominantly biliary excretion (>70%).

Dosage Regimen for Cardiopulmonary Bypass

■ Administration of an initial IV bolus of 10 μg/kg should be followed by an infusion of 0.15 μg/kg/minute started 10 minutes before heparin.
■ Standard heparin dosage can be administered 5 minutes post bolus dose to achieve an ACT >480 seconds.
■ Infusion should be stopped 1 hour before the end of surgery.
■ Heparin is reversed with protamine.
■ Postoperative anticoagulation is achieved with lepirudin.

This regimen has been used in a study of ten patients who had renal impairment as well as HIT-2 in which r-hirudin was contraindicated. All these patients underwent successful surgery with CPB, no patient required re-exploration for bleeding and postoperative chest-tube drainage was not increased. There was no clinical evidence of arterial thrombosis or embolism, or myocardial infarction. None of these patients developed thrombocytopenia postoperatively.

CONCLUSION

At present, there is no single drug regimen that is exclusively recommended for the treatment of HIT. The choice of selecting a drug should be based on the availability of a specific alternative anticoagulant, experience with its use, and the ability to monitor its anticoagulant effects.

SUGGESTED READINGS

Brieger DB, Mak KH, Kottke-Marchant K, et al. Heparin-induced thrombocytopenia. *J Am Coll Cardiol*. 1998;31:1449–1459.

Doherthy DC, Ortel TI, De Bruijn N, et al. "Heparin free" cardiopulmonary bypass first reported use of heparinoid (org 10172) to provide anticoagulation for cardiopulmonary bypass. *Anesthesiology*. 1990;73:562–565.

Follis F, Schmidt CA. Cardiopulmonary bypass in patients with heparin-induced thrombocytopenia and thrombosis. *Ann Thorac Surg*. 2000;70:2173–2181.

Harenberg J, Jörg I, Fenyvesi T. Heparin-induced thrombocytopenia: pathophysiology and new treatment options. *Pathophysiol Haemost Thromb*. 2002;32:289–294.

Hirsh J, Heddle N, Kelton JG. Treatment of heparin-induced thrombocytopenia. *Arch Intern Med*. 2004;164:361–369.

Jeske WP, Walenga JM. Antithrombotic drugs for the treatment of heparin-induced thrombocytopenia. *Curr Opin Investig Drugs*. 2002;3(8):1171–1180.

Murcebe L, Silver D. Heparin-induced thrombocytopenia: pathophysiology and management. *Vasc Endovascular Surg*. 2002;36:163–170.

Potzsch B, Iverson S, Riess FC, et al. Recombinant hirudin as an anticongulant in open-heart surgery: a case report [abstract]. *Ann Hematol*. 1994;68:A53.

Reilly RF. The pathophysiology of immune-mediated heparin-induced thrombocytopenia. *Semin Dial*. 2003;16(1):54–60.

Warkentin TE. Current agents for the treatment of patients with heparin-induced thrombocytopenia. *Curr Opin Pulm Med*. 2002;8:405–412.

Warkentin TE. Management of heparin-induced thrombocytopenia: a critical comparison of lepirudin and argatroban. *Thromb Res*. 2003;110:73–82.

Warkentin TE, Greinacher A. Heparin-induced thrombocytopenia and cardiac surgery. *Ann Thorac Surg*. 2003;76:2121–2131.

Chapter 20

Management of the Cardiac Surgical Emergency

Ravi Taneja

CORONARY REVASCULARIZATION FOR FAILED PERCUTANEOUS CORONARY INTERVENTION

Over the last 25 years, advances in percutaneous coronary interventions (PCIs) have contributed substantially to the care of the patient with a cardiac disorder. Improvements in operator experience and techniques have led to considerable reductions in failed or complicated PCI requiring urgent surgery. However, the acuity and risk profile of patients have also increased, thereby resulting in a greater proportion of high-risk patients undergoing complex procedures.

- Vascular injuries are more common with therapeutic interventional procedures (such as percutaneous transluminal coronary angioplasty [PTCA] and percutaneous balloon valvuloplasty) than with diagnostic cardiac catheterizations.
- Patients requiring emergency coronary artery bypass grafting (CABG) are more likely to be women, have complex coronary lesions, have intra-aortal balloon pumps (IABPs) inserted within 48 hours before PCI, and have acute myocardial infarction as an indication for the PCI. Patients on platelet glycoprotein IIb/IIIa inhibitors (see Chapter 2) and with prior CABG or PTCA may be less likely to require emergency CABG.
- Decisions for emergency surgical revascularization are based on comprehensive clinical, angiographic, and electrocardiogram (ECG) assessment. Recognition of procedural failure and poor response of accompanying pharmacomechanical therapy may prompt the interventional cardiologist to seek consultations from cardiac surgery and anesthesiology. Common indications include:
  - Uncontrolled angina and ischemia.
  - Acute or impending vessel closure (not managed by stenting).

- Perforation/dissection of coronary artery.
- Tamponade (not managed by pericardiocentesis).
- Severe hemodynamic instability (not responding to inotropes/IABP).
- Severe arrhythmias (ventricular fibrillation [VF] or ventricular tachycardia [VT], not managed by pharmacotherapy in the catheterization laboratory).
- Broken guide wires.
- Loss of stent (causing decreased flow or impending thrombotic occlusion).
- Worsening cardiac status, pulmonary edema, or shock.

Although the incidence of emergency CABG following contemporary PCI is low (0.14% to 2%), it is associated with an increased incidence of stroke, bleeding, renal failure requiring dialysis, and in-hospital mortality (up to 20%). It is generally accepted that delay in surgery worsens overall outcome.

Assessment and management ideally begins in the catheterization laboratory—rapid assessment of hemodynamic stability and the degree of myocardial ischemia is necessary to plan preoperative management (see Fig. 20-1).

Hemodynamically Stable, Nonischemic Patient

If there is no damage to coronary arteries, revascularization can proceed as an elective CABG with no unique considerations.

If, however, arterial damage is present, revascularization is carried out as an emergency. However, sufficient time may be given for the stomach to empty before surgery.

- Complete history and physical examination are usually possible.
- Optimize cardiovascular function preoperatively as appropriate.
- Patients may be anticoagulated or have received thrombolytic therapy preoperatively.
- Routine institution and emergence from cardiopulmonary bypass (CPB) may be possible.
- Postoperative coagulopathy and organ dysfunction may impede institution of fast-track program in the intensive care unit (ICU).

Hemodynamically Stable, Ischemic Patient

Prompt restoration of myocardial blood flow during the early phase of myocardial infarction remains the most effective therapy for reducing morbidity and mortality (Fig. 20-1). Emergency coronary revascularization has been advocated for salvage of myocardial function when performed within 4 to 6 hours of symptoms of acute myocardial infarction.

Preoperative Assessment

- Patients may be transferred to the ICU or coronary care unit (CCU) while awaiting entry into the operating room (OR). Expedited management will require coordinated effort between surgical, anesthesiology, and intensive care teams.
- Rapid preoperative assessment is usually possible and should be performed simultaneously with efforts to stabilize and transfer the patient to the OR. The anesthesiologist may have to limit assessment to essential history and physical examination,

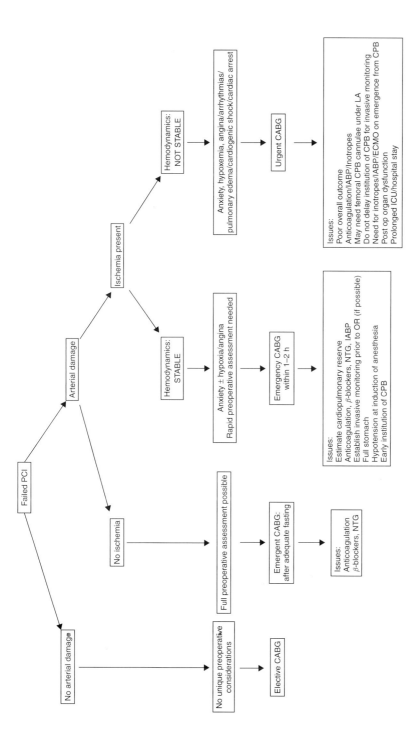

FIGURE 20-1. A synopsis of preoperative clinical scenarios that may manifest after a failed percutaneous coronary intervention. PCI, percutaneous coronary interventions; CABG, coronary artery bypass graft; NTG, notroglycerin; IABP, intra-aortic balloon pump; OR, operating room; CPB, coronary bypass; ABP, aortic balloon pump; LA, lupus anticoagulant; ECMO, extracorporeal-membrane oxygenation; ICU, intensive care unit.

187

and evaluate cardiopulmonary reserve, nature of lesion, extent of collaterals, and degree of left ventricular (LV) function.

- Active angina may necessitate intravenous nitroglycerin (NTG), heparin, and thrombolytic therapy, and narcotics.
- Hypoxemia may be related to the presence of LV dysfunction and pulmonary edema, requiring supplemental oxygen.
- Anxiety may be alleviated by reassurance. Confusion or combativeness may be associated with cerebral hypoperfusion and hypoxemia. Drugs such as benzodiazepines/ narcotics may jeopardize cardiopulmonary status and should be given only under invasive monitoring.
- Invasive monitoring preoperatively should be established where possible.
- Aspiration prophylaxis should be given if patients are not fasting.
- Cardiac status, optimizing fluids, and/or vasoactive medications should be improved. Many of these patients may already have IABP *in situ* and need monitoring during transport to the OR.

Intraoperative Considerations and Management

- Extra vigilance should be exercised during insertion of invasive monitoring in the patient on anticoagulants. Central venous access should not delay institution of CPB.
- Induction and maintenance: The goals are to prevent hypertensive responses to intubation and surgical stimulation as well as to prevent excessive myocardial depression and peripheral vasodilatation. There are no outcome data to support the selection of any particular anesthetic agents for these patients. Oxygen–narcotic-based techniques may be suitable; however, reduced doses of analgesics and anesthetics may be required in patients with borderline hemodynamic instability. Etomidate, with low doses of narcotics, may be used for rapid sequence induction.
- Obstruction of coronary blood flow commonly occurs because of angioplasty devices or elevated intimal flaps following coronary artery dissection. Coronary perfusion pressure must be maintained by optimizing systemic and filling pressures especially for right-sided lesions.
- Full-dose aprotinin (6 million KIU) is given routinely in our center.
- Prophylactic antiarrhythmic therapy with magnesium is recommended.
- Emergence from CPB is usually attempted with pharmacologic and mechanical support (IABP) to the myocardium. Commonly used drugs include milrinone and/or a combination of epinephrine/norepinehrine/vasopressin, with or without diastolic augmentation with IABP.
- Mediastinal bleeding may be common after discontinuation of bypass and usually requires blood products (as determined by coagulation results).

Hemodynamically Unstable, Ischemic Patient

Here, the clinical scenario may range from a patient who has mild LV dysfunction to cardiogenic shock and even cardiac arrest. Nothing should interfere with the institution of CPB. Surgery should proceed in a rapid but organized fashion.

Preoperative Considerations

- Prompt management of hemodynamically unstable patients with ischemia will optimally require sufficient anesthesia personnel to manage airway and hemodynamic issues efficiently. The members of the surgical team may need to be scrubbed and have to be ready to start, and the perfusionists need to be fully equipped to initiate CPB.
- Patients with a low cardiac output, accompanying pulmonary edema, and inadequate tissue perfusion will require very small and incremental doses of anesthetics. Hypotension is tolerated poorly and leads to worsening coronary hypoperfusion and subendocardial ischemia. Occasionally, femoral arterial and venous cannulas may have to be inserted under local anesthesia before induction of general anesthesia. This may facilitate rapid institution of CPB in case the patients become profoundly unstable.
- Patients who have already been intubated and ventilated before transfer may just need a low-dose inhalation agent and a nondepolarizing muscle relaxant. Narcotics, such as fentanyl, may be titrated later to effect once the response to surgical stimulus has been ascertained.
- Patients with cardiac arrest will need continued cardiac massage. Chest compressions should not be interrupted for >15 to 20 seconds and should be continued during skin preparation and draping. Internal cardiac compression must be commenced following sternotomy.
- Invasive monitoring may be established using the cannulas inserted for PCI and should not delay incision.

Intraoperative Management

- Chaos and confusion are inevitable when a patient who is critically ill suddenly reaches the OR. The anesthesiologist plays a crucial role not only in managing clinical issues but also in supervising the other teams in the OR. Good communication between the anesthesiologist, surgeon, and perfusionist is mandatory.
- Maintenance of systemic blood pressures should be the primary goal before institution of CPB.
- Heparin needs to be given early, primarily to ensure anticoagulation in anticipation of deteriorating hemodynamics and the need for urgent CPB.
- Most often, patients will receive hypothermic CPB with judicious warm/cold cardioplegia.
- The choice of arterial or venous conduits depends upon the urgency of the clinical scenario.
- CPB time is usually long. The anesthesiologist must oversee the maintenance of heparin, glucose, hemoglobin, metabolic status, and urine output during the bypass period.
- Emergence from CPB can be arduous and may require repeated attempts; it is customarily associated with the need for vasoactive medications, IABP, and mediastinal bleeding.

Postoperative Care

Risk factors for preoperative death after CABG for failed angioplasty include previous myocardial infarction, need for cardiopulmonary resuscitation (CPR), cardiogenic shock, compromised LV function, multivessel coronary artery disease, advanced age, and previous coronary artery surgery.

- Patients are usually sedated and ventilated in the immediate postoperative period. The initial and primary goals in the ICU are correction of coagulopathy, optimizing preload, and improving peripheral perfusion.
- As a general rule, most clinicians expect to see a period of cardiovascular stability along with improving peripheral organ function before any cardiopulmonary support is weaned. Sedation may be weaned off temporarily in the early postoperative period to assess neurologic status.
- There is no data to support weaning from vasoactive drugs with a specific protocol. However, while doing so, it is important to proceed in a stepwise fashion, evaluate the patient's response to decreasing cardiovascular support, and proceed cautiously with necessary monitoring.

  Postoperatively, patients are at a high risk of preoperative myocardial infarction, multiple organ dysfunction syndrome, and increased hospital mortality.

SURGERY FOR ACUTE AORTIC INSUFFICIENCY

Acute aortic insufficiency is an acquired cardiac disease and poses a unique challenge to the clinician. Common causes of this grave condition are endocarditis, aortic dissection, and prosthetic valve dehiscence.

- Development of acute insufficiency of the aortic valve results in a sudden volume overload of the otherwise normal left ventricle. Precipitous increase in the left ventricle end diastolic pressure (LVEDP) is initially associated with the premature closure of the mitral valve and may shield the pulmonary vessels from fluid overload; however, increasing LV distention soon leads to mitral annular enlargement and a functional mitral insufficiency, eventually jeopardizing right ventricular function. The reduction in stroke volume and increased LVEDP leads to low cardiac index, decreased coronary perfusion pressures, and pulmonary edema that is refractory to medical therapy.
- The only definitive treatment for acute aortic insufficiency is prompt aortic valve replacement.
- Goals of hemodynamic management are as follows:
  - Maintain sinus rhythm and a heart rate 80 to 90 beats per minute (bpm). External or transvenous pacing may be used if necessary. Bradycardia is associated with low cardiac index and a greater regurgitant flow.
  - Decrease afterload (cautiously because precipitous reduction may be associated with decreased coronary and peripheral perfusion pressures). Sodium nitroprusside (SNP), NTG, and hydralazine have been used.
  - Maintain and, if necessary, augment preload. Swan-Ganz measurements may underestimate preload, especially when acute increases in LVEDP prompt early mitral closure, or overestimate it in the event of pulmonary venous overload.

- Minimize myocardial depression. Positive inotropes are beneficial with heart rate and myocardial contractility but should be used with caution in cases of aortic dissection.
- IABP is contraindicated because diastolic augmentation leads to increased regurgitant fractions. Similarly, femoro–femoral bypass is also inappropriate.
- Induction of anesthesia may be extremely difficult in the orthopneic, hypoxic, hypotensive, and combative patient with pulmonary edema. Even small doses of anesthetics/analgesics may induce precipitous decreases in blood pressure.

SURGERY FOR COMPLICATIONS OF ACUTE MYOCARDIAL INFARCTION

Acute Ventricular Septal Defect

Ventricular septal infarction usually occurs within 2 to 6 days after acute myocardial infarction and is responsible for 1% to 5% of all infarction-related deaths. Septal rupture most commonly occurs in patients undergoing their first transmural infarction in whom the collateral circulation is limited or absent. The most common defect is in the anteroseptal position; posterior defects are associated with right ventricular infarction and have a worse prognosis.

- Development of a septal defect is associated with left to right shunt leading to acute right ventricular volume overload, pulmonary edema, biventricular failure, and, eventually, cardiogenic shock.
- Diagnosis is made by clinical suspicion, a step-up increase in oxygen saturation from the right atrium to the pulmonary artery, or by echocardiography. If possible, coronary angiography may be performed because myocardial revascularization is needed in more than one fourth of patients.
- Management involves stabilization of patient and preparation for surgery. Prognosis is done with medical therapy alone, but for the patients with small defects without evidence of hypoxemia and worsening peripheral perfusion, prognosis is dismal. The degree of left to right shunting helps decide the urgency of surgery.
- Most patients will need intra-aortic balloon counterpulsation and inotropic/vasodilator therapy as preparation for surgery. Goals of preoperative management are as follows:
  - Maintenance of preload and myocardial contractility.
  - Afterload reduction with maintenance of perfusion pressures.
  - Avoid myocardial depression.
  - Avoid maneuvers that increase or decrease pulmonary vascular resistance.
  - Thermodilution measurements of cardiac output may not be accurate (left to right shunt) and Swan-Ganz catheters may be relatively contraindicated for concerns of paradoxical embolism.
  - Maintain afterload reduction after bypass to limit intraventricular pressures.
- Operative mortality is related to the state of cardiac function at the time of operation. Persistence of severe cardiogenic shock in the postoperative period is associated with poor outcome.

Acute Mitral Regurgitation

Acute ischemic mitral regurgitation (MR) occurs in 0.5% of patients with symptomatic coronary artery disease and in 0.45% to 0.9% of patients following acute myocardial infarction. Acute MR may occur as a result of destruction of the valve itself (acute endocarditis), annular enlargement or ischemia and rupture of the papillary muscles, and distortion of accompanying subvalvular structures. Posteromedial papillary muscle ischemia is more common because it receives its sole blood supply from the angiographically dominant coronary artery (commonly the right coronary artery).

- The acute regurgitation results in distention of a noncompliant left atrium, thereby leading to a sudden increase in left atrial and pulmonary artery pressures. This, along with LV dysfunction, clinically manifests in pulmonary edema, hypoxia, hypotension, and, commonly, cardiogenic shock. Patients deteriorate rapidly and commonly require aggressive treatment with vasoactive medications and intraaortic counterpulsation before surgery, which remains the most definitive treatment modality. Most surgeons have traditionally advocated valvular replacement, although undersized ring annuloplasty and chordal preservation techniques have also been tried with encouraging results.
- Goals for management in the preoperative period include the following:
  - Stabilization and cardiac catheterization (if possible) before surgery.
  - Transesophageal echocardiography to monitor cardiac and valvular function/repair.
  - Maintenance of heart rate and preload.
  - Maintenance/increase in myocardial contractility and reduction in afterload (to decrease regurgitant fraction).
- Low cardiac output syndrome is common on emergence from CPB and is the most common cause of morbidity and mortality postoperatively. Mechanical circulatory assistance plays an important role in supporting patients until the myocardium recovers.

SUGGESTED READINGS

Cohen LH, Edmunds LH Jr, eds. *Cardiac surgery in the adult*. New York: McGraw-Hill; 2003.
Estafanous FG Barash PG, Reves JG, eds. *Cardiac anesthesia. Principles and clinical practice*. Philadelphia, PA: JB Lippincott Co., 1994.
Kaplan JA, Reich DL, Konstadt SN, eds. *Cardiac anesthesia*. 4th ed. Philadelphia, PA: WB Saunders; 1999.

Surgical Technique and Postoperative Consideration

Chapter 21

Myocardial Protection During Cardiac Surgery

Shafie Fazel and Richard D. Weisel

The operative mortality and morbidity of cardiac surgeries have decreased steadily. Improved myocardial protection has enabled surgeons to undertake more complex surgical procedures on patients who are extremely ill to have improved outcomes. Improved methods of intraoperative myocardial protection increases the early postoperative myocardial performance and long-term outcomes. Adequate myocardial protection requires the balancing of myocardial oxygen supply and demand with cardioplegic arrest or hypothermic fibrillation.

MYOCARDIAL OXYGEN DEMAND

In a loaded and beating state, myocardial oxygen demand is directly proportional to the heart rate and stroke work. Stroke work, the area within the pressure–volume loop, is dependent on ventricular preload, afterload, and contractility. Inotropic state is estimated by evaluating end or maximal systolic elastance or preload recruitable stroke work. In the normal heart, oxygen consumption (Mvo_2) approaches 8 mL/100g/minute. Cardiopulmonary bypass unloads the ventricles and decreases the Mvo_2 by approximately 20%. Reducing the heart temperature from 37°C to 22°C decreases the Mvo_2 by another 50%, but cardioplegic arrest decreases Mvo_2 by approximately 80%. Therefore, Mvo_2 is lower in the arrested heart even at normothermia (37°C) than in the hypothermic (22°C) heart.

MYOCARDIAL OXYGEN SUPPLY

Oxygen extraction in the normal beating heart approaches 80%. Oxygen extraction is marginally higher in pathologic conditions. Myocardial oxygen supply is, therefore, directly proportional to the coronary blood flow, which is directly dependent on the aortic root pressure and is inversely proportional to the venous pressure, intraventricular pressure, and the resistance of the coronary arterioles. Ventricular distention, either because of aortic valve incompetence or because of excessive pulmonary venous drainage, increases intraventricular and coronary venous pressure and limits myocardial perfusion.

HYPOTHERMIC FIBRILLATION

Less commonly used by cardiac surgeons today, hypothermic fibrillation is an effective method of myocardial protection. Dr. C.W. Akins has the largest reported experience with hypothermic fibrillation for routine coronary artery bypass grafting (CABG). He describes several principles that are necessary for successful application of hypothermic fibrillation. First, ventricular fibrillation at normothermia has high oxygen consumption compared to the empty beating heart, emphasizing the importance of achieving hypothermia for adequate myocardial protection. Second, regional myocardial blood flow is reduced when ventricular fibrillation is sustained electrically, as compared to spontaneous ventricular fibrillation. Third, optimal myocardial protection can only be achieved with meticulous attention to the aortic root and ventricular pressures to maintain an adequate perfusion pressure gradient across the fibrillating myocardium. Systemic pressures between 80 and 100 mm Hg are necessary for adequate cardiac perfusion. The ventricle must be decompressed with a left ventricular vent, which is usually introduced through the right superior pulmonary vein. Fourth, aortic cross clamping and global myocardial ischemia should be avoided to reduce the possibility of infarct expansion in regionally ischemic hearts. To aid surgical visualization, local vessel occlusion after arteriotomy may be necessary. Fifth, according to Akins, aggressive β blockade aids in the recovery of function after hypothermic fibrillation and is recommended routinely. The advantages and disadvantages of hypothermic fibrillation for CABG are listed in Table 21-1.

Hypothermic fibrillation is particularly suitable for patients in whom the surgeon wishes to avoid cross clamping the aorta because of severe atherosclerosis of the aorta. Under such circumstances, aortic cannulation may be guided by epiaortic ultrasound scanning to identify a "soft spot," or alternate arterial inflow sites such as the axillary artery may be used. After cooling the patient on cardiopulmonary bypass, spontaneous or induced fibrillation may be used with intermittent short periods of circulatory arrest to allow the construction of the bypass conduits. This technique can also be employed in redo patients with a patent left internal mammary artery to the left anterior descending artery bypass when the surgeon is unable to isolate or dissect the mammary artery free for clamping. Hypothermic fibrillation obviates the need to gain control of the patent mammary artery graft.

CARDIOPLEGIA

Hyperkalemic arrest of the heart lowers myocardial oxygen consumption to <80% of loaded beating conditions and affords excellent myocardial protection. The cardioplegic solution may be delivered as a buffered crystalloid solution or as a blood-based solution.

▌ **TABLE 21-1** Advantages and Disadvantages of Hypothermic Fibrillation

Advantages	*Disadvantages*
Aortic cross clamping is avoided, minimizing aortic manipulation	Retraction of the heart for the exposure of lateral and posterior wall coronary arteries may be more difficult in the fibrillating heart
Bypass grafts may be performed in any sequence, particularly the internal mammary artery grafting does not have to be delayed until the last anastomosis	Partial occlusion of the ascending aorta or intermittent hypothermic circulatory arrest are required for the completion of the proximal anastomoses
Myocardial protection in reoperative cases, in the face of patent bypass grafts (in particular, the patent internal mammary artery) is less complicated	Distal conduit to coronary artery anastomosis requires local occlusion of the coronary artery with attendant risk of injury to the artery
Fluid and potassium loads of cardioplegia solution are avoided	The operative field is more bloody

We routinely use blood-based cardioplegia because blood cardioplegia improves postoperative ventricular function by increasing oxygen delivery and oxygen consumption and preserves myocardial high-energy phosphate stores when compared to crystalloid cardioplegia. Our current cardioplegia system (myocardial protection system [MPS]) accomplishes arrest with a high concentration of potassium and magnesium in a very small volume of crystalloid. For maintenance of cardioplegic arrest, the lowest concentration of potassium, which maintains electrical silence, is employed. The MPS system (Quest Medical, Inc.) reduces the amount of crystalloid infused to a minimum and maintains the hemoglobin concentration ("microplegia").

Temperature

The standard method of delivering either blood or crystalloid cardioplegia consists of intermittent hypothermic infusions at 10°C (see Table 21-2). Cold blood cardioplegia is the preferred technique for most surgeons because it provides excellent protection even when homogeneous delivery is limited. Cold blood cardioplegia offers consistent myocardial protection particularly in high-risk patients. Unfortunately, hypothermia reduces myocardial metabolism not only during cardioplegic arrest but also during reperfusion after cross clamp removal. Delayed recovery of aerobic myocardial metabolism due to hypothermia frequently delays the recovery of ventricular function because of inadequate mitochondrial energy production. Cold blood cardioplegia may be particularly useful in patients who require prolonged aortic cross clamping. To reduce the duration of metabolic and functional dysfunction after cross clamp release, a terminal infusion of warm blood cardioplegia ("hot shot") prolongs electromechanical arrest and allows the recovery of temperature-dependent mitochondrial respiration.

With the advent of near continuous cardioplegia delivery systems and the inherent issues with hypothermic cardioplegia, warm cardioplegia technique was developed. If warm cardioplegia is given continuously during the cross clamp period,

▶ **TABLE 21-2 Advantages and Disadvantages of Warm versus Cold Cardioplegia**

Temperature	Advantages	Disadvantages
Cold	Lowest myocardial metabolism allowing the safe conduct of complex surgical procedures	Delays recovery of ventricular function by delaying recovery of cardiomyocyte mitochondrial metabolism
Warm	Rapid recovery of myocardial metabolism	Increases risk of neurologic injury; requires near continuous delivery

then the temperature-dependent mitochondrial enzymatic function could be preserved during cardioplegic arrest. On the other hand, in cases where cardioplegic delivery is not homogenous, as in patients with coronary artery disease, the surgeon risks possible normothermic ischemia of the underperfused regions. The warm heart trial investigators addressed these issues and found that warm or tepid cardioplegia was associated with improved early ventricular function and increased late event-free survival in >6,000 isolated patients with CABG. However, both warm and tepid cardioplegia must be delivered nearly continuously and can result in increased ischemic injury if cardioplegia cannot be delivered homogeneously. Tepid cardioplegia (28°C) provides some degree of cooling and protection from inhomogeneous delivery. Tepid and warm cardioplegia provide excellent protection if continuous and homogeneous delivery can be anticipated.

Combining warm cardioplegia with systemic warming to 37°C resulted in an increased risk of neurologic adverse events, as reported by investigators at Emory University in Atlanta, Georgia. Although warm (or tepid) heart surgery may have advantages, warm systemic perfusion had no substantial advantages. Therefore, most surgeons have adopted "tepid" systemic perfusion. The cardiopulmonary circuit is allowed to drift and then rewarmed slowly to avoid hyperthermic brain perfusion.

Delivery

Cardioplegia may be delivered antegrade either into the aortic root proximal to an aortic cross clamp or directly into the coronary ostia, retrograde into the coronary sinus, or by a combined approach of antegrade and retrograde. The advantages and disadvantages of each cardioplegic delivery method are listed in Table 21-3.

Antegrade cardioplegia is simple to use and provides predictable myocardial protection. In patients with total occlusion or tight coronary artery stenosis, distal perfusion and myocardial protection may be difficult to achieve with antegrade cardioplegia, with the exception of chronic lesions in patients with extensive collaterals. Antegrade delivery of cardioplegia should be undertaken with caution in redo CABG cases. Diffuse and friable atherosclerosis in patent, older vein grafts may embolize into the coronary circulation during dissection of the heart and manipulation of the grafts, an issue that persists during antegrade cardioplegia delivery. Retrograde cardioplegia both prevents embolization and washes out previously embolized debris during administration. Retrograde cardioplegia, however, faces the major disadvantage that the right ventricle

▶ **TABLE 21-3** Advantages and Disadvantages of Various Cardioplegia Delivery Techniques

Delivery	Advantages	Disadvantages
Antegrade	Simple to use; Predictable delivery of cardioplegia	Ventricular distention with aortic valve incompetence
		Risk of coronary embolization in redo CABG
		Requires frequent interruptions during CABG
		Decreased perfusion distal to coronary stenosis/occlusions
		Cumbersome during AV surgery
Retrograde	Near continuous delivery	Decreased perfusion to the RV and posterior septum, and unpredictable perfusion to the LV
Combined	Maximizes myocardial perfusion	Complex and cumbersome delivery system

CABG, coronary artery bypass grating; AV, aortic valve; RV, right ventricular; LV, left ventricular.

and posterior septum may be inadequately protected, and the nutritive flow to the left ventricle may be unpredictable because of the presence of Thebesian channels and ven-ovenous shunts. Antegrade delivery may also lead to ventricular distention in the presence of aortic valve incompetence, which may be caused by retraction of the heart during the operation. Ventricular distention decreases transmyocardial perfusion pressure gradient, and decreases cardioplegia delivery and myocardial protection. Ventricular distention may require placement of a left ventricular vent. Antegrade delivery during aortic valve procedures may be cumbersome but may be achieved by individual cannulation of the coronary ostia. Anterior wall circulation may be severely compromised in the presence of a short left main artery because of cannulation of the ongoing circumflex and inadequate or absent perfusion into the left anterior descending artery. Near continuous retrograde cardioplegia may be used in such cases as well as during the implantation of a cardiac transplant, but there are two major disadvantages. First, given that coronary sinus pressures >40 mm Hg may cause coronary sinus rupture, myocardial protection of a hypertrophied heart in patients with aortic stenosis may be increasingly difficult with retrograde cardioplegia. Second, in cases where severe left heart failure has led to pulmonary hypertension and right ventricular hypertrophy, protection of the critical right ventricle may not be achieved with retrograde cardioplegia.

For routine CABG cases, we have developed the technique of combined cardioplegia whereby near continuous retrograde cardioplegia is complemented with intermittent antegrade cardioplegia delivered through each constructed bypass graft. This technique ensures maximal distribution of cardioplegia and affords optimal myocardial protection but is cumbersome.

FUTURE DIRECTIONS

Previous research has focused on delivering cardioplegia at the right temperature to as much myocardium as possible. Current and future research is focused on developing substrate-enhanced cardioplegia to decrease cardiac injury during cross clamp-induced ischemia-reperfusion injury. Promising additives include L-arginine $\pm$ tetrahydro-biopterin to enhance nitric oxide production by the endothelium, adenosine to effect the protective consequences of ischemic preconditioning, insulin to facilitate resumption of aerobic metabolism, and Na^+/H^+ exchange pump inhibitors such as cariporide to limit reperfusion-related calcium overload.

SUGGESTED READINGS

Akins CW. Hypothermic fibrillatory arrest for coronary artery bypass grafting. *J Card Surg.* 1992;7:342–347.

Buckberg GD, Brazier JR, Nelson RL, et al. Studies of the effects of hypothermia regional myocardial blood flow and metabolism during cardiopulmonary bypass. I. The adequately perfused beating, fibrillating, and arrested heart. *J Thorac Cardiovasc Surg.* 1977;73:87–94.

Fremes SE, Christakis GT, Weisel RD, et al. A clinical trial of blood and crystalloid cardioplegia. *J Thorac Cardiovasc Surg.* 1984;88:726–741.

Mallidi HR, Sever J, Tamariz M, et al. The short-term and long-term effects of warm or tepid cardioplegia. *J Thorac Cardiovasc Surg.* 2003;125:711–720.

The Warm Heart Investigators. Randomized trial of normothermic versus hypothermic coronary bypass surgery. *Lancet.* 1994;343:559–563.

On-pump Coronary Artery Bypass Surgery

Terrence M. Yau

Coronary artery bypass surgery has for many years been the single most commonly performed major surgical procedure. It achieves the maximal possible myocardial revascularization, and despite being performed on many patients who are extremely ill, it has generally superb outcomes. These outcomes depend, however, on meticulous attention to detail not only during the operation but also in all aspects of care during the perioperative period.

DIAGNOSIS

Clinical history will often reveal a typical history of angina or an anginal equivalent, but diabetic or female patients are more likely to present with atypical or no symptoms. Physical examination is often noncontributory, unless the patient has sequelae of a prior myocardial infarction (MI) resulting in decreased ventricular compliance, left ventricular (LV) dilatation, or mitral regurgitation.

Noninvasive testing with perfusion imaging will define areas of fixed or reversible ischemia, wall thickening, and endocardial excursion. Echocardiography or stress echocardiography will delineate global and regional wall motion abnormalities and valvular disease. In severely dysfunctional ventricles, delayed thallium imaging or fluorodeoxyglucose position emission tomography (FDG-PET) may visualize areas with residual viability.

Coronary angiography is the definitive invasive modality to define coronary anatomy. Left ventriculography is usually performed unless contraindicated, and is of particular importance in patients with LV aneurysms or significant regional dysfunction. Although newer techniques to evaluate coronary anatomy, utilizing electron beam angiography or magnetic resonance, are being developed, spatial resolution with the equipment available in most hospitals is as yet insufficient to direct surgery.

INDICATIONS FOR SURGERY

Class I, IIa, and IIb indications for coronary artery bypass grafting (CABG), as recommended by the American College of Cardiology (ACC)/American Heart Association (AHA) task force on practice guidelines, are summarized in Table 22-1.

SURGICAL APPROACH

Conduits

The left internal thoracic artery (LITA), grafted to the left anterior descending (LAD) coronary artery, has the greatest long-term patency of any graft-target combination, approximately 90% at 10 years, and is associated with improved survival and freedom from repeat revascularization and late cardiac events. LITA use is universal unless contraindicated by previous chest wall irradiation, left subclavian artery stenosis, or rarely, inadequate flow after harvesting. Its use in octogenarians varies between surgeons.

The right internal thoracic artery (RITA) is the preferred second arterial conduit and is usually grafted to the circumflex system. Nonrandomized studies have demonstrated further improvements in freedom from reoperation, and, to a lesser degree, late survival, in patients receiving two internal thoracic artery (ITA) grafts rather than one. When possible, the *in situ* RITA is brought through the transverse sinus to a proximal obtuse marginal or intermediate coronary artery, where it will not be jeopardized if repeat sternotomy is required in the future. If this is not possible, it is generally used as a free graft based on the LITA, but the flow capacity of the bilateral ITA Y-graft relative to the requirements of the target coronary beds must be assessed carefully. Grafting the *in situ* RITA to the LAD permits use of an *in situ* LITA to the circumflex, but increases the risk of injury to the RITA if repeat sternotomy is required.

Skeletonization of the LITA and RITA may preserve sternal blood flow and reduce the rate of sternal osteomyelitis when bilateral ITA grafting is performed. Skeletonization also results in greater length of conduit and increases the range of the *in situ* ITA. Skeletonization has not been conclusively shown to affect late patency either favorably or unfavorably.

The radial artery is our third choice of arterial conduits. Although harvesting is easy and can be performed concurrently with that of the ITAs, radial artery grafts are extremely sensitive to competitive flow and their use is generally reserved for target coronaries with a proximal stenosis of at least 90%. Use of the radial artery is safe but has not yet been shown to improve late survival or freedom from reintervention in a randomized trial.

The right gastroepiploic artery (RGEA) is used rarely and, when employed, is usually anastomosed to the posterior interventricular artery (PIV). Harvesting must be meticulous to maximize conduit length and prevent spasm, and subsequent upper abdominal surgery may jeopardize this graft. Use of the RGEA has not been demonstrated to improve survival or late cardiac events.

Greater and lesser saphenous vein grafts (SVGs) are still employed in most patients, and their use increases in elderly patients or those with hemodynamic instability. Previous

▶ TABLE 22-1 Class I, IIa, IIb Indications for Coronary Artery Bypass Graft as Defined by the American College of Cardiology/American Heart Association Task Force on Practice Guidelines

Anatomy/Clinical Scenario	No/Mild Angina	Stable Angina	Unstable Angina/Non-STEMI	STEMI	Poor LV	Ventricular Arrhythmias	Failed PTCA	Previous CABG
Left main stenosis	—	—	—	—	—	—	—	—
Prox LAD and prox Cx	—	—	—	—	—	—	—	—
3VD	—	—	—	—	I if 2-3VD	—	—	—
Prox LAD and 1-2VD	IIa	I if 2VD and EF <50% or + perfusion scan	IIa	—	—	IIa	—	—
1-2VD, no prox LAD	IIb	I if high-risk perfusion scan, extensive ischemia, IIa if moderate ischemia	IIb	—	—	IIa if bypassable	—	—
Prox LAD only	—	IIa, I if EF <50%, extensive ischemia	—	—	—	—	—	—
Disabling angina or ongoing ischemia on maximal medical Rx	—	I if operative risk acceptable	I	IIa	—	—	—	—
Progressive LV pump failure, extending infarct	—	—	—	IIb	—	—	—	—
Primary reperfusion (<6-12 h) after MI	—	—	—	IIb	—	—	—	—

continued

TABLE 22-1 (Continued)

Anatomy/Clinical Scenario	No/Mild Angina	Stable Angina	Unstable Angina/Non-STEMI	STEMI	Poor LV	Ventricular Arrhythmias	Failed PTCA	Previous CABG
Any coronary anatomy	—	—	—	—	IIa if significant viable, non-contractile, revascularizable myocardium	—	I if hemodynamic compromise; becomes IIa if impaired coagulation, no previous sternotomy; or IIb if impaired coagulation, previous sternotomy	IIa if bypassable vessel(s) and large area of ischemia
Patent IMA to LAD, ischemia in other territories, without maximal medical Rx or PCI								IIb
Foreign body in crucial anatomic position	—	—	—	—	—	—	IIa	—

ACC, American College of Cardiology; AHA, American Heart Association; Prox, proximal; Cx, circumflex; LAD, left anterior descending; VD, vessel disease; Rx, treatment; LV, left ventricular; MI, myocardial infarction; EF, ejection fraction; IMA, internal mammary artery; PCI, percutaneous coronary intervention; STEMI, ST-elevation myocardial infarction; PTCA, percutaneous transluminal coronary angioplasty; CABG, coronary artery bypass graft.

data suggests a 10-year patency of approximately 50%, with only 25% of grafts remaining free of angiographic disease, but it seems likely that the contemporary patency of SVGs has been improved by aggressive use of cholesterol-lowering agents.

Cryopreserved allograft or xenograft veins or polytetrafluroethylene (PTFE) prosthetic conduits have been associated with dismal patency rates and are used only as a last resort.

Cannulation

Epiaortic echocardiography is generally performed in patients in whom significant aortic atherosclerosis has been visualized radiographically or by transesophageal echocardiography, in those with risk factors for aortic disease, or when palpable aortic atherosclerosis is discovered after sternotomy.

In most patients, cannulation of the distal ascending aorta is performed, but the lesser curvature of the distal arch is an attractive alternative when atherosclerotic or aneurysmal disease of the ascending aorta is present. Arch cannulation has been shown to reduce transcranial Doppler high-intensity transient signals in the middle cerebral artery, but its effect on perioperative stroke has not yet been defined.

The right axillary artery is usually free of atherosclerosis and is another alternative when ascending aortic cannulation is inadvisable. End-to-side anastomosis of an 8-mm Dacron graft to the axillary artery, instead of direct cannulation, permits simultaneous perfusion of both the right common carotid artery and the arm, and the graft is easily stapled and amputated at the conclusion of the procedure.

Femoral arterial cannulation is performed rarely, and generally when there is a considerable risk of injury to the heart, great vessels, or patent grafts at the time of repeat sternotomy. Femoral arterial cannulation is never indicated when ascending aortic atherosclerosis is detected because descending thoracic atherosclerosis is virtually guaranteed and will result in retrograde cerebral embolization.

Cannulation of the right atrium with a single two-stage venous cannula is performed for patients undergoing isolated coronary bypass surgery, with biatrial or bicaval cannulation reserved for those undergoing concomitant mitral valvular or right heart procedures.

Cardiopulmonary bypass is carried out with a heparin-coated or standard circuit and centrifugal or roller pumps, allowing systemic temperatures to drift to 34°C. Careful attention is paid to minimize gaseous microemboli from entrainment of air in the venous line or from medication injection into the bypass circuit. Although shed mediastinal blood can be processed in a cell saver and reinfused, we have generally found that the volume of shed blood in primary CABG is insufficient to process and therefore do not routinely employ a cell saver.

Endarterectomy of the right coronary artery (RCA) and proximal PIV is carried out in a few patients, but can generally be performed safely with minimal impact on the rate of perioperative MI. Endarterectomy of the LAD or circumflex systems, however, is a marker of advanced coronary atherosclerosis and is associated with increased perioperative MIs and morbidity.

Sequential grafting with either an ITA or SVG has the theoretical advantage of increasing graft flows and, perhaps, patency of grafts to target coronaries with limited outflow. However, if the more distal coronary anastomoses are those with limited outflow, graft flow will be increased only in the proximal portion of the sequential graft, and the distal portion will still be in jeopardy. Only if the most distal anastomosis is constructed to a target coronary with the best outflow will the theoretical advantage of the sequential graft apply. Because sequential grafts necessarily jeopardize multiple distal anastomoses if problems occur in the proximal graft, they are used at our institution only in specific anatomic situations or when the length of conduit is inadequate for separate grafts.

The Atherosclerotic Aorta

Management of the atherosclerotic aorta is required in a steadily increasing proportion of patients. The most crucial aspect of managing this disease is early recognition of the problem and selection of an alternative surgical technique.

- If cannulation of the ascending aorta, aortic arch, or right axillary artery cannot be performed safely, off-pump CABG may be the only option. Inflow for bypass conduits may be taken from the ITAs, from the innominate artery, or from the aorta with a proximal anastomotic device without aortic clamping if a suitable area for deployment can be identified.
- If arterial cannulation can be performed safely but not aortic clamping, another alternative is to use cardiopulmonary bypass, using ventricular fibrillation or an off-pump coronary artery bypass (OPCAB) stabilizer device to perform the distal anastomoses. Proximal graft inflow can be achieved through the same options listed above, but construction of hand-sewn proximal anastomoses under hypothermic low-flow cardiopulmonary bypass (approximately 200 mL/minute for 3 to 4 minutes, to keep air from entering the aortotomy) without aortic clamping is also feasible.
- When arterial cannulation can be performed, replacement of the ascending aorta may also be undertaken, with an open distal anastomosis performed under hypothermic circulatory arrest before cross clamping of the graft and resumption of cardiopulmonary bypass. In our experience, replacement of the atherosclerotic ascending aorta has been associated with a greater risk of perioperative stroke than "no-touch" techniques. Although replacement of the ascending aorta has been theorized to eliminate a potential source of future embolic strokes, this future benefit must be weighed carefully against the immediate neurologic risks of this procedure. If replacement is carried out, SVGs based on the Dacron conduit should be constructed with a large button to minimize the potential for pannus formation to obstruct the orifice.

Potential Reoperation

Preparation for a potential reoperation is an essential part of the procedure. It is our practice to close the pericardium in all patients, irrespective of age, unless the hemodynamics are adversely affected. Pericardial closure has been shown to reduce cardiac output slightly, but it increases the distance from the posterior table of the sternum to the anterior wall of the right ventricle (RV). *In situ* LITA grafts are mobilized to the level of the superior edge of the subclavian vein, so that they can be directed posterior to the left upper lobe and enter the pericardium through a lateral slit, keeping them well away from the initial dissection at reoperation. Meticulous attention to hemostasis will minimize adhesions.

Reoperative surgery carries increased risks due to more advanced coronary atherosclerosis, a greater likelihood of incomplete revascularization, and the potential for injury to patent grafts at the time of repeat sternotomy.

- Careful review of the previous operative note, angiogram, plain radiographs of the chest, and, in some patients, a computerized tomography (CT) scan of the thorax will reveal the course of patent LITA or RITA grafts and the proximity of the RV to the sternum.
- If the LITA graft is close to the midline, angling the blade of the oscillating saw so that the anterior table of the sternum is incised to the left of the midline and the posterior table is incised to the right, will keep the saw further away from the LITA. Incising the sternum at the usual perpendicular angle but to the right of the midline will also reduce the risk to the LITA but may render the right hemisternum excessively thin and fragile. An *in situ* RITA graft directed across the midline to the LAD is at particular risk.
- Exposure of the femoral vessels, and on occasion initiation of femoral–femoral cardiopulmonary bypass, may be warranted when the risk of compromise to patent grafts, the RV, or a dilated aorta is particularly high.
- Retrograde cardioplegia is used in most reoperations and is an independent predictor of mortality in redo coronary surgery; it is often combined with antegrade perfusion of a vein graft to the RCA.
- Diseased vein grafts are excised or ligated. The hood of an old vein graft, which usually remains patent even when the body of the graft is occluded, can be used as the site of a new proximal anastomosis when space on the ascending aorta is limited.

OUTCOMES

Mortality

Operative mortality has declined steadily over the last decade despite a progressive increase in the risk profile of patients referred for surgery. Overall mortality for isolated CABG in the Society of Thoracic Surgeons (STS) National Database fell from approximately 3.6% in 1992 to 2.6% in 2001, and risk-adjusted mortality fell from 4.3% to 2.4%. At our institution, overall mortality fell from 2.4% in 1990 to 1993 (N = 5,171, including emergent or repeat revascularization) to a consistent 1.2% (N = 9,937, January 1998 to June 2004).

In 18,041 consecutive patients, hospital mortality was independently predicted by LV dysfunction, increasing age, female gender, hypertension, diabetes, cardiogenic shock, congestive heart failure, peripheral vascular disease, reoperative surgery, left main disease, and urgent surgery.

The influence of severe LV dysfunction and reoperative surgery on mortality has declined with time as outcomes have improved. Severe LV dysfunction (EF <20%), formerly the most common predictor of mortality, no longer had a statistically significant impact on death in a recent cohort of 6,893 patients. Emergency surgery is required less frequently than in previous years, but because patients referred emergently now represent a subgroup not rescued after repeated and sometimes prolonged attempts at percutaneous salvage, the requirement for emergent surgery still carries a substantial risk for mortality.

Morbidity

Stroke remains a devastating complication of CABG and a major cause of morbidity and increased resource utilization. Its prevalence has been reported to be as high as 3.8% in a contemporary cohort. At our institution, stroke occurred in 1.3% of patients undergoing CABG from January 2002 to June 2004.

In contrast, low cardiac output syndrome (defined as the requirement for an intra-aortic balloon pump or inotropic support for more than 30 minutes to maintain a cardiac index >2.0 L/minute/m^2 despite appropriate preload and afterload) is significantly less common than in previous years and occurred in only 3.5% of patients after 2002.

The length of stay in the hospital after CABG has fallen from a median of 7 days in 1992 to 5 days in 2001 (STS National Database).

SUGGESTED READINGS

The BARI Investigators. The Influence of diabetes on 5-year mortality and morbidity in a randomized trial comparing CABG and PTCA in patients with multivessel disease: the Bypass Angioplasty Revascularization Investigation (BARI). *Circulation*. 1997;96:1761–1769.

Eagle KA, Guyton RA, Davidoff R, et al. ACC/AHA guidelines for coronary artery bypass graft surgery: executive summary and recommendations: a report of the American College of Cardiology/American Heart Association Task Force on Practice Guidelines. *Circulation*. 1999; 100:1464–1480.

Ferguson TB Jr, Hammill BG, Peterson ED, et al. A decade of change—risk profiles and outcomes for isolated coronary artery bypass grafting procedures, 1990-1999: a report from the STS National Database Committee and the Duke Clinical Research Institute. *Ann Thorac Surg*. 2002;73:480–489.

Loop FD, Lytle BW, Cosgrove DM, et al. Influence of the internal-mammary-artery graft on 10-year survival and other cardiac events. *N Engl J Med*. 1986;314:1–6.

Lytle BW, Blackstone EH, Loop FD, et al. Two internal thoracic artery grafts are better than one. *J Thorac Cardiovasc Surg*. 1999;117:855–872.

Off-pump Coronary Revascularization Surgery

Richard J. Novick

Although conventional coronary artery bypass grafting using cardiopulmonary bypass has long been a "gold standard" for surgical myocardial revascularization, off-pump coronary artery bypass grafting (OPCAB) has experienced a resurgence since the early 1990s and is now practiced by a significant minority of cardiac surgeons. This chapter reviews the scientific evidence comparing outcomes after on-pump coronary artery bypass grafting (ONCAB) and OPCAB; it also reviews techniques to facilitate the intraoperative conduct of OPCAB, explores the issue of the learning curve of this procedure, and highlights the importance of avoiding an emergent conversion to cardiopulmonary bypass. Although beating heart coronary revascularization includes not only OPCAB via a sternotomy but also the use of limited access incisions such as a left anterior or posterior minithoracotomy or a subxiphoid approach (for isolated access to the left anterior descending [LAD], circumflex, and distal right coronary artery territories, respectively), the focus of this chapter is on the full sternotomy-OPCAB approach, which provides simultaneous, unimpeded access to all coronary artery territories. The tremendous advances in robotic coronary artery bypass that have occurred during the past 5 years are reviewed in Chapter 24 of this book.

EVIDENCE-BASED ASSESSMENT OF OFF-PUMP CORONARY ARTERY BYPASS

During the past decade, the scientific assessment of OPCAB has progressed from anecdotal cases and single institutional case series to multi-institutional prospective cohort studies to well-designed randomized controlled trials and, finally, to a comprehensive meta-analysis. A single institutional series reflecting an initial experience of OPCAB in the mid to late 1990s demonstrated that complete myocardial revascularization can be routinely achieved using OPCAB techniques, with the construction of an average of three grafts per patient (Cartier et al., 1999 and 2000). In 2001 and 2002, three large prospective cohort studies showed a reduced risk-adjusted morbidity and mortality rate in OPCAB, as opposed to ONCAB patients (Plomondon et al., 2001; Cleveland et al., 2001; Mack et al., 2002). A follow-up study including a cohort of 8,449 patients used propensity score analytical methods to demonstrate that the elimination of cardiopulmonary bypass resulted in improvement in early survival after multivessel coronary artery bypass surgery (Magee et al., 2002).

The first randomized controlled trials comparing OPCAB and ONCAB included the Beating Heart Against Cardioplegic Arrest Studies (BHACAS) I and II trials conducted by Angelini et al. in Bristol, England. The pooled results of these two studies demonstrated a significant reduction of in-hospital morbidity (but not mortality) in OPCAB patients without a compromise to intermediate-term outcomes. A subsequent randomized controlled trial by the Emory University group demonstrated that OPCAB patients experienced a similar completeness of revascularization, similar in-hospital and 30-day outcomes, but less myocardial injury, a reduced transfusion requirement, and a shorter length of stay as compared to ONCAB patients (Puskas et al., 2003). A recent comprehensive meta-analysis of 37 randomized trials including 3,369 patients demonstrated that OPCAB provided no significant improvement in mortality, stroke, perioperative myocardial infarction, or renal failure compared to ONCAB (Cheng et al., 2005). However, OPCAB significantly decreased the incidence of atrial fibrillation, transfusion, inotrope requirement, respiratory infection, ventilation time, intensive care unit (ICU) and hospital length of stay, and hospital costs, while the impact on neurocognitive function was inconclusive. Early and intermediate-term graft patency was reported in four randomized trials comparing OPCAB and ONCAB. As noted in our recent meta-analysis, the time point to angiography and the completeness of follow-up varied considerably among these trials. One trial reported decreased patency at 3 months in the OPCAB group, compared to ONCAB patients (Khan et al., 2004). Three larger trials, however, reported no significant differences in patency at varying time points (Lingaas et al., 2004; Nathoe et al., 2003; Puskas et al., 2003). The long-term angiographic follow-up of OPCAB and ONCAB patients participating in these randomized trials is imperative so that the impact of the surgical approach to myocardial revascularization on long-term graft patency can be definitively ascertained.

OPERATIVE TECHNIQUES OF OFF-PUMP CORONARY ARTERY BYPASS SURGERY

The anesthetic management of patients undergoing OPCAB is reviewed in Chapter 3 of this book. Optimal management includes the use of a pulmonary artery catheter to measure pulmonary artery pressures and cardiac index as well as the use of transesophageal echocardiography to identify regional myocardial wall motion abnormalities and the severity of mitral regurgitation. In addition, the patient should be kept warm during the procedure to prevent myocardial hypothermia and lessen the incidence of intraoperative arrhythmias. Whereas during the initial experience with OPCAB the heart rate was pharmacologically slowed and periods of ischemic preconditioning of the coronary circulation were employed, these methods are no longer used by the vast majority of OPCAB surgeons.

Specific techniques to expose and stabilize the coronary vessels during OPCAB surgery have been extensively reviewed in the literature and summarized in individual case series as well as in recent review articles (Cartier et al., 2004). Although we formerly invariably revascularized the LAD territory first, our more recent practice has been to revascularize the coronary vessel with the highest degree of stenosis and the largest degree of collateralization at the outset. Either a traction or suction-type stabilizer can be used; the former results in significant financial savings, but coronary exposure with it can occasionally be difficult in patients with a very deep chest or a large heart.

Table positioning is an important technical detail to enhance visibility for the surgeon during OPCAB. The LAD, diagonal, and circumflex vessels are best visualized with the patient in a reverse Trendelenburg position with the table rotated toward the right side, whereas the distal right coronary artery territory is better exposed by rotating the table toward the left. The placement of several deep posterior pericardial retraction sutures on the left side helps to "verticalize" the heart and facilitates exposure of the anterior and lateral wall coronary circulation, especially when traction stabilizers are used. In addition, a "hernia sling" that is sutured to the diaphragmatic pericardium and passed around the distal lateral ventricular wall before being tacked to the right side of the operative table can facilitate exposure to the distal circumflex territory when traction stabilizers are used. On the other hand, use of an apical suction device in concert with the suction-type stabilizers can greatly facilitate lateral and inferior wall coronary artery exposure without the need for a sling retractor or extensive verticalization maneuvers.

Prior to proceeding with OPCAB, the surgeon must make certain that no relative or absolute contraindications to this procedure exist. Key contraindications include deeply buried coronary vessels (especially the LAD) and the presence of significant mitral regurgitation that may require a mitral valve repair procedure. Relative contraindications include severe hemodynamic instability at the outset that cannot be reversed by the anesthetist or the presence of dense ascending aortic calcification that precludes aortic side clamping. The former problem can sometimes be managed by the targeted use of adrenaline and milrinone, with the occasional placement of an intra-aortic balloon pump in patients who are in a particularly precarious condition. The latter issue can be addressed via the use of clampless proximal anastomotic connectors, although the long-term patency of grafts anastomosed to the aorta with these connectors may be suboptimal (Carrell, 2003). If a patient does develop increasing pulmonary artery pressure during the conduct of OPCAB despite inotropic support (including the use of phosphodiesterase inhibitors), an intermittent inferior vena cava snaring maneuver can be used to temporarily limit the right and left ventricular preload. Proactive surgical judgment and careful anesthetic management of the OPCAB patient is necessary in order to avoid an urgent or emergent conversion to ONCAB, with its potential deleterious effect on patient outcome, as noted below. Furthermore, current standard practice involves the careful documentation of graft flow (and, if possible, the pulsatility index) after the completion of each coronary anastomosis and following the administration of protamine sulfate prior to chest closure.

TRANSGRESSING THE LEARNING CURVE IN OFF-PUMP CORONARY ARTERY BYPASS

A significant number of cardiac surgeons are still reluctant to perform OPCAB because of the perception of a higher likelihood of adverse outcomes during the learning phase.

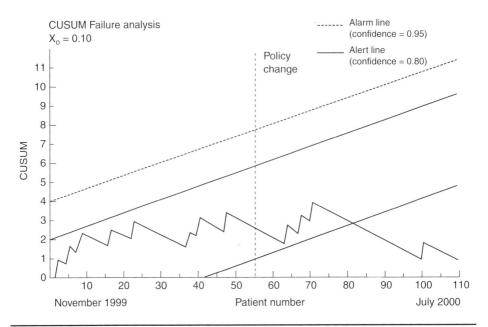

FIGURE 23-1. Cumulative sum failure analysis of clinical experience before and after a policy change from routine on-pump to off-pump coronary artery bypass grafting. The X-axis denotes consecutive first-time coronary artery bypass patients from November 1999 to July 2000; the Y-axis denotes the number of adjusted cumulative failures (death or any of nine prespecified major postoperative complications), assuming a total "acceptable failure rate" of 10%. CUSUM, cumulative sum. (Reprinted with permission from Novick RJ, Fox SA, Stitt LW, et al. Cumulative sum failure analysis of a policy change from on pump to off pump coronary artery bypass grafting. *Annals of Thoracic Surgery.* 2001;72[Suppl.]:S1016–S1021.)

This is a veritable concern, given the high level of scrutiny and public reporting of outcomes that has become the norm in coronary artery bypass surgery. The importance of a dedicated operating room (OR) nursing, anesthesiology, and surgical team cannot be overemphasized and is a key determinant of success. The teaching of OPCAB techniques is now a standard part of most cardiac surgery residency programs, and studies have shown that OPCAB can be safely taught to cardiothoracic trainees (Caputo et al., 2001). We have formally studied the impact of a policy change from ONCAB to OPCAB using cumulative sum (CUSUM) failure methods and have documented an improvement in patient outcomes as manifested by a less steep CUSUM curve after a policy change from routine ONCAB to OPCAB (see Fig. 23-1). The importance of proactive planning of the details of each OPCAB operation and very close communication between all members of the operative team are key features to ensure a low rate of conversion to ONCAB and the best possible outcomes in OPCAB surgery.

CONVERSION FROM OFF-PUMP CORONARY ARTERY BYPASS TO ON-PUMP CORONARY ARTERY BYPASS GRAFTING

The reported incidence of conversion from OPCAB to ONCAB has ranged from 1% to almost 20%, but the operational definition of "conversion" has differed in these studies. A useful paradigm for assessing the impact of conversion is to determine both the timing and patient status during this process. Edgerton et al. have defined "early" and "late" conversion as occurring prior to or after the commencement of any coronary anastomosis, respectively. In addition, they have defined conversion as "elective" if the maneuver was planned and unhurried versus "urgent or emergent" if the patient was hemodynamically unstable or experiencing life-threatening cardiac arrhythmias. In the experience of this group, as well as our own, the impact of an early, elective conversion was minimal, illustrating that patients who are booked for OPCAB can safely be converted to ONCAB at the initial stages of the procedure, if the judgment of the surgeon and anesthesiologist so dictate. On the other hand, late conversions, especially when the patient is hemodynamically and/or electrically unstable, are associated with high morbidity and mortality rates. This illustrates the importance of proactive patient management by the surgeon and anesthesiologist so that any conversions from OPCAB to ONCAB that do occur are early and unhurried.

FUTURE DIRECTIONS

To date, the vast majority of randomized controlled trials comparing OPCAB and ONCAB have included mainly low-risk patients. To our knowledge, only one published study has included "high-risk patients," defined as having at least three of the following characteristics: age >65 years, high blood pressure, diabetes, serum creatinine levels >133 μmol/L, ejection fraction <45%, chronic pulmonary disease, unstable angina, congestive heart failure, repeat bypass surgery, anemia, and significant carotid atherosclerosis (Carrier et al., 2003). Given the fact that these characteristics are very common among patients routinely referred for coronary artery bypass surgery at present, further randomized controlled trials need to target patients at even higher operative risk (e.g., age >75 or 80 years with significant baseline renal dysfunction and peripheral vascular disease). Such studies will need to involve multiple centers in order to increase the rate of recruitment and enable the study results to have wide generalizability.

In addition, because it is highly likely that multivessel coronary artery bypass grafting will soon be able to be conducted using robotic surgical techniques, randomized controlled trials comparing outcomes in these patients, versus those undergoing OPCAB via sternotomy, should be performed. Furthermore, long-term angiographic follow-up of grafts that have been constructed via conventional ONCAB versus OPCAB versus robotic surgical techniques is essential in order to determine the risk versus benefit ratios over the long term of these different surgical approaches to myocardial revascularization.

SUGGESTED READINGS

Angelini GD, Taylor FC, Reeves BC, et al. Early and midterm outcome after off-pump and on-pump surgery in Beating Heart Against Cardioplegic Arrest Studies (BHACAS 1 and 2): a pooled analysis of two randomised control trials. *Lancet.* 2002;359:1094–1119.

Caputo M, Chamberlain MH, Ozalp F, et al. Off-pump coronary operations can be safely taught to cardiothoracic trainees. *Ann Thorac Surg.* 2001;71:1215–1219.

Carrel TP, Eckstein FS, Englberger L, et al. Pitfalls and key lessons with the symmetry proximal anastomotic device in coronary artery bypass surgery. *Ann Thorac Surg.* 2003;75:1434–1436.

Carrier M, Perrault LP, Jeanmart H, et al. Randomized trial comparing off-pump to on-pump coronary artery bypass grafting in high-risk patients. *Heart Surg Forum.* 2003;505–508.

Cartier R. From idea to operating room: surgical innovation, clinical application and outcome. *Semin Cardiothorac Vasc Anesth.* 2004;4:103–109.

Cartier R, Blain R. Off-pump revascularization of the circumflex artery: technical aspect and short-term results. *Ann Thorac Surg.* 1999;68:94–99.

Cartier R, Brann S, Dagenais F, et al. Systematic off-pump coronary artery revascularization in multivessel disease: experience of three hundred cases. *J Thorac Cardiovasc Surg.* 2000;119: 221–229.

Cheng DC, Bainbridge D, Martin JE, et al. Does off-pump coronary artery bypass reduce mortality, morbidity and resource utilization when compared to conventional coronary artery bypass? A meta-analysis of randomized trials. *Anesthesiology.* 2005;102:188–203.

Cleveland JC Jr, Shroyer ALW, Chen AY, et al. Off pump coronary artery bypass grafting decreases risk-adjusted mortality and morbidity. *Ann Thorac Surg.* 2001;72:1282–1289.

Edgerton JR, Dewey TM, Magee MJ, et al. Conversion in off-pump coronary artery bypass grafting: an analysis of predictors and outcomes. *Ann Thorac Surg.* 2003;76:1138–1143.

Kahn NE, DeSouza A, Mister R, et al. A randomized comparison of off-pump and on-pump multivessel coronary artery bypass surgery. *N Engl J Med.* 2004;350:21–28.

Lingaas PS, Hol PK, Lundblad R, et al. Clinical and angiographic outcome of coronary surgery with and without cardiopulmonary bypass: a prospective randomized trial. *Heart Surg Forum.* 2004;7:37–41.

Mack N, Bachand D, Acuff T, et al. Improved outcomes in coronary artery bypass grafting with beating-heart techniques. *J Thorac Cardiovasc Surg.* 2002;124:598–607.

Magee MJ, Jablonski KA, Stamou SC, et al. Elimination of cardiopulmonary bypass improves early survival for multivessel coronary artery bypass patients. *Ann Thorac Surg.* 2002;73:1196–1203.

Nathoe HM, V an Dijk D, Jansen EWL, et al. The comparison of on-pump and off-pump coronary bypass surgery in low-risk patients. *N Engl J Med.* 2003;348:394–402.

Novick RJ, Fox SA, Stitt LW, et al. Cumulative sum failure analysis of a policy change from on pump to off pump coronary artery bypass grafting. *Ann Thorac Surg.* 2001;72(Suppl.):S1016–S1021.

Plomondon ME, Cleveland JC Jr, Ludwig ST, et al. Off pump coronary artery bypass is associated with improved risk-adjusted outcomes. *Ann Thorac Surg.* 2001;72:114–119.

Puskas JD, Williams WH, Duke PG, et al. Off-pump coronary artery bypass grafting provides complete revascularization with reduced myocardial injury, transfusion requirements and length of stay: a prospective randomized comparison of 200 unselected patients undergoing off-pump versus conventional coronary artery bypass grafting. *J Thorac Cardiovasc Surg.* 2003;125:797–808.

Puskas JD, Williams WH, Mahoney EM, et al. Off-pump versus conventional coronary artery bypass grafting: early and one year graft patency, cost, and quality-of-life outcomes: a randomized trial. *JAMA.* 2004;291:1841–1849.

Chapter 24

Robotic Coronary Artery Revascularization Surgery

Bob Kiaii, R. Scott McClure, and W. Douglas Boyd

During the last quarter of the 20th century, and especially during the last decade, there has been a paradigm shift in the methods by which surgery is performed. The "invasiveness" of many procedures has been considerably reduced, and the outcomes significantly improved, as evidenced by better survival, fewer complications, and faster return to functional health and productive life.

In the late 1980s, great enthusiasm and momentum was initiated by laparoscopic cholecystectomy. For the first time, it was possible for surgeons neither to look directly at nor touch the tissues or organs that they operated on. Hence, endoscopic surgical techniques were adopted by several different surgical disciplines because of the decreased morbidity and shorter recovery times. Most of these surgical procedures have been excisional in nature and not reconstructive and microsurgical. Unfortunately, the resounding success of this excisional procedure led to unrealistic expectations of the early conversion of other surgical procedures, such as microvascular reconstructive cardiac surgery, to less invasive approaches as well. Initially, this was not possible because of the limitations of conventional endoscopic instruments. Hence, until recently, endoscopic approaches have not been successful in cardiac surgery. Many of the limitations of conventional endoscopic approaches have been overcome with the development of robotic surgical systems or computer-assisted surgical systems.

Robotic surgery allows a digital interface between the surgeon's hands and the instruments. This interface enhances dexterity, allows scaling of motions, provides tremor filtering, and enables the performance of endoscopic microsurgery. Therefore, the use of robotic surgical systems over the last few years has enabled cardiac surgeons to perform minimally invasive endoscopic coronary artery bypass grafting (CABG) on the beating heart. This advantage eliminates the need for cardiopulmonary bypass (CPB) and sternotomy, and reduces tissue trauma, which translates into decreased patient morbidity, increased patient satisfaction, shorter hospital stay, and potentially reduced healthcare costs.

TELEMANIPULATION SYSTEMS

Initially, two telemanipulation systems were available—the ZEUS (Computer Motion, Goleta, California) and the da Vinci Surgical System (Intuitive Surgical, Sunnyvale, California). However, recently, these two companies have merged, and only the da Vinci Surgical System is commercially available and is the system used for robotic coronary revascularization by most health-care centers worldwide. The da Vinci Surgical System consists of a surgeon console, a surgical cart, and the vision system.

The surgeon console includes the display system, master handles, user interface, and the electronic controller. The surgeon at the console is able to view the transmitted image of the surgical field through a high-resolution three-dimensional display. The system projects the image of the surgical site, while the controller transforms the spatial motion of the tools into the camera frame of reference. Hence, the system provides natural hand–eye coordination. Motion scaling allows for various ratios for master and instrument motions. The camera can be controlled by activating a foot pedal at the console. By activating another foot pedal (clutch), the surgeon is able to temporarily uncouple and reposition the master control arms in the working field to achieve a better ergonomic position, while the instrument in the operating field remains stationary (indexing). The tremor filter minimizes the involuntary tremors.

The surgical cart is stationed at the side of the operating table and consists of four robotic arms. One central arm is for the endoscope and the other three arms are for the surgical instruments. The instruments (end effectors) are attached to the three instrument arms and are recognized automatically by the system. The instruments can easily be interchanged. Because of the EndoWrist feature of the instruments, a total of six degrees of freedom is possible.

EVOLUTION OF ROBOT-ASSISTED CORONARY BYPASS SURGERY

Over the last 4 years, cardiac surgeons have recognized the importance of achieving video dexterity and have been adopting video-assisted techniques in increasing numbers. The early work by Drs. Nataf in Paris, France, Mayfield in Atlanta, Georgia, and Wolf in Cincinnati, Ohio, laid the groundwork for an endoscopic minimally invasive revolution. The development of video-assisted techniques and the use of new equipment in cardiac procedures represented a paradigm shift and a quantum leap in our efforts to provide a less traumatic coronary revascularization procedure. In parallel to these developments, new robotic technology was emerging and was demonstrating efficacy in endoscopic surgery in other disciplines.

There are presently four levels of robotic coronary surgery that are being practiced.

1. Robotic camera control and video assistance with manual conduit harvesting: The surgeon harvests the arterial conduit with robotic camera control and performs the anastomosis through a minithoracotomy.
2. Telerobotic conduit harvesting and manual anastomosis: The surgeon harvests the internal thoracic artery (ITA) from the master console and performs a manual anastomosis through a minithoracotomy.
3. Computer-assisted endoscopic coronary anastomosis: The surgeon harvests the ITA manually through a conventional sternotomy and performs the coronary anastomosis on the arrested or the beating heart through a sternotomy or minithoracotomy.
4. Totally endoscopic coronary artery bypass: The surgeon performs conduit harvesting, preparation, target vessel preparation, control, and anastomosis remotely from the master console through port access.

This chapter focuses on levels 2 and 4.

INDICATIONS FOR ROBOTIC REVASCULARIZATION

- Single- or double-vessel coronary artery disease with Grade I–II left ventricular function.
- Coronary arteries, left anterior descending (LAD) coronary artery, with ostial stenosis not amenable to percutaneous coronary intervention (PCI).
- Multivessel disease utilizing hybrid technique (single or bilateral ITA grafting with PCI of other diseased vessels).
- High risk for open sternotomy approach.
  - Ascending aortic atheroma or calcified aorta.
  - Comorbid conditions making a conventional surgery high risk.

PATIENT SELECTION

In addition to understanding the standard contraindications to surgical coronary artery revascularization, patient selection for robotic coronary artery revascularization involves a history and physical examination, heavily weighted on uncovering factors that affect the external and internal thoracic structures. Anatomy hindering preoperative port placement, limiting robotic arm movement, or reducing the already limited field of view inside the thorax will lead to considerably increased chances of surgical error and will expose the patient to unnecessary risk.

- Absolute contraindication:
  - Extensive pleural symphysis.
- Relative contraindications:
  - Severe obesity.
  - Substantial cardiac enlargement (insufficient space in thoracic cavity).
  - Excessive mediastinal, pericardial, and chest wall fat.
  - Narrow intercostals spaces.
  - Thick chest wall.

- Previous history of coronary surgery.
- Diffuse distal coronary disease.
- Severe pulmonary disease (intolerance to single lung ventilation).

OPERATIVE TECHNIQUES

Anesthesia Considerations

- Paravertebral block for postoperative pain control.
- Double lumen end tracheal tube or bronchial blocker.
- Central venous pressure/Swan-Ganz catheter.
- Carbon dioxide (CO_2) insufflations of the thoracic cavity during the procedure.
  - Intrathoracic pressures 5 to 15 mm Hg.
- Maintenance of normothermia with warming and forced air blankets.

Preparation, Positioning, and Draping

Initial positioning of the patient can have a considerable effect on the operative procedure because proper positioning minimizes interference from internal and external body structures with the robotic equipment. Judicious care at this stage ensures that the necessary landmarks for port placement are easily accessible to maximize robotic arm maneuverability intraoperatively.

The patient is positioned at the left edge of the operating room table. A comfortable support is placed under the distal two thirds of the left side of the patient's thorax. This support usually takes the form of a rolled up towel and elevates the patient's thorax 6 to 8 inches superiorly. The left arm is positioned at the side of the operating room (OR) table to allow the left shoulder to drop downward. The table is rotated 30 degrees up so that the patient is in the partial left lateral position (see Fig. 24-1).

Leads and external defibrillator pads are positioned on the patient's chest away from the left lateral and midclavicular areas of the thorax so as not to interfere with port

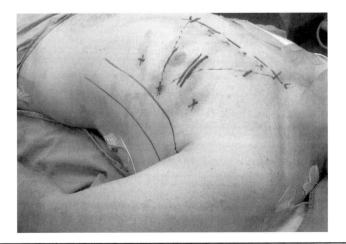

FIGURE 24-1. Proper patient positioning.

placement. One pad is placed on the right anterior lateral thorax and the other is placed on the left posterior thorax. The patient is prepped in a routine manner for conventional CABG and saphenous vein harvesting, safeguarding against the possibility of having to convert the case to an open procedure. The only variation in the preparation is the exposure of the patient's thorax and axilla on the one side for port placement.

Port Placement

Proper port placement is fundamental to the success of the operation. Placement of each port is centered on constructing an ideal configuration that ensures mobilization of the ITA from the first rib to the sixth rib with the least amount of impedance to the robotic arms. It is imperative that the surgeon be meticulous with each individual patient, taking the necessary time needed to ensure proper completion of port placement before moving forward with the operation.

Lack of intrathoracic visualization is the premier challenge in determining port placement. Careful review of the coronary angiogram and chest radiographs preoperatively, along with direct examination of the anatomic structures of the individual patient in the operating room, help alleviate this problem.

- Chest radiograph:
  - Evaluate the chest radiograph in an orderly manner. Identify pertinent thoracic landmarks.
    - ▲ Suprasternal notch.
    - ▲ Angle of Louis.
    - ▲ Xiphoid.
    - ▲ Second, third, fourth, and fifth intercostal spaces (ICS).
    - ▲ Left internal thoracic artery (LITA) and right internal thoracic artery (RITA) locations—1 to 3 cm lateral to the sternum.
  - Note the position of the heart in the mediastinum.
  - Note the size of the heart in relation to the pleural space on the port-access side of the chest.
  - Lateral view: Observe the degree of space between the anterior surface of the heart and underside of the thorax.
- Direct examination of patient's thorax:
  - Evaluate the external anatomic characteristics of the patient's thorax and conceptualize the internal anatomic characteristics on the basis of the previously viewed chest radiograph and preoperative coronary angiogram.
- Outline with a felt marker precisely where each port is to enter the thoracic cavity using the standardized guidelines discussed subsequently. Make necessary adjustments for individual patients on the basis of the information acquired from diagnostic imaging and patient examination.

Standardized Guidelines for Port Placement
- Triangle model of configuration:
  - Proximal to distal end of LITA is one side of triangle (surgical area).
  - Position endoscope at the fifth ICS in axillary line (one vertex of triangle).

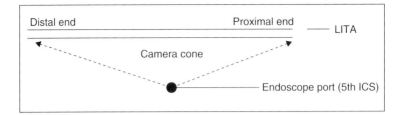

FIGURE 24-2. Triangle model of configuration. LITA, left internal thoracic artery; ICS, intercostal space. (Adapted from Falk V, Loulmet D, Wolf RK. *Procedural guide. Robotically assisted IMA harvest.* Mountain View, CA: Intuitive Surgical; 2001.)

- Lines from endoscope port extend to both proximal and distal ends of the LITA (triangle formed).
- Create the "camera cone" (see Fig. 24-2).
- Place the instrument ports outside the camera cone (see Figs. 24-1 and 24-3).
- Place ports a few centimeters off the line of the defined triangle.
- Allow 7 to 10 cm between ports to ensure robotic arms have full range of motion without collision.
- Create a circle from the camera port (7 to 10 cm) and avoid placing ports inside this circle.
■ Common port locations:
   - Port site will vary on the basis of body habitus. A larger thorax would require more obtuse angles in order to visualize the entire anatomy, whereas a small thorax would require more acute angles for the same reason.
   - Endoscope port: fifth ICS anterior axillary line (AAL) or slightly medial to this point, depending on body habitus.
   - Right and left instrument ports: third and seventh ICS, respectively; 2 to 3 cm medial to the AAL or midway between AAL and midclavicular line (MCL).

Takedown of Left Internal Thoracic Artery

Once the robotic instruments are adequately positioned within the thoracic cavity, the surgical workspace for harvesting the LITA is maximized using single lung ventilation

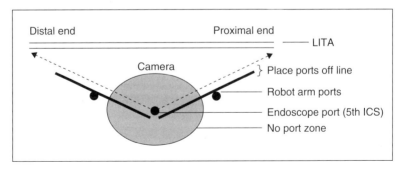

FIGURE 24-3. Port placement positioning based on triangle model. LITA, left internal thoracic artery; ICS, intercostal spaces. (Adapted from Falk V, Loulmet D, Wolf RK. *Procedural guide. Robotically assisted IMA harvest.* Mountain View, CA: Intuitive Surgical; 2001.)

and continuous CO_2 insufflation. The surgeon must be overtly sensitive to visual cues throughout the surgical procedure compensating for a lack of haptic feedback with robotic assistance. This prevents unnecessary tension or trauma occurring to the arterial conduit during mobilization. Using a 30-degree endoscope angled up and inserted into the camera port, an initial inspection of the internal mammary artery and its relation to surrounding anatomic structures within the thorax is performed.

- Request single lung ventilation and inform the anesthesia team of initiation of insufflation.
- Insert the endoscope port. Insufflate the thoracic cavity with CO_2 through the insufflation port on the endoscope cannula keeping insufflation pressures between 6 and 10 mm Hg, unless blood pressure requires more conservative levels.
- Insert the endoscope and move it freely through its full range of motion with your hands. Locate the distal and proximal ends of the LITA and ensure that the endoscope does not collide with external body parts such as the hip or shoulder (occasionally, to reach the lower third aspect of the ITA through the same port incision, the port is "punched down" to the fourth ICS).
- Inspect the inner cavity with the endoscope to be certain that there is a clear path for insertion of instrument ports.
- Observe insertion of instrument ports with direct view from the endoscope.
- Dock the robot and adapt the robotic arms to the appropriate endoscopic ports.
- Insert the instruments through the ports and attach to the instrument arms.
- Insert a Verres needle at approximately the sixth ICS MCL and attach it to low suction for venting.
- Initial inspection of the LITA.
  - Locate the LITA (most visible at the second rib).
  - Follow the LITA proximally to its origin at the subclavian artery and distally to the sixth ICS. Arterial pulsation is a beneficial guide. Adipose tissue and muscle obscure the artery at the mid and lower one thirds, respectively.
  - Locate and be conscious of the presence of the phrenic nerve at all times. It should be clearly visible traversing the pericardium. Follow it proximally toward the origin of the ITA.
- Key points to remember for successful robotic-assisted takedown of the ITA:
  - Progress in a slow and controlled manner maintaining hemostasis.
  - Identify the ITA and vein and work from the known to the unknown.
  - Keep the ITA and robotic instruments in view at all times.
  - Use the "no-touch" technique to mobilize the ITA to reduce pedicle trauma.
- With the cautery/spatula blade in the right arm and a DeBakey forceps in the left arm, incise the parietal pleura at the most visible point. This is 1 cm medial to the artery at the second rib. Use a low monopolar electrocautery setting at 10 to 15 watts.
- Begin the dissection by scoring the fascia with the spatula 1 cm lateral and medial to the LITA. Continue with a lateral to medial technique and slowly take down the LITA with a combination of spatula blade blunt dissection and electrocautery. Move proximal to the top of the first rib and then distal to the sixth ICS. Be careful not to put undue tension on the pedicle during mobilization. Mobilization to the top of the first rib provides an additional 3 to 4 cm of length to the pedicle and makes distal anastomosis easier.

- Small branches off the LITA are cauterized at a safe distance from the vascular pedicle. Larger branches require instrument interchange and clips to be applied.
- Once the adequate length of LITA has been harvested, the vessel is skeletonized distally.
- Heparin is given and the distal LITA is clipped and left attached to the chest wall.
- For bilateral ITA harvesting, the right pleural space is entered and the RITA is dissected first. Occasionally, there is a need to switch to zero-degree endoscope.

Hemostasis Management

To maintain hemostasis when bleeding occurs, evaluate the severity of the bleed in relation to the increased magnification of the image projected by the endoscope. When small venous or arterial branches are responsible, apply gentle pressure to the area for 2 to 3 minutes with the tip of the robotic instruments. Often, this is all that is required. If bleeding continues and if the site of bleeding is in clear view, apply a clip to the vessel and cauterize the distal end. A handheld thoracoscopic bipolar instrument may be helpful. Surgicel hemostasis gauze is also effective if needed.

If bleeding is felt to be of a high severity or if the patient shows signs of hemodynamic instability, remove the robotic instrumentation immediately and convert to a conventional CABG via sternotomy.

Left Internal Thoracic Artery to Left Anterior Descending Anastomosis

In the second intercostal space MCL, a fourth endoscopic port is inserted and adapted to the fourth robotic arm. A nontraumatic tissue grasper is placed in this port.

- Pericardiotomy:
  - Pericardiotomy is performed 2 to 3 cm anterior to the phrenic nerve.
  - Using the fourth arm, the pericardial fat is first removed.
  - The pericardium is opened.
  - LAD artery identified on the basis of its location on the ventricular septum and its path to the apex.

- Anastomosis:
  - If anastomosis is to be performed endoscopically, the ITA pedicle is not detached from the chest wall until anastomosis is performed to avoid torsion of the graft.
  - If anastomosis is to be performed through minianterior thoracotomy, ITA pedicle transected, and to avoid torsion, it is attached to the edge of the pericardium, using a clip, in the normal anatomic orientation at the site where the anastomosis is to be performed.

LEVEL 2: MINI-ANTERIOR THORACOTOMY APPROACH OR ATRAUMATIC CORONARY ARTERY BYPASS

- Insert a long needle under the direct visualization of the endoscope to identify the optimal ICS to perform thoracotomy for the best exposure of the LAD.
- Insufflation can be momentarily stopped to take away the shift in the mediastinum.

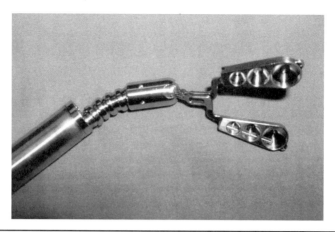

FIGURE 24-4. Octopus TE endoscopic stabilizer.

- Mark the intercostal space from inside using electrocautery.
- Undock the robot and remove the instrument ports.
- Perform a minianterior thoracotomy.
- Identify the pericardiectomy site and the ITA pedicle.
- Detach the ITA and deliver through the incision, and immediately place two suspension sutures to prevent the pedicle from twisting.
- Assess ITA length and flow, and prepare for anastomosis.
- Select port site for the endoscopic Octopus TE stabilizer (Medtronic, Minneapolis, Minnesota) (see Fig. 24-4).
- Achieve stabilization.
- Apply proximal and distal occlusion snares or an intravascular shunt depending on the patient's hemodynamics.
- Perform anastomosis in the usual fashion.
- Check graft flow using an intraoperative flow measuring device.
- Intraoperative angiography is performed to check the ITA patency, and PCI of other coronary vessels is performed at the same time in the specialized hybrid operating room (see Fig. 24-5).

LEVEL 4: TOTALLY ENDOSCOPIC CORONARY ARTERY BYPASS

- Once the site of anastomosis on the LAD is identified, occlusion silastic snares are placed proximally and distally.
- The suture to be used for anastomosis is placed in the thoracic cavity to avoid CO_2 leaks during the procedure.
- The Octopus TE endoscopic stabilizer (Fig. 24-4) is inserted through a subxiphoid port, and stabilization of the selected area is achieved with the help of the robotic instruments.
- The anastomosis is begun in the usual fashion by inserting the first stitch in the ITA while still attached to the chest wall.

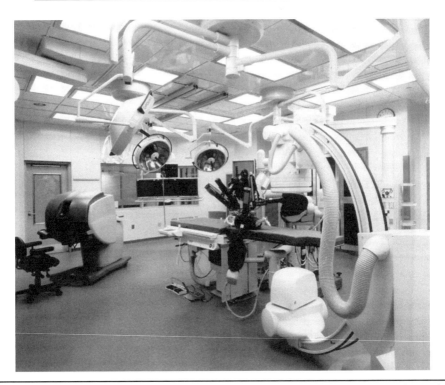

FIGURE 24-5. Hybrid cardiac operating room at the London Health Sciences Centre and Canadian Surgical Technologies & Advanced Robotics (CSTAR). The room is fully equipped for robotic surgery, angiography, and percutaneous coronary intervention.

- After this stitch, the ITA is detached and held by the fourth arm and placed in the second midclavicular line (MCL) ICS.
- Irrigation or a blower is used during the anastomosis to keep the vessel clear of blood and provide adequate visualization of the LAD.
- At the completion of anastomosis, the pedicle is anchored to the surface of the heart to prevent twisting.
- Intraoperative angiography is performed to check ITA patency and PCI of the other vessels at the same time, if needed, in the hybrid operating room (Fig. 24-5).

FUTURE DIRECTIONS

In the future, we must be ready to adapt what is best from other fields. The introduction of drug-eluting stents will surely have a considerable impact on "best revascularization" strategies. In the future, it is likely that optimal revascularization strategies for patients will involve a combination of facilitated endoscopic robot-assisted arterial grafting and catheter-based interventions (Fig. 24-5) in addition to the real-time image-guided application of transmyocardial laser therapy, angiogenic factors, or stem cells to nonrevascularizable areas of the myocardium. To accommodate this approach efficiently, new ORs have to be designed to allow the integration of space-consuming robotic systems and imaging and guidance systems as part of a complete hybrid OR. The continued advance of computers, imaging, and robotic technology has the potential to revolutionize both the OR and the cardiac surgery speciality. Many of these emerging technologies have dedicated research and development groups working zealously on the next stage of evolution. For these developments to be truly relevant in surgery, however, they will require input and guidance from the clinical community. Surgical robotic technology is still in its infancy. Much as airplanes now perform tasks never imagined by the Wright brothers, it is likely that the medical robots of tomorrow will deliver functionality and breadth of utility beyond our imagination.

SUGGESTED READINGS

Boyd WD, Kiaii B, Novick RJ, et al. RAVECAB: Improving outcome in off-pump/minimal access surgery with robotic assistance and video enhancement. *Can J Surg*. 2001;44:45–50.

Falk V, Loulmet D, Wolf RK. *Procedural guide. Robotically assisted IMA harvest*. Mountain View, CA: Intuitive Surgical; 2001.

Franco KL, Verrier ED, eds. *Advanced therapy in cardiac surgery*. 2nd ed. Ontario: BC Decker, Inc.; 2003.

Ohtuska T, Wolf RK, Hiratzka LF, et al. Thoracoscopic internal mammary artery harvest for MICABG using the harmonic scalpel. *Ann Thorac Surg*. 1997;63:S107–S109.

Chapter 25

Surgery of the Aortic Valve

Tirone E. David

ANATOMY

The aortic valve is better described as an aortic root because its function depends on more than just the aortic cusps. The aortic root has four anatomic components: aortic annulus, aortic cusps, aortic sinuses or sinuses of Valsalva, and sinotubular junction. The aortic annulus attaches the aortic root to the left ventricle, and it has a scalloped shape that serves for insertion of the aortic cusps, which are semilunar in shape. The aortic annulus is attached to the interventricular septum in approximately 45% of its circumference and to fibrous tissue in 55% of its circumference. The segment of arterial wall delineated by the annulus proximally and the sinotubular junction distally is the aortic sinus. There are three aortic sinus and three cusps: right, left, and noncoronary. The left coronary artery arises from the left aortic sinus and the right coronary artery arises from the right aortic sinus.

The highest point of the aortic cusps where two of them come in proximity is called the *commissure*. There are three commissures, and the triangular spaces underneath them are called *subcommissural triangles*. These triangular spaces are also important for aortic valve function. The subcommissural triangle between the left and right cusps is made of myocardium, whereas the other two are made of fibrous tissue.

The sinotubular junction is a ridge that demarcates the end of the aortic sinuses and the beginning of the ascending aorta. The commissures of the aortic valve are located immediately below the sinotubular junction.

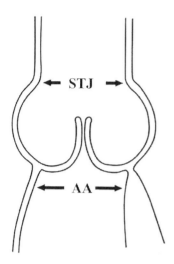

FIGURE 25-1. The transverse diameter of the aortic annulus (AA); it is 15% to 20% larger than the diameter of the sinotubular junction (STJ) in children but tends to equalize in adults.

Although the aortic cusps are the most important component of the aortic valve, the other cusps also affect its function. Therefore, dilation of the aortic annulus or of the sinotubular junction causes aortic insufficiency (AI) because of displacement of the aortic cusps. The aortic sinuses are important to facilitate opening and closure of aortic cusps and minimize the mechanical stress during the cardiac cycle, but isolated anatomic abnormalities of the aortic sinuses do not cause AI. That is the reason why children with rupture of an aortic sinus into another cardiac chamber may have an entirely competent aortic valve.

The aortic root and the ascending aorta are structures that contain a large amount of elastic fibers in young patients. Consequently, these structures distend and shorten during the cardiac cycle. The number of elastic fibers decreases with aging, and the aortic root and ascending aorta become progressively less compliant. The transverse diameter of the aortic annulus at the nadir of the cusps is 15% to 20% larger than the diameter of the sinotubular junction in children. In adults, these two diameters tend to equalize and sometimes even reverse (see Fig. 25-1).

PATHOLOGY

Anatomically, the normal tricuspid aortic valve may become calcified late in life and may cause aortic stenosis (AS). This lesion is called *dystrophic calcification*, senile calcification, or degenerative calcification. The pathogenesis of this lesion is complex and poorly understood, but it appears to be related to inflammation, infiltration of lipoproteins, and ossification. Statins (3-hydroxy-3-methyl-glutamyl coenzyme A reductase inhibitors) are effective in retarding calcification of the aortic cusps.

A bicuspid aortic valve (BAV) occurs in approximately 1% to 2% of the population and is the most common aortic valve disease. It may function well until late in life when it may become calcified and stenotic. BAV can also cause AI, AS, and mixed lesions in younger patients. Most BAVs have three aortic sinuses, and the larger one of the two cusps has a raphe instead of a commissure. The right coronary artery is usually nondominant and small.

A unicusp aortic valve is relatively less common in comparison with the BAV and usually causes AS.

Patients with unicusp and BAV frequently have premature degenerative changes of the media of the aortic root and ascending aorta and are at risk of developing an aneurysm and dissection of the ascending aorta.

A quadricusp aortic valve is rare and causes AI. Three cusps are usually of similar size and one is hypoplastic.

A subaortic ventricular septal defect can cause AI because of the distortion of the aortic annulus and cusp prolapse. Another congenital anomaly of the aortic root is supra-aortic stenosis, which consists of a very narrow sinotubular junction, dilated aortic sinuses, and redundant cusps. The cusps may be thickened in some patients, thereby causing restriction. The coronary artery orifices may also be stenotic.

Dilation of the aortic root is the most common cause of AI in North America. Dilation of the sinotubular junction causes AI because of outward displacement of the aortic cusps (see Fig. 25-2). This lesion is often seen in older patients with an ascending aortic aneurysm. Dilation of the aortic annulus causes AI by changing the geometric relation of the cusps along the subcommissural triangles (see Fig. 25-3). These triangles tend to become more obtuse with dilation of the aortic annulus. The aortic valve may be tricuspid or bicuspid in patients with a dilated aortic root. Young patients with aortic root aneurysms may or may not have Marfan syndrome.

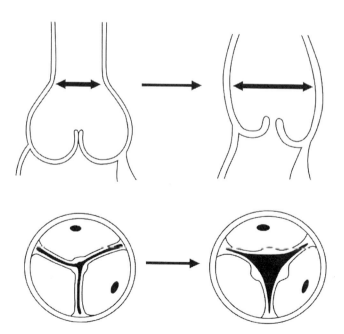

FIGURE 25-2. Dilation of the sinotubular junction causes aortic insufficiency.

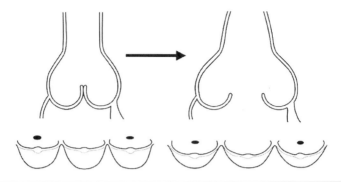

FIGURE 25-3. Dilation of the aortic annulus causes aortic insufficiency.

Marfan syndrome is an autosomal dominant variably penetrant inherited disorder of the connective tissue in which the cardiovascular, skeletal, ocular, and other systems may be involved. The prevalence is estimated to be in 1:5,000 people. The clinical features are the result of a weakening of the supporting tissues owing to defects in fibrillin 1, a glycoprotein and an important component of the microfibril. The gene for fibrillin 1 (FBN1) is located in chromosome 15. Several hundred mutations have been documented. The diagnosis of Marfan syndrome is made on clinical grounds. These patients often develop aortic root aneurysm, which may cause rupture or aortic dissection. Myxomatous degeneration of the mitral valve with consequent annular enlargement and mitral regurgitation may also be present. The prognosis of patients with Marfan syndrome is largely determined by the aortic root aneurysm, which, if left untreated, will rupture, dissect, or cause AI and consequent heart failure.

Aortic dissection involving the ascending aorta can cause AI because of detachment of one or more commissures of the aortic valve.

Rheumatic aortic valve is still seen in North America, but largely in immigrants. This disease causes fibrosis, commissural fusion, thickening, and contraction of the aortic cusps; it may also calcify in the later stages. This disease can cause AS and AI.

Infective endocarditis of the aortic valve usually occurs in patients with pre-existing aortic valve disease, particularly BAV, but it may also occur in patients with normal valves. The infection destroys one or more cusps and causes AI.

There are also several connective tissue disorders that can cause AI: ankylosing spondylitis, Reiter syndrome, osteogenesis imperfecta, rheumatoid arthritis, systemic lupus erythematosus, and others.

An increasingly more common cause of aortic valve disease is prosthetic and biologic valve disease. The mechanical aortic valve may become stenotic because of pannus or thrombosis. The bioprosthetic valves and aortic valve homograft may become stenotic or incompetent because of tissue degeneration, which is frequently associated with calcification and/or cusp tear. Finally, the pulmonary autograft (Ross procedure) may become incompetent because of cusp prolapse and/or dilation of the root, and tissue degeneration.

PATHOPHYSIOLOGY

Acquired AS develops gradually and the left ventricle adapts itself by replication of sarcomeres and concentric hypertrophy. As the ventricular mass increases, compliance decreases with consequent increase in left ventricular end-diastolic pressure and left atrial pressure. The degree of AS is considered severe when the aortic valve area is <0.5 cm²/m² of body surface area or the peak systolic gradient exceeds 50 mm Hg with normal cardiac output.

The hemodynamic consequences of AI in the left ventricle depend on its severity and chronicity. Acute severe AI is poorly tolerated by the left ventricle, and heart failure and shock are usually inevitable. Chronic progressive AI results in a gradual increase in left ventricular end-diastolic volume with consequent rise in end-diastolic pressure. These changes in volume and pressure promote replication of the sarcomeres in series with consequent eccentric left ventricular hypertrophy. Because of this hypertrophy, left ventricular ejection fraction is maintained in spite of a large left ventricular end-diastolic volume, but eventually the ventricle fails.

NATURAL HISTORY

Asymptomatic patients with AS have a good prognosis. Sudden death is rare among asymptomatic patients. The prognosis becomes poor once symptoms develop, and more than two thirds of the patients die within a couple of years.

Patients with chronic AI remain asymptomatic for many years but also have a poor prognosis when symptoms develop.

DIAGNOSIS

The classic symptoms of AS (i.e., congestive heart failure, angina pectoris, and syncope) usually occur late in the course of the disease. Most patients are diagnosed during a routine physical examination before symptoms develop. On auscultation, there is a harsh systolic murmur, sometimes with a thrill along the left sternal border, often radiating to the neck. The second heart sound is soft, absent, or paradoxically split. The carotid pulses are diminished and delayed. The electrocardiogram (ECG) may show signs of left ventricular hypertrophy. Echocardiography establishes the diagnosis and provides information regarding its severity, ventricular size and thickness, and pulmonary hypertension. Coronary angiography should be performed in patients older than 45 years, or even in younger patients if they have coronary artery risk factors.

AI is not as readily diagnosed, and many patients escape clinical detection before it becomes symptomatic. Palpitations and head pounding may occur during exertion. Angina pectoris may occur, but less commonly than in AS. Syncope is rare. Symptoms of congestive heart failure are usually an indication of left ventricular dysfunction. On examination, there is a wide pulse pressure. Echocardiography establishes the diagnosis and also provides other important information about the mechanism of AI and left ventricular function. The severity of AI decreases as the left ventricular end-diastolic pressure increases because of a lower pressure gradient between the aorta and left ventricle.

INDICATIONS FOR SURGERY

Patients with asymptomatic severe AS (aortic valve area < 0.50 cm^2/m^2) should be considered for surgery when the left ventricle begins to become hypertrophic. Surgery should also be considered in all symptomatic patients.

Patients with asymptomatic severe AI should have assessment of left ventricular function, and surgery should be considered when systolic left ventricular function begins to deteriorate. All symptomatic patients should be considered for surgery.

Patients with aortic root aneurysm should have surgery when the diameter of the aortic root exceeds 50 mm. Patients with Marfan syndrome and a family history of aortic dissection should be operated on when the aortic root reaches 45 mm in diameter.

The indications for surgery in patients with prosthetic aortic valve dysfunction are similar to those of native valve, but the clinical presentation is broader and more complex. Patients with small paravalvular dehiscence that causes hemolysis and anemia should be considered for reoperation. Mechanical valve stenosis by pannus or thrombus is also an indication for reoperation. Bioprosthetic and biologic valves should be replaced when there is echocardiography evidence of moderate or severe dysfunction.

SURGICAL OPTIONS

Aortic Valve Repair

Patients with AI are candidates for aortic valve repair as long as the aortic cusps are reasonably normal by echocardiography. Most aortic valve repairs are performed in patients with degenerative diseases of the aortic root, such as aneurysms with dilation of the sinotubular junction and/or aortic annulus, and in patients with congenital disorders, such as BAVs and subaortic ventricular septal defect with prolapse of the right coronary cusp.

Aortic Valve Replacement

There are mechanical and tissue valves for aortic valve replacement (AVR). Mechanical valves are durable but require lifelong anticoagulation with warfarin sodium to prevent valve thrombosis and thromboembolism. There are various mechanical valves, and they are grouped as bileaflet, single leaflet, and ball valves. Bileaflet mechanical valves are the most commonly used. Tissue valves can be obtained from a variety of sources. Aortic valve homografts have been used since the early days of heart surgery. The pulmonary valve of the patient can be transferred into the aortic position and a biological valve such as a pulmonary homograft can be implanted in the place of the pulmonary valve (Ross procedure). Finally, xenograft valves are commercially available for AVR. These valves are usually made from porcine aortic valves or bovine pericardium. In either case, the xenograft tissue is chemically treated with glutaraldehyde to render it less antigenic and more resistant to fatigue. Bioprosthetic valves are available mounted in a stent and without a stent. Tissue valves usually have a limited durability, but they do not require anticoagulation with warfarin sodium.

Aortic Root Replacement

Patients with abnormal aortic roots may require replacement of the aortic cusps and aortic sinuses with reimplantation of the coronary arteries. This operation is often referred to as *Bentall procedure*, although it is no longer performed as originally described. Aortic root replacement can be performed with mechanical and tissue valves.

Matching the Prosthesis to the Patient

It is not always simple to match the patient to the type and size of heart valve. Mechanical valves are durable, but because oral anticoagulation is mandatory, patients have a constant risk of bleeding. Tissue valves do not require anticoagulation but may have limited durability. Therefore, patients who are likely to outlive their tissue valves may require reoperation. Bioprosthetic valves are ideal for patients who are as old as 70 years or older because the probability of reoperation for valve failure is very low. An aortic valve homograft is ideal for patients with active infective endocarditis, particularly if they have an aortic root abscess. The Ross procedure is ideally suited for children and young adults, although some surgeons use this procedure in older patients also. The main characteristic of this valve in children is that the valve increases in size as the child grows.

Another important aspect of AVR is that an implanted prosthetic aortic valve has to have an adequate orifice to prevent the so-called "patient-prosthesis mismatch." Ideally, the effective orifice area of a prosthetic valve should exceed $0.85 \text{ cm}^2/\text{m}^2$ of the patient's body surface area. If the aortic annulus is too small, it is possible to implant a larger valve by replacing the aortic root with a stentless valve or by enlarging the aortic annulus with a patch. There are basically two techniques to enlarge the aortic annulus. In the first, the aortic annulus is incised along its fibrous portion, usually along the sub-commissural triangle between the left and noncoronary sinuses and into the base of the anterior leaflet of the mitral valve. This technique allows for implantation of a valve one size larger than the original diameter of the aortic annulus without causing distortion of the outflow tract. Another technique, the Konno procedure, consists in incising the aortic annulus along the subcommissural triangle between the left and right aortic sinuses. In this procedure, the right ventricle has to be opened and the interventricular septum incised 1 to 3 cm, depending on how much enlargement is desirable. Two separate patches are needed to reconstruct the interventricular septum and the right ventricle. The Konno procedure allows the implantation of a valve two or three sizes larger than the original size of the annulus, but it is a more complicated procedure and is associated with a septal infarct because the first septal perforator is often severed.

OPERATIVE TECHNIQUES

Aortic Valve Replacement

AVR is usually performed through a 15- to 20-cm long incision in the skin over the sternum and full median sternotomy. It can also be performed through a limited skin incision (7 to 10 cm) and a partial or full sternotomy (minimal access AVR). AVR requires cardiopulmonary bypass, clamping and opening the ascending aorta, and protecting

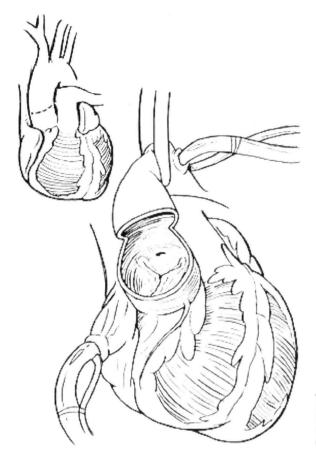

FIGURE 25-4. Aortic valve replacement: the aorta is opened through a transverse incision made 5 mm above the sinotubular junction.

the myocardium with cardioplegia during the aortic clamping (see Fig. 25-4). The diseased aortic valve is completely excised and the aortic annulus is cleared from any calcification. The aortic annulus is measured with a specific manufacturer's valve sizer, and the largest possible valve should be implanted to avoid patient-prosthesis mismatch. The prosthetic valve is secured to the aortic annulus according to the manufacturer's specifications. We prefer to secure mechanical valves with 20 to 30 simple interrupted sutures of 2-0 polyester, depending on the valve size (see Fig. 25-5). Currently used stented bioprosthetic valves are designed to be implanted in the supra-annular position, and, for this reason, 10 to 12 horizontal mattress sutures with pledgets on the ventricular side of the annulus are used (see Fig. 25-6).

There are basically three methods to implant stentless biologic valves: subcoronary implantation, aortic root inclusion, and aortic root replacement. In the subcoronary implantation, the bioprosthetic aortic valve is supported by the patient's aortic root, and matching the size of the valve with the size of the aortic root is crucial for proper function of the stentless valve (see Fig. 25-7). In the aortic root inclusion technique, the donor root is secured inside the recipient aortic root. These two methods are technically demanding, and most surgeons prefer to implant stentless valves using the technique of aortic root replacement.

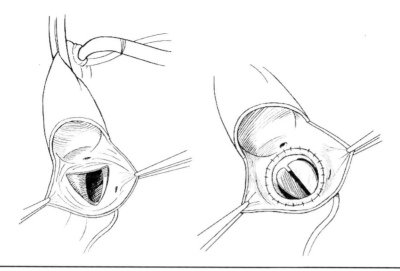

FIGURE 25-5. Aortic valve replacement with a mechanical valve.

Aortic Root Replacement

The ascending aorta is transected immediately above the sinotubular junction and the diseased aortic cusps are excised. The coronary arteries are detached from the aortic root leaving 4 to 6 mm of aortic sinus wall around their orifices. When a mechanical valve is used, a conduit of Dacron graft containing a valve is secured to the aortic annulus using 20 to 30 simple sutures, as described for AVR, or if the aortic annulus is dilated, multiple horizontal mattressed sutures of 2-0 polyester with pledgets, which

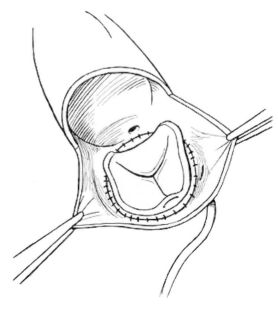

FIGURE 25-6. Aortic valve replacement with a bioprosthetic valve.

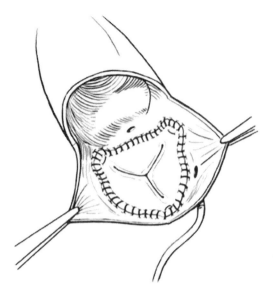

FIGURE 25-7. Aortic valve replacement with a stentless valve in the subcoronary position.

are left on the aortic side of the annulus, should be used (see Fig. 25-8). The coronary arteries are reimplanted into this graft, and its distal part is anastomosed to the ascending aorta.

A similar technique is used for aortic root replacement with pulmonary autograft, aortic valve homograft, or xenograft (see Fig. 25-9).

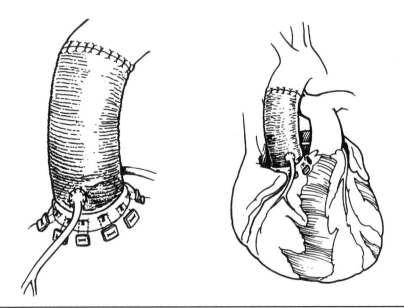

FIGURE 25-8. Composite replacement of the aortic valve and ascending aorta with a mechanical valve.

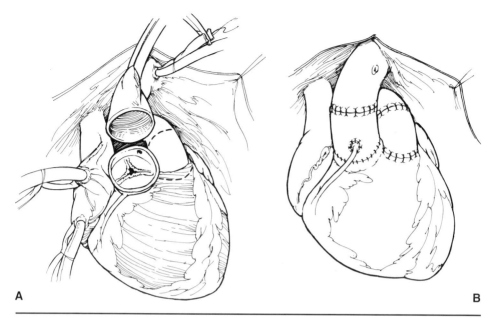

A   **B**

FIGURE 25-9. Aortic root replacement with pulmonary autograft. The pulmonary root is transferred to the aortic position and a pulmonary homograft is implanted in the right side of the circulation.

Reimplantation of the coronary arteries is the Achilles heel of aortic root replacement. In addition to performing a hemostatic anastomosis between the coronary arteries and the aortic root graft, it is also extremely important to align them correctly to prevent kinking with consequent myocardial ischemia. The latter is more common with the right coronary artery.

Aortic Valve Repair and Reconstruction of the Aortic Root

Patients with aortic root aneurysm often have normal or near normal cusps, and reconstruction of the aortic root with preservation of the aortic cusps is often feasible. There are basically two techniques: remodeling of the aortic root and reimplantation of the aortic valve. In the first, the aortic sinuses are excised leaving 4 to 5 mm of arterial wall attached to the aortic annulus. A tubular Dacron graft is tailored to recreate the three aortic sinuses as illustrated in Figure 25-9. The diameter of the graft is estimated by placing the three commissures into an imaginary circle that allows the three cusps to coapt centrally. Three neoaortic sinuses are created in one of the ends of the graft and then sutured to the aortic annulus and remnants of the aortic sinuses (see Fig. 25-10). The coronary arteries are reimplanted into their respective sinuses.

In the technique of reimplantation of the aortic valve, the sinuses are excised as described earlier, and a graft of diameter that exceeds the double of the height of the aortic cusps is sutured to the left ventricular outflow tract along a single horizontal plane immediately below the lowest level of the aortic annulus, except in the commissural area between the left and right cusps where it follows the scalloped shape of the

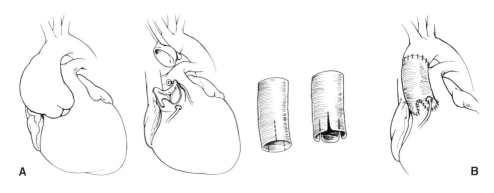

FIGURE 25-10. Aortic valve sparing operation: remodeling of the aortic root.

aortic annulus (see Fig. 25-11). The three commissures are suspended inside the graft and the aortic annulus, and remnants of the aortic sinuses are sutured to the graft. The coronary arteries are reimplanted into their respective sinuses. Darts are placed in between commissures to create neoaortic sinuses. If one or more cusps are prolapsing, the free margin can be shortened by plicating the central portion along the nodule of Aranti.

AI due to BAV can also be corrected by means of aortic valve repair as long as the cusps are of good quality and only one cusp is prolapsing. If the aortic annulus is dilated, which is often the case, the technique of aortic valve reimplantation provides the best long-term results.

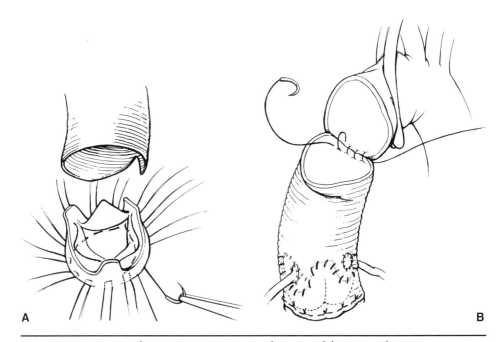

FIGURE 25-11. Aortic valve sparing operation: reimplantation of the aortic valve.

OPERATIVE MORTALITY AND MORBIDITY

The operative mortality for AVR varies with the patient's age and cardiac and non-cardiac comorbidity. First-time, isolated elective AVR in otherwise healthy patients is associated with an operative mortality of 1% or less. The risk increases in patients with coronary artery disease; in reoperations; in elderly patients; in active infective endocarditis, particularly if there is a paravalvular abscess; and in patients with other systemic diseases such as peripheral vascular disease, renal failure, and severe chronic obstructive lung disease. In the Society of Thoracic Surgeons National Database, which contains tens of thousands of patients, the operative mortality is approximately 4% for isolated AVR and 7% for AVR combined with coronary artery bypass.

The operative mortality associated with aortic valve repair and reconstruction of the aortic root is reportedly low at 1% to 3%, depending on the patient's clinical presentation.

Excessive postoperative bleeding may require re-exploration of the mediastinum in 2% to 5% of the patients. Perioperative myocardial infarction occurs in 1% to 2% of patients, particularly if coronary artery disease is present. Myocardial infarction can cause life-threatening ventricular dysrhythmias and/or heart failure. The risk of perioperative stroke varies with a patient's age, the presence of coronary artery disease, and ascending aorta and arch atherosclerosis. It is rare in young patients but it rises up to 10% or more in the elderly. Other complications such as renal and respiratory failure are uncommon and usually predictable. Sternal wound infection is rare if meticulous aseptic operative and intensive care unit (ICU) techniques are exercised. Patients with prosthetic aortic valves have a constant risk of developing prosthetic valve endocarditis, which is highest during the few months after surgery when it reaches 1% to 2%. For this reason prophylactic antibiotics should be given during the first 2 days after surgery or longer if the patient has a lung or wound infection.

Patients with mechanical valves should be started on heparin a couple of hours after removal of the chest drains and on warfarin sodium as soon as they can swallow. We do not believe that patients with tissue valves need warfarin sodium unless they are in atrial fibrillation. We give these patients only aspirin, but other surgeons recommend oral anticoagulation for the first 3 months.

Although AVR is performed with intraoperative echocardiography, a postoperative echocardiogram should be obtained before discharge to rule out pericardial effusion and assess valve and ventricular function.

LATE OUTCOMES

Patients who have had AVR must remain under the surveillance of a cardiologist and have an ECG and echocardiogram annually. Prosthetic valve dysfunction is best treated while ventricular function is normal. Therefore, patients with a failing bioprosthetic valve should have elective reoperations while they are well, instead of waiting until severe symptoms of heart failure ensue.

Long-term survival after AVR depends on the patient's age, functional class at the time of surgery, left ventricular function, coronary artery disease, and other systemic diseases. The type of valve implanted does not seem to affect long-term survival. Adults who have AVR have a mean age of 65 years, and the 10-year survival is approximately 60%; it ranges from 40% to 80% depending on comorbidities.

The risk of thromboembolic events, usually transient ischemic attacks or strokes, is approximately 1% to 2% per year, but it varies with the patient's age and associated diseases. Therefore, in young patients with tissue valves, the risk of thromboembolism is practically nil, whereas in older patients the risk is approximately 2% per year. The same is true for mechanical valves. Atherosclerosis increases the risk of thromboembolic stroke.

The risk of hemorrhage caused by oral anticoagulants varies with international normalized ratio (INR) level and by patient. The recommended level of anticoagulation for mechanical valves in the aortic position is an INR of 2.0 to 3.0. At this level of anticoagulation, the risk of major bleeding is approximately 1% per year. The risk of bleeding increases with a higher INR.

The risk of developing prosthetic infective endocarditis is approximately 0.3% to 1.0% per year. Patients with prosthetic valves need antibiotic prophylaxis when exposed to bacteremia.

Other valve-related problems are bioprosthetic valve failure, prosthetic valve dehiscence, hemolysis, prosthetic valve stenosis due to pannus, or thrombosis. Most of these complications need surgical reintervention.

The long-term results of aortic valve repair with reconstruction of the aortic root have been excellent in experienced centers. Late development of AI is the main problem with these operations. In our experience with more than 200 patients operated on during the past 15 years, the need for reoperation in the aortic valve was only 5% at 10 years. Other valve-related complications were rare among these patients.

SUGGESTED READINGS

Cohen G, David TE, Ivanov J, et al. The impact of age, coronary artery disease, and cardiac comorbidity on late survival after bioprosthetic aortic valve replacement. *J Thorac Cardiovasc Surg.* 1999;117:273–234.

David TE. Surgery of the aortic valve. *Curr Probl Surg.* 1999;36:421–504.

Khan SS, Trento A, DeRobertis M, et al. Twenty-year comparison of tissue and mechanical valve replacement. *J Thorac Cardiovasc Surg.* 2001;122:257–269.

Sioris T, David TE, Ivanov J, et al. Clinical outcomes after separate and composite replacement of the aortic valve and ascending aorta. *J Thorac Cardiovasc Surg.* 2004;128:260–265.

Chapter 26

Surgery of the Mitral Valve

Tirone E. David

ANATOMY OF THE MITRAL VALVE

The mitral valve is a complex structure with the following components: mitral annulus, leaflets, chordae tendineae, papillary muscles, and left ventricular wall. The mitral annulus is an extension of the central fibrous body of the heart from the lateral to the medial fibrous trigones. The posterior leaflet is attached to the posterior wall of the left ventricle and the anterior leaflet is attached to the intervalvular fibrous body that separates the mitral from the aortic valve. The mitral annulus has a sphincterlike function because the posterior leaflet is attached to the basoconstrictor muscles (bulbo and sinospiral muscle bundles). The area of the mitral valve is reduced by approximately 25% during systole. The mitral annulus is circular in late diastole and becomes flatter in systole.

The mitral valve leaflets are a single structure but function as two structures, the anterior and posterior leaflets. The length of the base of the anterior leaflet corresponds to approximately one third of the circumference of the mitral annulus and of the base of the posterior leaflet to the remaining two thirds. The anterior leaflet is narrower and longer than the posterior leaflet, but the areas of the two leaflets are similar.

The areas where the two leaflets join each other are called *commissures*. There are two commissures, an anterior and a posterior. The posterior leaflet also has two false commissures that divide it into three segments: lateral, central, and medial scallops.

The chordae tendineae are extensions of the leaflets that reach the papillary muscles. These extensions originate from the free margins of the leaflets and from the

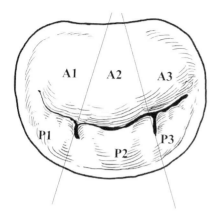

FIGURE 26-1. Carpentier's classification of the various segments of the mitral valve.

ventricular surface. The chordae tendineae in the free margins of the leaflets are primary chordae, those in the ventricular surface of the leaflets are secondary chordae, and chordae that attaches the leaflets to the ventricular wall directly are tertiary chordae.

There are two papillary muscles: anterior and posterior. The anterior papillary muscle anchors the lateral half of the mitral valve and the posterior papillary muscle anchors the medial half. The anterior papillary muscle receives its blood supply from branches of the left anterior descending and circumflex arteries, whereas the posterior papillary muscle has a single blood vessel that comes from the posterolateral branch of the right coronary artery. The papillary muscles are an extension of the ventricular wall.

Figure 26-1 shows a sketch of the atrial view of the mitral valve and its various segments according to Carpentier's classification. Surgeons often use this classification to describe anatomic and functional abnormalities of the mitral valve.

PATHOLOGY OF THE MITRAL VALVE

Rheumatic fever remains a common problem in the third world and in developing countries, and it can cause severe mitral valve dysfunction. During its acute phase, rheumatic fever causes mitral regurgitation (MR) and later may cause mitral stenosis (MS), MR, or both. Fibrosis of all components of the mitral valve is the principal pathologic feature of chronic rheumatic valve disease. The leaflets thicken, the commissures fuse, and the chordae tendineae thicken, fuse, and shorten. The commissures and other parts of the valve may become calcified. The papillary muscles become bulky and hypertrophic. The left atrium is often dilated and the appendage may be filled with clots in cases of MS.

Degenerative diseases of the mitral valve include various entities that range from ruptured chordae tendineae of a grossly normal valve to various degrees of myxomatous degeneration to heavy calcification of the mitral annulus, chordae tendineae, and, sometimes, even the papillary muscle heads. Myxomatous degeneration is the most common form of degenerative disease of the mitral valve. The mitral annulus dilates, the leaflets become voluminous and billowing, and the chordae tendineae may thicken, elongate, or rupture. These abnormalities can cause leaflet prolapse with consequent MR. Mitral valve prolapse is the most common cause of MR in North America.

Distrophic calcification of the mitral annulus may occur in isolation but may also be present in patients with mitral valve disease such as in myxomatous disease and less commonly in rheumatic disease. It occurs more often in older patients, and more often in women than in men.

Ischemic MR is defined as a valve dysfunction caused by coronary artery disease. The leaflets and chordae tendineae are usually normal and the mechanism of MR is based on abnormal ventricular muscle mechanics due to papillary muscle/ventricular wall ischemia or infarction. The MR can be acute or chronic and caused by dysfunction of the ventricular wall or rupture of a papillary muscle head.

Congenital mitral valve disease is far less common than acquired diseases (see Chapter 37).

PATHOPHYSIOLOGY OF MITRAL VALVE DISEASE

Mitral Stenosis

MS is usually caused by rheumatic fever. The normal mitral valve orifice in adults ranges from 4 to 6 cm^2. MS occurs when the mitral valve area is <2 cm^2, and it becomes crucial when the orifice is reduced to 1 cm^2. Reduction in the mitral valve orifice causes a rise in the left atrial pressure, which in turn raises pulmonary venous and capillary pressure with consequent dyspnea. This problem is aggravated by exercise, stress, and atrial fibrillation (AF). The left ventricle is small in size in patients with MS.

Mitral Regurgitation

The pathophysiology of MS is complicated because the regurgitant mitral valve orifice is functionally in competition with the aortic valve orifice. A regurgitant orifice larger than the aortic orifice is not compatible with life. The regurgitant mitral flow depends on the combination of the instantaneous size of the regurgitant orifice and the pressure gradient between the left ventricle and left atrium. MR may be acute or chronic. In acute MR, the left ventricle compensates by emptying more completely, with consequent reduction in wall tension and by increasing preload. As the regurgitant volume becomes chronic, the ventricle dilates, and according to the Laplace principle, wall tension increases to normal and eventually to supranormal levels. Dilation of the left ventricles causes dilation of the mitral annulus with consequent increase in the regurgitant orifice, creating a vicious circle in which "MR begets more MR." The compliance of the left atrium and pulmonary venous bed is an important determinant of hemodynamic and clinical presentation of MR.

NATURAL HISTORY

The onset of symptoms of MS is insidious, and patients tend to modify their activities to minimize them. Most patients are in advanced functional classes when they seek medical assistance, particularly in countries where rheumatic fever is still a major health problem. In the presurgical era, the 5-year survival of patients with MS in the New York Heart Association (NYHA) functional classes III and IV was 62% and 15%, respectively.

The natural history of MR depends on the severity of regurgitant volume, left ventricular function, and the cause of mitral valve dysfunction. Patients with severe MR and impaired ventricular function do not live long whether they are symptomatic or not. Chronic MR due to mitral valve prolapse is usually well tolerated for many years before left ventricular function becomes impaired, but currently most patients are operated on before reaching that point if the valve can be repaired. Ischemic MR has a poor prognosis, and surgery may alter only the symptoms and may have no effect on survival if left ventricular ejection fraction is low.

CLINICAL MANIFESTATIONS AND DIAGNOSIS

The principal symptom of MS is dyspnea. Other symptoms are fatigue, decreased exercise tolerance, hemoptysis, and chest pain. Depending on the stage of the disease, these patients may develop pulmonary hypertension and tricuspid regurgitation with symptoms and signs of venous hypertension such as hepatomegaly, peripheral edema, ascites, and pleural effusion.

Patients with chronic MR remain asymptomatic for a long time, and by the time symptoms become apparent, left ventricular dysfunction may already be present. Decreased exercise tolerance and fatigue are the early symptoms. Acute MR causes pulmonary congestion and dyspnea, and, depending on the severity, it may cause cardiogenic shock.

The diagnosis of mitral valve disease can be made by a careful physical examination and can be confirmed by echocardiography. If the images obtained by a transthoracic echocardiogram are inadequate to establish the diagnosis, a transesophageal echocardiogram (TEE) can be done, which will certainly establish the diagnosis and provide information about the mechanism of valve dysfunction. If surgical treatment is indicated, coronary angiography should be performed in patients older than 45 years to rule out the presence of coronary artery disease.

TREATMENT

Mitral Stenosis

Symptomatic patients experience considerable improvement with diuretics and with restriction of sodium intake. Digitalis glycosides are only valuable in patients with AF. β-Blockers may increase exercise tolerance by reducing heart rate. Patients in AF should be anticoagulated with warfarin sodium to reduce the risk of thromboembolism. Symptomatic patients should be investigated, and if appropriate, percutaneous balloon valvotomy or mitral valve repair should be performed.

The feasibility of mitral valve repair, as well as of percutaneous balloon valvotomy, can usually be determined by preoperative TEE. Stenotic valves with thin and pliable leaflets and chordae tendineae that are at least 1 cm long are usually suitable for percutaneous balloon valvotomy or surgical repair. Surgical repair consists of performing a commissurotomy and maneuvers to increase mobilization of fused chordae tendineae such as chordal resection and papillary muscle splitting.

Stenotic valves with more advanced fibrotic changes are best managed by valve replacement. The valve should be completely excised and a prosthetic valve secured to the mitral annulus. We believe that resuspension of the papillary muscles with 4-0 Gore-Tex sutures reduces the risk of atrioventricular separation after mitral valve replacement, and it may preserve the left ventricular systolic function.

Mitral Regurgitation

Afterload reduction is beneficial in patients with both acute and chronic MR. Afterload reduction with nitroprusside is lifesaving in patients with acute MR and cardiogenic shock. The intra-aortic balloon pump is also of value to stabilize patients for angiography and surgery. The condition of symptomatic patients with chronic MR also improves with afterload reduction using an angiotensin inhibitor or oral hydralazine. The cause of MR should be established and symptomatic patients should be subjected to surgery. If mitral valve repair is feasible, even asymptomatic patients with severe MR should be considered for surgery if they are young and if the operative risk is very low (under 1%). Mitral valve replacement is reserved for patients in NYHA functional classes III and IV in whom repair is not feasible.

The feasibility of mitral valve repair for MR depends on the pathology of the mitral valve and on the surgeon's experience. Although rheumatic MR can be corrected by means of valvuloplasty by performing maneuvers to increase mobility of the leaflets and by means of a ring annuloplasty, the long-term results are suboptimal, and repair should be reserved only for young patients with thin and pliable leaflets. MR due to mitral valve prolapse secondary to ruptured chordae tendineae or myxomatous degeneration is ideal for mitral valve repair. TEE can determine the segment of prolapse, the thickness of the leaflets, and the presence or absence of calcium in the annulus and in other parts of the valve. In experienced hands, mitral valve repair is feasible in >90% of patients. Repair consists of segmental leaflet resection, chordal transfer or chordal replacement with Gore-Tex sutures, edge-to-edge suturing, and ring annuloplasty.

Ischemic MR remains a challenging surgical problem. The pathophysiology is complex and is best studied by TEE in the echo lab. The most common mechanism of MR is tethering of the medial half of the mitral valve because of dysfunction of the posterior papillary muscle and the corresponding ventricular wall. Papillary muscle elongation with consequent prolapse of a segment of the leaflets may also be a cause of MR. A combination of these two main mechanisms is also responsible for the MR. The mitral annulus may also be dilated. Valve repair should be tailored to correct the abnormal pathophysiology. For patients with MR due to tethering of the medial half of the mitral valve, a simple reduction annuloplasty may resolve the problem. Recently, some investigators have proposed severance of the secondary chordae tendineae on the area of the leaflet that is involved by the abnormal tethering combined to annuloplasty. Papillary muscle elongation is corrected by shortening of the muscle and by annuloplasty. If repair is not feasible, mitral valve replacement should be performed, with preservation of the attachments between the mitral annulus and papillary muscles.

PROSTHETIC MITRAL VALVES

If the mitral valve cannot be repaired, replacement with a mechanical or bioprosthetic valve is necessary. Mechanical valves are durable but require lifelong anticoagulation with warfarin sodium. Bioprosthetic valves have limited durability but do not require anticoagulation in patients in sinus rhythm. The durability of bioprosthetic valves in the mitral position is not as good as in the aortic position. Age plays a role in bioprosthetic valve durability—the freedom from failure is approximately 80% in patients older than 65 years and is approximately 60% in younger patients.

The choice of valve is not always simple, and the patient should be consulted before surgery. If a patient is in chronic AF and is already taking warfarin sodium, a mechanical valve may be more appropriate. However, if the patient's expected life span is lower than that of the bioprosthetic valve, the use of a bioprosthesis is justifiable even if the patient is in AF because anticoagulants can be maintained at a lower level with bioprosthesis than be done with mechanical valves. Moreover, there is now an operative procedure to treat AF.

OPERATIVE TECHNIQUES

Mitral Valve Repair for Degenerative Mitral Valve Disease

Prolapse of the central portion of the posterior leaflet (P2 of Carpentier's classification) is the most common cause of MR. It may present in isolation or in combination with prolapse of other segments. P2 often becomes elongated before prolapsing. A quadrangular, rectangular, or triangular resection of the prolapsing segment is performed as illustrated in Figure 26-2. The height of the leaflet is reduced to no more than 1 cm. The margins are approximated with inverting interrupted 4-0 polyester sutures. The leaflet is reattached to the annulus. A mitral annuloplasty is necessary because patients with myxomatous disease have a dilated mitral annulus (see Fig. 26-3). A posterior band suffices in most cases.

Prolapse of the anterior leaflet is corrected by chordal transfer or chordal replacement with Gore-Tex sutures as illustrated in Figure 26-4. Some surgeons use an edge-to-edge repair to correct prolapse of the anterior leaflet (see Fig. 26-5), and this technique is known as the *Alfieri stitch*.

Mitral Valve Replacement

If the posterior leaflet is normal, it should be preserved during mitral valve replacement as shown in Figure 26-6. Preservation of the attachments between the mitral valve and papillary muscles may preserve left ventricular function and prevents spontaneous rupture of the posterior wall of the left ventricle, a rare but dreadful complication of mitral valve replacement. If the leaflets that require mitral valve replacement are excessively diseased, as usually is the case, the valve is completely excised and the papillary muscles are resuspended with Gore-Tex sutures as shown in Figure 26-7.

POSTOPERATIVE CARE

After mitral valve surgery, patients are treated in an intensive care unit (ICU) during the first postoperative day (see ICU care for valve surgery). All patients should be anticoagulated with warfarin sodium if any prosthetic device was placed in the mitral valve

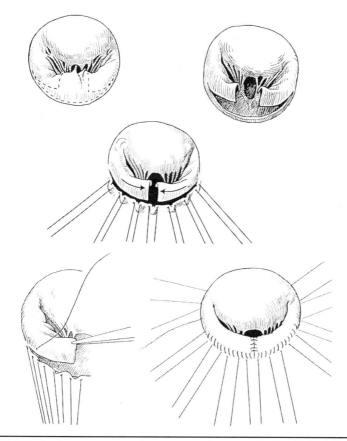

FIGURE 26-2. Mitral valve repair: correction prolapse of posterior leaflet.

(artificial valve or annuloplasty ring/band). The international normalized ratio (INR) should be maintained between 2 and 3 for patients who have had valve repair or bioprosthetic valves and between 2.5 and 3.5 for those who have had mechanical valves. Anticoagulation is discontinued after 3 months in patients who have had valve repair or replacement with bioprosthetic valves if they are in sinus rhythm.

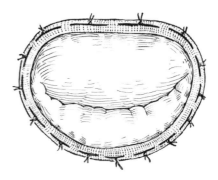

FIGURE 26-3. Mitral valve annuloplasty.

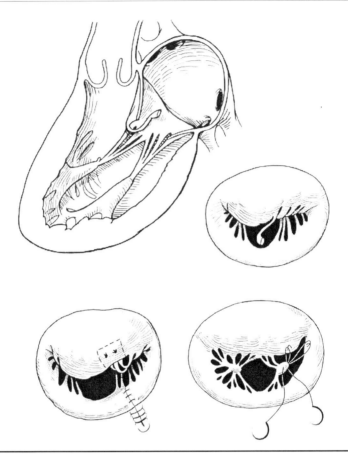

FIGURE 26-4. Mitral valve repair: correction of prolapse of anterior leaflet by chordal transfer or chordal replacement with Gore-Tex sutures.

Diuretic, angiotensin inhibitor, and antidysrhythmic drugs are prescribed as needed.

An echocardiogram should be obtained 1 week postoperatively to assess valve and ventricular function, as well as to rule out pericardial effusion.

CLINICAL OUTCOMES

The operative mortality for isolated mitral valve repair for MS or MR due to rheumatic or degenerative disease is low and is usually approximately 1% at experienced centers. It is slightly higher for ischemic MR or if coronary artery disease is present. The operative mortality for mitral valve replacement depends on the patient's clinical presentation, ventricular function, coronary artery disease, and comorbid conditions. Elective procedures in stable patients can be performed with operative mortality of 3% to 10%, depending on whether it is an isolated problem or is concomitant with other problems such as tricuspid valve repair and coronary artery disease. In the Society of Thoracic Surgeons National Database, the operative mortality for isolated mitral valve replacement is approximately 6%, and combined with coronary artery bypass, it is approximately 12%.

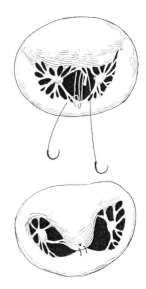

FIGURE 26-5. Mitral valve repair: Alfieri's edge-to-edge repair of leaflet prolapse.

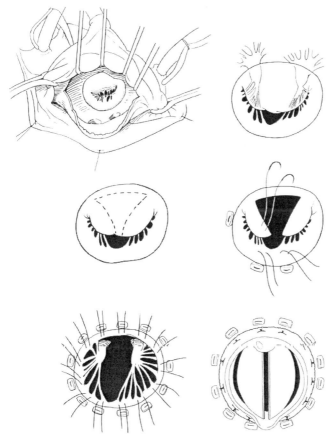

FIGURE 26-6. Mitral valve replacement with preservation of the chordae tendineae.

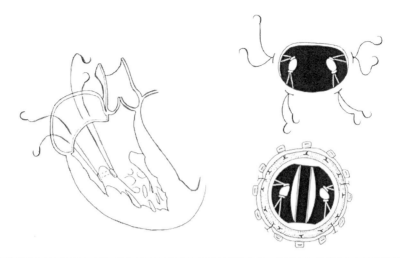

FIGURE 26-7. Mitral valve replacement with resuspension of the papillary muscles with Gore-Tex sutures.

Patients in cardiogenic shock due to acute MR secondary to myocardial infarction have a high operative mortality, and it ranges from 25% to 50% in most reports.

The long-term survival after mitral valve surgery depends on a patient's age, left ventricular function, and coronary artery disease. The 10-year survival after mitral valve repair for degenerative disease is approximately 70% to 80% and after mitral valve replacement for all pathologies is approximately 50%. The long-term survival after mitral valve repair or replacement for rheumatic or degenerative mitral valve disease is much better than for ischemic MR.

Patients who undergo mitral valve surgery must see a cardiologist annually and have a complete physical examination, as well as an electrocardiogram and an echocardiogram. As with all patients with heart valve disease, they are at risk of developing valve-related complications such as endocarditis, thromboembolism, valve dehiscence with MR, valve stenosis due to thrombus or pannus, and valve degeneration in those with bioprosthetic valves.

MAZE PROCEDURE FOR ATRIAL FIBRILLATION

The maze procedure was developed by James Cox to treat AF. The operation evolved over a couple of decades and it is currently performed in isolation to treat patients with lone AF or, more commonly, it is combined with mitral valve surgery in patients with chronic or paroxysmal AF. The original operation is described as "cut and sew" maze whereby a set of incisions is made in both atria and cryolesions in areas that cannot be cut to ablate the atrial tissue to prevent re-entry. Because the pulmonary veins are the most common foci of AF, most surgeons perform the maze only in the left atrium.

Several newer techniques of tissue ablation were introduced into surgery during the last decade as an alternative to the "cut and sew" maze. Radiofrequency is the most commonly used technique for tissue ablation. Other methods are microwave, laser, and ultrasound.

The rate of elimination of AF with the "cut and sew" maze is higher than the other techniques. Most surgeons report at least an 80% freedom of AF at 1 year. The results are better for paroxysmal AF than for permanent AF. The long-term efficacy of newer methods of tissue ablation to perform the maze is presently unknown.

SUGGESTED READINGS

Ad N, Cox JL. Combined mitral valve surgery and the Maze III procedure. *Semin Thorac Cardiovasc Surg.* 2002;14:206–209.

David TE, Ivanov J, Armstrong S, et al. Late outcomes of mitral valve repair for floppy valves: implications for asymptomatic patients. *J Thorac Cardiovasc Surg.* 2003;125:1143–1152.

Gillinov AM, Wierup PN, Blackstone EH, et al. Is repair preferable to replacement for ischemic mitral regurgitation? *J Thorac Cardiovasc Surg.* 2001;122:1125–1141.

Hellgren L, Kvidal P, Horte LG, et al. Survival after mitral valve replacement: rationale for surgery before occurrence of severe symptoms. *Ann Thorac Surg.* 2004;78:1241–1247.

Chapter 27

Tricuspid Valve Surgery

Tirone E. David

ANATOMY

The functional anatomy of the tricuspid valve is complex and is not well understood. This atrioventricular valve has three leaflets: septal, anterior, and posterior. The base of the septal leaflet is attached to the interventricular septum through fibrous strands (annulus), and its free margin is attached directly to the interventricular septum through chordae tendineae. The base of the anterior leaflet is attached to the anterior wall of the right ventricle by a fibrous annulus and its free margin is anchored by chordae tendineae, which are attached mostly to the anterior papillary muscle and in the area adjacent to the septal leaflet, to the septal band of the interventricular septum. The base of the posterior leaflet is attached to the posterior (diaphragmatic) wall of the right ventricle by a fibrous annulus and to the posterior and anterior papillary muscles through chordae tendineae. This anatomic configuration of the three leaflets makes the function of the tricuspid valve more complex than that of the mitral valve. In adults, the orifice of the tricuspid valve is around 8 cm^2 and the perimeter of the annulus is 11 to 14 cm.

PATHOLOGY

Tricuspid regurgitation (TR) due to dilation of the tricuspid annulus is the most common abnormality of this valve. The dilation is asymmetric because of the anatomy of the leaflets, and it involves mostly the commissural area between the anterior and posterior leaflets (see Fig. 27-1). This type of lesion is referred to as "functional TR" because the leaflets and chordae tendineae are usually normal. It is often associated with mitral valve disease and pulmonary hypertension.

Congenital anomalies, rheumatic fever, myxomatous degeneration, endocarditis, ischemia, trauma, and tumors are the usual causes of organic tricuspid valve disease. Rheumatic involvement of the tricuspid valve never occurs in isolation, and it is often

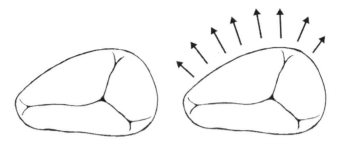

FIGURE 27-1. Functional tricuspid regurgitation is due to dilation of the annulus along the anterior and posterior leaflets.

associated with rheumatic mitral valve disease. It causes fibrosis of the leaflets with fusion of the commissures and with shortening and fibrosis of the chordae tendineae. It usually causes a mixed lesion with stenosis and regurgitation. Myxomatous degeneration causes billowing of the leaflets and elongation of the chordae tendineae, with consequent TR. Endocarditis of the tricuspid valve is usually seen in intravenous drug users. Papillary muscle infarction/rupture is a rare cause of TR. Papillary muscle rupture may also occur as a consequence of trauma. The tricuspid valve may become stenotic and regurgitant in patients with carcinoid syndrome due to fibrosis of the leaflets and chordae tendineae.

PATHOPHYSIOLOGY

TR causes dilation of the right cardiac chambers and eventually impairs right ventricular contractility. Venous hypertension is the hallmark of severe tricuspid valve disease. In addition to damaging the heart, it causes hepatomegaly, peripheral edema, and ascites. If left untreated, cardiac cirrhosis may ensue. Tricuspid stenosis causes venous hypertension and its sequelae.

DIAGNOSIS

Because isolated tricuspid valve disease is rare, symptoms of left-sided heart failure may prevail. However, patients may also complain of peripheral edema, increased abdominal girth, and sensation of fullness, all consequent to venous hypertension. The diagnosis is confirmed by echocardiography. Most patients with tricuspid valve disease also had mitral valve disease and pulmonary hypertension. If surgery is indicated, coronary angiography should be performed in patients older than 45 years.

TREATMENT

Diuretics and restriction of sodium intake are the principal means to reduce peripheral edema and ascites. Patients with severe TR and pulmonary hypertension should be treated surgically. If the TR is functional, tricuspid valve annuloplasty should be done at the time of the left-sided valve operation (e.g., mitral valve surgery). If it is due to rheumatic disease, repair is more difficult and involves mobilization of the leaflets by commissurotomy and chordal resection and by ring annuloplasty. If the leaflets are excessively fibrotic, tricuspid valve replacement is necessary.

Infective endocarditis of the tricuspid valve usually responds to appropriate antibiotic therapy. *Staphylococcus aureus* and fungi are more difficult to eradicate with antibiotics alone and there may also be lung abscesses in these patients. Surgery of the tricuspid valve may be necessary. Repair or replacement is performed depending on how extensive the leaflets destruction is. Valvulectomy alone is not a good alternative in our experience because most patients develop low cardiac output syndrome and ascites.

Isolated TR after trauma is usually well tolerated for many years but right ventricular function must be carefully monitored. Valve repair should be performed before the right ventricle dilates excessively. Once the right ventricle becomes hypokinetic, valve repair does not change the symptoms or prognosis.

Tricuspid Valve Annuloplasty

Functional TR can be corrected by simple reduction of the annulus along the anterior and posterior leaflets, mostly along the commissural area of these two leaflets. There are various commercially available annuloplasty rings, some rigid and others flexible. Sizing of the annuloplasty ring and distribution of the sutures are crucial to correct the deformity caused by dilation. A simple rule is to have an orifice no larger than the area of the anterior leaflet of the tricuspid valve.

The De Vega annuloplasty consists of reducing the length of the annulus of the anterior and posterior leaflets using a double layer of nonabsorbable suture material. We believe that this suture should be buttressed with Teflon pledgets to prevent cutting through the annulus and leaflets in patients with increased right ventricular pressure, as illustrated in Figure 27-2. Annuloplasty rings are believed to provide more stable repairs than the De Vega annuloplasty (see Fig. 27-3).

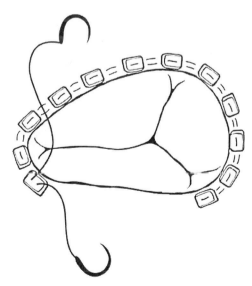

FIGURE 27-2. Modified De Vega annuloplasty.

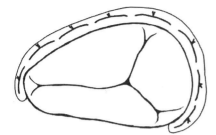

FIGURE 27-3. Annuloplasty with Cosgrove band.

Tricuspid Valve Replacement

Both mechanical or bioprosthetic valves can be used for tricuspid valve replacement. There is no proof that one type of valve is better than the other in the tricuspid position. Both types of valves are associated with more complications in the right side of the circulation than in the left, likely because of the anatomy and blood flow characteristics of the right ventricle. Mechanical valves are associated with risk of valve thrombosis and tissue valve with pannus and stenosis. Permanent epicardial pacemaker leads should be inserted at the time of surgery after tricuspid valve replacement because of the risk of heart block or the future need for an implantable pacemaker.

CLINICAL OUTCOMES

Patients who have had tricuspid valve surgery have a tendency to retain fluids for several months and even years and require diuretic therapy. Mechanical valves in the tricuspid position require higher levels of anticoagulation with warfarin sodium than in the mitral position. The international normalized ratio (INR) should be maintained between 3 and 4.

Tricuspid valve surgery is seldom performed in isolation; it is sometimes done late after correction of mitral and aortic valve lesions, and the operative mortality is usually in the double digits because of the preoperative status of the patients. TR after correction of mitral valve dysfunction is usually managed conservatively for many years, and by the time the patients are referred to surgery, they are in an advanced New York Heart Functional class and the right ventricle is already impaired. For this reason alone, even moderate TR should be corrected at the time of mitral/aortic valve surgery to prevent the development of severe TR and eventual deterioration of right ventricular function. Tricuspid valve repair has no effect on the long-term survival after mitral valve surgery, but if TR is not corrected at the time of the mitral/aortic surgery, it may adversely affect functional class and survival. On the other hand, if the tricuspid valve has to be replaced, long-term survival is reduced.

SUGGESTED READINGS

McCarthy PM, Bhudia SK, Rajeswaran J, et al. Tricuspid valve repair: durability and risk factors for failure. *J Thorac Cardiovasc Surg.* 2004;127:674–685.
Cox J. Surgery of the tricuspid valve. *Op Tech Thorac Cardiovasc Surg.* 2003;4:167–212.

Chapter 28

Robotic Cardiac Valvular Surgery

Alan H. Menkis

Heart surgery is a recent addition to the field of video-assisted or endoscopic surgery. These techniques have been in routine use in gynecology, orthopaedics, and general surgery for more than two decades. The requirement of microsurgical techniques for cardiac surgical procedures such as coronary revascularization necessitated greater dexterity than that afforded by the typical endoscopic hand instruments.

Two devices evolved from the seminal idea that surgery might be performed with the surgeon being at a remote location from the patient so that the possibilities of surgery on distant space missions or in remote locations or in dangerous military situations could be addressed. At the present time, the Intuitive Surgical "da Vinci" device dominates the robotics field. This robotic surgical device has two main components—a surgeon's control console, which has a real-time three-dimensional camera and viewer; and hand controls for the surgeon to manipulate controls that filter and scale the motions. The surgeon views the operative field in a high-resolution three-dimensional image.

INDICATIONS FOR ROBOTIC CARDIAC SURGERY

■ Endoscopic internal thoracic artery harvest for minimally invasive direct coronary bypass (MIDCAB), totally endoscopic coronary artery bypass (TECAB), or multiple vessel small thoracotomy procedures (MVST).
■ Robotic-assisted mitral valve repair.
■ Robotic-assisted atrial septal defect repair.

Only robotic mitral valve repair for nonischemic mitral regurgitation is discussed in this chapter. Earlier referral for mitral valve repair is preferred on an elective basis in asymptomatic or mildly symptomatic patients who have severe mitral regurgitation and a repairable valve.

PATIENT INCLUSION CRITERIA

- Patients with isolated primary mitral valve disease are ideal candidates.
- Most body types are suitable.
- Most adult patients are suitable, including patients older than 70 years.
- Small atrial septal defect or patent foramen ovale may be incidentally repaired and are acceptable findings.

PATIENT EXCLUSION CRITERIA

- Anticipated complex bileaflet repair (relative exclusion criterion).
- Calcified mitral annulus.
- Severe pulmonary hypertension.
- Coronary artery disease.
- Previous right thoracotomy.
- Peripheral vascular disease.
- Other concomitant cardiac conditions requiring sternotomy approach.

SURGICAL TECHNIQUE

Setup

- Transesophageal echocardiography (TEE).
- Single or double lung ventilation.
- Regional block anesthesia strategy (e.g., paravertebral).
- Patient position: right side 30-degree upward position.
- Femoral arterial and venous cannulation; isolated vessels percutaneous style over the wire insertion.
- 3 to 5 cm skin incision on fourth intercostals space.
- Chitwood transthoracic aortic clamp.
- Aortic root cardioplegia to be directed.
- Chest cavity to be filled with carbon dioxide (CO_2).
- Two robotic arm 1- to 2-cm incisions on third and fifth intercostals space triangulated with camera position in working incision.

Valve Repair

Valve repair uses the same techniques as with open repair: partial resection of the posterior leaflet, triangular resection of the anterior, chordal transfer or chordal replacement with Gore-Tex sutures, edge-to-edge repair, and annuloplasty.

General

- Attention should be paid to hemostasis due to small access for possible postoperative bleeding emergencies.
- TEE control should be performed to assess the valve intraoperatively pre- and postrepair and for insertion and placement of femoral arterial and venous catheters.
- Left atrial appendage orifice is oversewn in all cases.
- Temporary right ventricular epicardial pacer wires should be placed before removing cross clamp.

DEVICES CURRENTLY AVAILABLE

- Aesop Robotic Voice Activated Camera Controller (Intuitive Surgical, Mountain View, California).
- Zeus Robotic Surgical Device (Intuitive Surgical, Mountain View, California).
- Da Vinci Robotic Surgical Device (Intuitive Surgical, Mountain View, California).

POSTOPERATIVE CARE

Analgesia

- Preoperative and intraoperative regional block (paravertebral).
- Intraoperative postprocedure intercostal nerve block (two spaces above and below anterior and posterior to the working incision).
- Use of postoperative narcotics as per routine.
- Use of nonsteroidal anti-inflammatory as per routine.

Ventilatory Support

- Early extubation protocol.

Anticoagulation

- Warfarin sodium for 3 months if in sinus rhythm.
- Long-term warfarin sodium if in atrial fibrillation.

OUTCOMES

There have been two multicenter U.S. Food and Drug Administration (FDA) safety efficacy robotic mitral valve trials. The initial trial in 2000 involved 20 patients. These initial studies were characterized by long operative times but good results. There were very few procedure-related complications. Average postoperative length of stay was 4 days, and no patient had more than a trace mitral regurgitation 3 months postoperatively. All were in functional class I after 1 month. The phase II U.S. FDA trial included 112 patients in ten centers. Operative times were shortened, however, nine patients

(8%) had grade II or higher mitral regurgitation and six (5.4%) of these patients had re-operations. There were no deaths, strokes, or major device-related complications. As a result, in November 2002, the U.S. FDA approved the da Vinci system for use in mitral valve surgery.

SUMMARY

Robotic mitral valve surgery has yet to achieve widespread use, primarily because of the capital cost of the robotic device and the lack of perceived advantages for the patient by the surgical community. However, the perception of patients undergoing this procedure is that they have received a superior procedure with less invasiveness. They are more likely to leave the hospital and return to normal activities sooner. The current application of robotics in mitral valve surgery still involves considerable conventional stages and minimally invasive stages to the operation. The technologic advances that are required for further use of robotics and cardiac valvular surgery are occurring at a rapid rate. The increased application of robotics has accompanied the dedication and increasing experience of those involved in this innovative endeavor.

The safety and effectiveness of these procedures remain paramount in this continually advancing field.

SUGGESTED READINGS

Kypson MD, Chitwood R Jr. Robotic mitral valve surgery. *Am J Surg*. 2004;188(Suppl. 4A):83S–88S.
Menkis AH, Kodera K, Kiaii B, et al. Robotic surgery, the first 100 cases. Where do we go from here? *Heart Surg Forum*. 2004;7:1–4.

Surgery of the Ascending Aorta

Tirone E. David

CHRONIC ANEURYSMS OF THE ASCENDING AORTA

The ascending aorta is the segment present between the sinotubular junction of the aortic root and the innominate artery. The wall of the aorta is composed of three layers: intima, media, and adventitia. The intima is a thin layer of ground substance lined by endothelium, and it is easily traumatized. The media is the thickest of the three layers and is made of elastic fibers, which are arranged in spiral fashion to increase the tensile strength. The adventitia is a thin fibrous layer that contains the vasa vasorum, which carries the nutrients to the media. The aorta is very compliant and expands and contracts during the cardiac cycle because of the elastic fibers in the media. Compliance decreases with aging because of fragmentation of the elastic fibers and an increase in the amount of fibrous tissue in the media. Hypertension, hypercholesterolemia, and coronary artery disease cause premature aging of the aorta. Exercise seems to protect the elasticity of the aorta.

Degenerative diseases of the media with aneurysm formation are the most common disorders of the ascending aorta. A broad spectrum of pathologic and clinical entities are grouped under degenerative disorders and include idiopathic ascending aortic aneurysms, which may rupture or may cause aortic dissection to mild dilation of the ascending aorta in elderly patients. Bicuspid and unicusp aortic valve disease are often associated with dilation of the aorta due to premature degenerative changes of the arterial wall. Degenerative aneurysms of the ascending aorta may occur in isolation or may be associated with aortic root aneurysm such as in patients with the Marfan syndrome. It may also be associated with dilation of the transverse arch and descending thoracic aorta, the so-called mega-aorta syndrome. Dilation of the ascending aorta can cause dilation of the sinotubular junction with consequent aortic insufficiency (see Fig. 29-1). Atherosclerosis, infectious and noninfectious aortitis, and trauma are other pathologic entities that cardiac surgeons must be familiar with. Primary tumors of the ascending aorta are rare.

Ascending aortic aneurysms tend to increase in size and eventually rupture or cause aortic dissection. The transverse diameter of the aneurysm is the most important predictor of rupture or dissection. The risk is low in aneurysms with diameters smaller

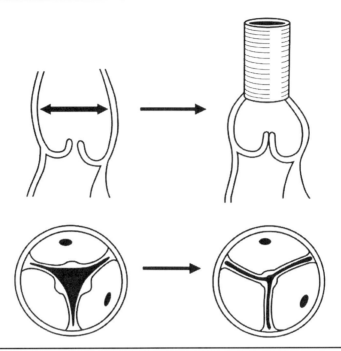

FIGURE 29-1. Replacement of the ascending aorta with correction of aortic insufficiency by reducing the diameter of the sinotubular junction.

than 5 cm. The median size of the ascending aortic aneurysm at the time of rupture or dissection was 5.9 cm.

The growth rates of thoracic aneurysms are exponential. The growth rate ranges from 0.08 cm/year for small aneurysms (<4 cm) to 0.16 cm/year for large (8 cm) aneurysms.

Most patients with ascending aortic aneurysms are asymptomatic, and the aneurysm is usually found during routine chest x-rays, which show widened mediastinum. A massive ascending aortic aneurysm can cause compression of the superior vena cava. If aortic insufficiency is present, there may be cardiac enlargement and the physical findings associated with it. The diagnosis of ascending aortic aneurysm can be confirmed by echocardiography, computerized tomography, magnetic resonance imaging (MRI), and angiography. Magnetic resonance angiography (MRA) has largely replaced contrast angiography.

An ascending aortic aneurysm may cause aortic insufficiency in patients with anatomically normal aortic valve cusps if the sinotubular junction becomes dilated (see Chapter 25).

Surgery is recommended when the transverse diameter of the ascending aorta exceeds 55 mm.

Operative Techniques

Surgery for an ascending aortic aneurysm is performed under cardiopulmonary bypass. Arterial return can be obtained by cannulating the transverse aortic arch, right axillary artery, or femoral artery. Venous drainage is obtained by placing a cannula into the right atrium. Because the aneurysm frequently extends up to the origin of the innominate artery, a brief period of circulatory arrest is necessary to resect the aneurysm and perform the distal anastomosis (see Chapter 30). For this reason, cannulation of the right axillary artery is the ideal site for arterial return because it can provide blood supply to the brain if circulatory arrest is needed while performing distal anastomosis. The proximal anastomosis should be performed at the level of the sinotubular junction. The Dacron graft used to replace the ascending aorta should not be too long or too large. It is important to remember that when the ascending aorta dilates to form an aneurysm, it also becomes elongated. Therefore, during its replacement, the graft should be much shorter than the aneurysm. Actually, a graft of 5 or 6 cm in length is all that is needed to replace the entire ascending aorta from sinotubular junction to origin of the innominate artery. The diameter of the graft should be between 24 to 30 mm, depending on the patient's body surface area. When the diameter of the graft used is larger than the diameter of the sinotubular by more than a couple of millimeters, its caliber should be reduced to that of the sinotubular junction at the level of the anastomosis. This is easily done by plication of that end of the graft. Matching the diameter of the graft to that of the sinotubular junction is important to prevent the development of aortic insufficiency. Conversely, if the patient has aortic insufficiency due to dilation of the sinotubular junction, reduction of its diameter corrects the valve dysfunction (Fig. 29-1).

If the aortic valve is diseased, such as in patients with bicuspid aortic valve, aortic valve replacement and supracoronary replacement of the ascending aorta can be done using either tissue or mechanical valve. If the aortic root is also aneurysmal, aortic root replacement should be performed (see Chapter 25).

Clinical Outcomes

Isolated replacement of the ascending aorta for chronic aneurysm is uncommon. Patients with an ascending aortic aneurysm often have aortic insufficiency or aortic valve disease that may also need surgical attention. Whether the operation is done in isolation or in combination with other procedures, the operative mortality for elective surgery is low. From 1990 to 2001, 79 patients with ascending aortic aneurysm and aortic insufficiency underwent surgery at Toronto General Hospital, and only one patient died perioperatively. During the same period, 133 patients had aortic valve replacement and supracoronary replacement of the ascending aorta and there were seven operative deaths. Both groups included patients with acute type A aortic dissection, reoperations, and patients with active infective endocarditis. Other surgeons report similar operative mortality rates. Age, functional class, and associated diseases play an important role in the operative risk.

Patients who had replacement of the ascending aorta with or without aortic valve surgery must be evaluated annually with echocardiography to assess the size of the retained aortic root if it was not replaced, and the function of the aortic valve. They should also have computerized tomography or MRI of the remaining thoracic and abdominal aorta. Aneurysms of the aortic root, false aneurysms, valve dysfunction, and infections in the graft or aortic valve are problems that may develop and require reoperation.

** *Section III Surgical Technique and Postoperative Consideration*

AORTIC DISSECTIONS

Aortic dissection occurs when blood enters the media of the aortic wall and extends for a variable length creating a false lumen. This false lumen may thrombose or may become permanent with continuous blood flow if it re-enters into the true lumen. Either way, the risk of rupture is high without treatment. Aortic dissections are classified according to their site of the intimal tear and extent of the dissection. In DeBakey type I, the intimal tear is in the ascending aorta and the dissection extends down into the thoracic and abdominal aorta; in type II, the dissection is limited to the ascending aorta; and in type III, the intimal tear is in the proximal descending thoracic aorta. The Stanford classification is used more often than the DeBakey classification. Stanford type A indicates dissection involving the ascending aorta with or without distal dissection, and in type B the dissection is in the descending thoracic aorta. Stanford type B dissections are discussed in more detail in Chapter 31.

Aortic root and/or ascending aortic aneurysm, bicuspid aortic valve, Marfan syndrome, and other connective tissue disorders are predisposing factors to type A aortic dissection. This type of dissection occurs at least twice more often in men than in women, and it may affect individuals of all ages, but the peak incidence is between 50 and 55 years of age. The prognosis for untreated aortic dissections is very poor. Collective autopsy data indicated that 50% of patients die within 48 hours, 84% within 1 month, and 90% within 3 months. For this reason, prompt diagnosis and immediate therapy is necessary to save these patients. Transesophageal echocardiography (TEE) has become the diagnostic tool of choice in patients with suspected aortic dissection. It is particularly useful in patients with type A aortic dissection because it can also give information about the aortic root and aortic valve function. Other useful diagnostic tools are computerized tomography, MRI, and angiography. These techniques are usually time consuming and should be used only when TEE is not diagnostic. If feasible, coronary angiography should be performed in patients with history of angina pectoris or myocardial infarction.

Patients with type A aortic dissection are best treated with immediate surgery. Cardiopulmonary bypass through the right axillary artery and right atrium is probably the best approach in these patients. Hypothermia and circulatory arrest should be employed to make sure there is no intimal tear in the transverse aortic arch or, if there is, the arch should be replaced with a Dacron graft. The aortic root can be preserved if normal, or it can be repaired or replaced if it has an aneurysm. Aortic valve–sparing operations are ideally suited for patients with type A aortic dissection and dilated aortic root because they remove all dissected tissues from the aortic root. If the aortic cusps are abnormal, aortic root replacement with a mechanical or tissue valve is performed.

The operative mortality for surgery for type A aortic dissection varies widely with the surgeon's experience and the timing of the operation. Experienced centers report operative mortality of 10% to 25%. Continued surveillance of the persistent false lumen and the aortic anastomoses is imperative in these patients. Therefore, TEE, and computed tomography or MRI, at 6 months postoperatively, and then annually, is necessary. Also, because many patients have systemic hypertension, it is imperative that the blood pressure is well controlled. β-Blockers are useful in patients with aortic dissections. Many patients will require reoperation in the aortic root for aortic insufficiency if the native valve was preserved. Others will require reoperations because of expansion of the false lumen of the dissected thoracic and abdominal aorta. The actuarial survival including operative mortality is around 50% to 60% at 10 years.

SUGGESTED READINGS

David TE, Armstrong S, Ivanov J, et al. Surgery for acute type A aortic dissection. *Ann Thorac Surg.* 1999;67:1999–2001.

David TE, Ivanov J, Armstrong S, et al. Aortic valve sparing operations in patients with aneurysms of the aortic root or ascending aorta. *Ann Thorac Surg.* 2002;74:S1758–S1761.

Lai DT, Miller DC, Mitchell RS, et al. Acute type A aortic dissection complicated by aortic regurgitation: composite valve graft versus separated valve graft versus conservative valve repair. *J Thorac Cardiovasc Surg.* 2003;126:1978–1986.

Sioris T, David TE, Ivanov J, et al. Clinical outcomes after separate and composite replacement of the aortic valve and ascending aorta. *J Thorac Cardiovasc Surg.* 2004;128:260–265.

Chapter 30

Surgery of the Transverse Aortic Arch and Cerebral Protection

Christopher M. Feindel

Operations on the distal ascending aorta and transverse aortic arch require temporary interruption of the blood supply to the brain. At normal body temperature, the human brain rapidly ceases to function within seconds of losing its blood supply, and, after 3 to 4 minutes without blood flow, permanent damage will likely occur. Because even the simplest operations cannot be performed within this time, a variety of methods have been developed over the years that allow surgeons to safely interrupt the cerebral blood supply for longer than 3 to 4 minutes to repair the distal ascending aorta and/or the aortic arch. However, all these methods have limitations, and cerebral injury, whether it is temporary or permanent, continues to be the most serious potential complication following surgery of the ascending aorta and transverse aortic arch. In addition to cerebral injury that can result from the interruption of cerebral blood flow (CBF), neurologic complications may also result from embolization of air and/or atherosclerotic debris into the cerebral vessels from a diseased aorta.

INDICATIONS FOR SURGERY

The two main indications for operating on the distal ascending aorta and transverse aortic arch include:

- Aortic aneurysms.
- Aortic dissection.

These surgeries include:

- Replacement of the ascending aorta including its junction with the proximal transverse aortic arch.
- Replacement of the ascending aorta and the inferior portion of the transverse aortic arch ("hemiarch" replacement).
- Replacement of the entire transverse aortic arch including the proximal portion of the descending thoracic aorta (in this case the arch vessels are reimplanted either individually or inclusively as a single island of aorta).

In all the above procedures, the surgeon must interrupt the circulation to the brain to allow an unobstructed view of the operative field. At systemic temperatures of <20°C, the brain can withstand approximately 30 minutes of circulatory arrest. This technique, known as *deep hypothermic circulatory arrest* (HCA), allows the surgeon enough time to complete the anastomosis of a graft to the distal part of the ascending aorta or the proximal part of the aortic arch, following which circulation can be re-established. However, longer periods are required for more complex operations involving the mid and distal transverse arch, especially for operations that involve the proximal descending aorta. Additional measures must be taken if irreversible brain damage is to be avoided. These include retrograde cerebral perfusion of the brain through the superior vena cava, as well as various methods of antegrade perfusion, which can be achieved either through the axillary artery or through one or more of the brachiocephalic arteries. Each of these will be described separately, although surgeons often will use a combination of these techniques depending on specific circumstances.

DEEP HYPOTHERMIA AND CIRCULATORY ARREST

Deep hypothermia is the mainstay of any operation that requires opening the distal ascending aorta or transverse aortic arch where blood flow to the brain must be interrupted. Although there may be controversy about the best method of cerebral perfusion during surgeries that involve the aortic arch, deep hypothermia alone will usually provide the surgeon with a safe arrest period of 30 minutes, provided the patient's brain is cooled to <20°C.

The technique of deep hypothermia and circulatory arrest is relatively straightforward and is easily implemented by any experienced cardiac surgeon. However, because these operations are not performed frequently in most centers, it is incumbent on the surgeon to first review exactly what is being planned with the other members of the operating room team. Excellent communication, attention to detail, and timing are vital. All necessary items such as tubing and cannulae should be organized ahead of time because time should not be wasted in searching for a crucial item during the actual period of circulatory arrest.

The specific circumstances of the patient will determine the location of the cannulation site for arterial inflow. The ascending aorta, aortic arch, and axillary or femoral artery in all possible sites and specific circumstances will determine the optimal site. In cases of aortic dissection, either the femoral or axillary artery must be used because the ascending aorta cannot be safely cannulated. Venous drainage is preferred by the right atrium but, if necessary, can also be achieved using the femoral vein or veins.

Cardiopulmonary bypass (CPB) is started and the patient is cooled to 18°C to 25°C depending on the anticipated duration of circulatory arrest. A correctly positioned nasopharyngeal temperature probe records the temperature. A rectal probe can be used; however, proper positioning tends to render these readings unreliable. If available, a bladder catheter with a temperature sensor is very useful. As the body temperature of the patient decreases, the heart will spontaneously fibrillate. At this time, a left ventricular sump is inserted through the right superior pulmonary vein to decompress the left ventricle. If the patient has an incompetent aortic valve, as may be the case in an aortic dissection, manual compression of the distending heart may be necessary at this time.

Once the patient's systemic temperature has been lowered to the desired level, CPB is stopped and venous blood is drained. The patient is positioned head down and the left ventricular sump is temporarily turned off. The ascending aorta is opened and the pathology inspected. A determination is then made as to what operation will be necessary and, more importantly, what will be the estimated arrest time required. For relatively short periods of arrest (i.e., <30 minutes), no additional measures are necessary, although many surgeons will start retrograde cerebral perfusion through the vena cava (see subsequent text). For longer periods of arrest, other measures involving some form of antegrade perfusion (see subsequent text) will need to be implemented in order to avoid brain damage. During the period of circulatory arrest, the anesthesiologist should encase the patient's head in ice packs in order to promote cerebral cooling. In addition, steroids may be given to help reduce cerebral edema, although there is little evidence that steroids are beneficial. Because the brain is far more sensitive to ischemia than the heart, valuable time should not be wasted in giving cardioplegia at this time.

In cases where only the distal ascending aorta or proximal aortic arch is being replaced, HCA provides enough time to complete the distal anastomosis. Once this is done, the arterial inflow cannula, if in the femoral artery, is re-positioned into the new graft. This is a very important step, especially in cases of aortic dissection where the possibility of a re-entry site exists in the descending aorta. There is no need to reposition the arterial cannula if the axillary artery was used. The pump is turned on slowly to de-air the graft and aortic arch. The open end of the graft is then clamped, and full antegrade pump flow is re-established. The patient is rewarmed, during which time the proximal end of the graft is connected to the proximal ascending aorta and any other necessary procedures in the aortic root are performed (e.g., aortic valve replacement, root replacement, and/or coronary artery bypasses). Cardioplegia is given at this time.

RETROGRADE CEREBRAL PERFUSION

Retrograde cerebral perfusion has been introduced as an adjunct to cerebral cooling as a means to protect the brain during periods of circulatory arrest. Although current evidence suggests that retrograde cerebral perfusion probably does not adequately perfuse the brain, it does have the advantage of washing out air and/or atherosclerotic debris that may have embolized to the arch vessels. Therefore, many surgeons use it even if the period of circulatory arrest is relatively short (i.e., 10 to 20 minutes). In this technique, the patient's body and brain temperature are cooled to 18°C to 20°C by CPB, as described in the previous text. After the heart-lung machine is turned off, a cannula (either the arterial cannula or a separate cannula) is placed directly into the superior vena cava. Blood, at 10°C, is then perfused in a retrograde manner at a rate of 300 to 500 mL/minute. With the observation of dark blood emanating from the origins of the cerebral vessels in the aortic arch, the surgeon confirms the presence of retrograde flow.

DEEP HYPOTHERMIA WITH ANTEGRADE CEREBRAL PERFUSION

Recent evidence suggests that the brain may be injured if the period of circulatory arrest extends beyond 30 minutes, even at temperatures <20°C. Therefore, there is renewed interest in methods to restore antegrade cerebral perfusion during operations on the aortic arch. Perfusion can be maintained through the axillary artery or directly into the aortic arch vessels.

Axillary Artery Perfusion

Although axillary artery cannulation is more difficult and time consuming than femoral cannulation, it offers a relatively easy way to maintain cerebral flow while operating on the aortic arch. While cooling the patient, the arch vessels and the innominate vein are carefully dissected. After shutting off the circulation and opening the aortic arch, the origin of the cerebral vessels is examined for loose debris and/or disease. If they are relatively clear, then all three arch vessels are gently clamped and antegrade perfusion is restarted through the axillary artery, taking care to de-air these vessels. Deep hypothermia is still maintained, as it is often necessary to shut off the circulation in order to avoid flooding the surgical field, especially in cases where a graft must be sewn deep in the chest to the proximal descending aorta.

Direct Aortic Arch Vessel Perfusion

If axillary artery cannulation is not possible, surgery of the transverse aortic arch must be planned to allow for early re-establishment of cerebral perfusion. Rather than performing the distal anastomosis to the proximal descending aorta as the initial step under circulatory arrest, a separate graft is first attached to the island of aorta that includes the arch vessels. Once completed, this graft is cannulated and cerebral perfusion re-established by the arch vessels, whereas a separate graft is sewn to the proximal descending aorta. Then, under another period of circulatory arrest, the arch graft is connected to the side of the graft going to the proximal descending aorta graft. Perfusion is again restarted and the proximal part of this composite graft is connected to the aortic root.

COAGULATION DEFECTS

Patients who undergo a period of circulatory arrest frequently experience considerable coagulation defects. Although these defects may be reduced by the use of aprotinin, the surgeon and the anesthesiologist should be prepared to use blood products. It is much better to give these early after coming off bypass, rather than after a prolonged period of attempting to control nonsurgical bleeding.

PHARMACEUTICAL AND OTHER NEUROPROTECTIVE ADJUNCTS

There is little clinical evidence of effective pharmacotherapy to limit the extent of neurologic injury resulting from HCA. However, there is a considerable amount of data to suggest that appropriate CPB management may help to minimize the negative neurologic and cognitive outcomes after cardiac surgery.

Acid-Base Control

The alpha stat (α-stat) method allows drift of blood pH toward more alkaline values as the patient's temperature drops. The α-stat method preserves cerebral autoregulation, resulting in reducing CBF at a lower temperature. The pH-stat method involves elevating and maintaining PCO_2 at 40 mm Hg to compensate for reduced activity of $[H^+]$ ion at lower temperatures. However, with the pH-stat method, cerebral autoregulation is lost and this results in a passive increase or decrease of cerebral flow in response to perfusion pressure changes. Clinical studies suggest that patients undergoing coronary artery bypass grafting (CABG) surgery have better neurologic and cognitive outcomes when α-stat of blood pH control is used compared to the pH-stat method. Therefore, α-stat is preferred for adult patients undergoing profound hypothermia and circulatory arrest.

Glucose Control

In the setting of global or focal brain ischemia, severe hyperglycemia has been demonstrated to be harmful and, during global ischemia, will exacerbate metabolic acidosis of the brain. It is not known what levels of glucose are acceptable, but it is important to treat hyperglycemia, particularly if it occurs before circulatory arrest.

TEMPERATURE MONITORING DURING THE REWARMING PHASE

Even short periods of perfusing the brain at temperatures >40°C to 41°C may result in cerebral injury, particularly if subjected to previous ischemic insult. Therefore, it is important to limit the rate of systemic rewarming in order to avoid cerebral hyperthermia. A small but important technical point is that blood temperature may exceed the measured nasopharyngeal temperature by as much as 3°C during the rewarming phase.

SUMMARY

Surgery of the transverse aortic arch presents numerous challenges for the cardiac surgeon and to the operative team. Attention to details is critical; however, with today's technical advances the opportunity for a successful outcome for the patient is relatively good.

SUGGESTED READINGS

Bachet J, Guilmet D, Goudout B, et al. Antegrade cerebral perfusion in operations on the proximal thoracic aorta. *Ann Thorac Surg.* 1999;67:1874–1878.

Hagl C, Ergin MA, Galla JD, et al. Neurological outcome after ascending aortic-aortic arch operations: effect of brain protection technique in high risk patients. *J Thorac Cardiovasc Surg.* 2001;121:1107–1121.

Kuroda Y, Uchimoto R, Kaieda R, et al. Central nervous system complications after cardiac surgery: a comparison between coronary artery bypass grafting and valve surgery. *Anaesth Analg.* 1993;76:222–227.

McCullough JN, Zhang N, Reich DL, et al. Cerebral metabolic suppression during hypothermic circulatory arrest in humans. *Ann Thorac Surg.* 1999;67:1895–1899.

Moshkovitz Y, David TE, Caleb M, et al. Cold retrograde cerebral perfusion with moderate systemic hypothermia: an alternative strategy during circulatory arrest. *Ann Thorac Surg.* 1998;66:1179–1184.

Murkin JM, Martzke JS, Buchan AM, et al. A randomized study of the influence of perfusion technique and pH management strategy in 316 patients undergoing coronary artery bypass surgery: II. Neurological and cognitive outcomes. *J Thorac Cardiovasc Surg.* 1995;110:349–362.

Strauch JT, Spielvogel D, Lauten A, et al. Technical advances in total aortic arch replacement. *Ann Thorac Surg.* 2004;77(2):581–589; discussion 589–590.

Wareing TH, Davila-Roman VG, Barzilai B, et al. Management of the severely atherosclerotic ascending aorta during cardiac operations. A strategy for detection and treatment. *J Thorac Cardiovasc Surg.* 1992;103:453–462.

Chapter 31

Surgery of the Descending Thoracic Aorta

Steve K. Singh and Michael A. Borger

INTRODUCTION

The descending thoracic aorta begins distal to the left subclavian artery and ends at the diaphragm. The pathology involving this area includes aneurysm, dissection, atherosclerotic ulcers, intramural hematoma (IMH), and traumatic injury. This chapter briefly outlines the etiology, pathophysiology, and natural history of each condition. The primary diagnostic modalities and principles of management are described. Lastly, clinical outcomes of the respective conditions are summarized.

Descending Thoracic Aortic Aneurysm

Aortic aneurysms are abnormal dilatations of the aorta. The incidence of descending thoracic aortic aneurysms (TAAs) is approximately 5 per 1,000 persons. Although associated with aneurysms, atherosclerosis is not a direct cause of aneurysm formation and growth. There is evidence suggesting a genetic predilection. Other risk factors include hypertension, chronic obstructive lung disease, chronic aortic dissection, and infections of the aortic wall.

Patients are usually asymptomatic but may present with signs and symptoms secondary to compression of surrounding structures. Hoarseness, stridor, dyspnea, dysphagia, and plethora may occur because of encroachment upon the left recurrent laryngeal nerve, trachea, esophagus, and superior vena cava. The natural history varies with the rate of growth. The risk of rupture is 16% at a diameter of 6 cm and is 31% at 7 cm.

Descending Thoracic Aortic Dissection

Aortic dissection is when an intimal disruption results in the entry of blood into the outer two thirds of the aortic media. When the intimal tear occurs in the descending aorta, it is classified as Stanford type B dissection. The prevalence is approximately 0.5% and affects men more than women. Hypertension is the most important risk factor. Connective tissue disorders (e.g., Ehlers-Danlos, Marfan syndrome), bicuspid aortic valve, aortic coarctation, pregnancy, and surgical manipulation of the aorta are also risk factors. The culprit intimal tear usually occurs just distal to the ligamentum arteriosum, the greatest point of hemodynamic stress.

If untreated, visceral and peripheral tissue malperfusion may occur. Aneurysmal dilation and rupture are late complications.

Penetrating Atherosclerotic Ulcer

A penetrating atherosclerotic ulcer (PAU) is most often found in the distal descending thoracic aorta. Large atherosclerotic plaques penetrate through the intima into the media. A hematoma subsequently develops within the wall of the aorta. Clinical presentation of PAU is similar to that of classic aortic dissection. The natural history is less well understood but the ulcer is thought to have a slow progression. PAU is associated with a low incidence of acute rupture. If left untreated, PAU may result in pseudoaneurysm and intramural thrombus formation.

Intramural Hematoma

IMH is thought to be the result of rupture of the vasa vasorum within the wall of the aorta. This leads to aortic wall disintegration and hematoma formation. The absence of an intimal tear is what distinguishes IMH from PAU. Regional thickening of the aortic wall with the absence of an intimal flap and no enhancement after contrast injection is considered diagnostic of IMH. Anecdotally, one third of IMHs enlarge and rupture, one third have no change in size and do not rupture, and one third regress with no sequelae.

Traumatic Injury of the Descending Thoracic Aorta

Traumatic injury of the aorta is infrequent but devastating, accounting for 10% to 25% of motor vehicle fatalities. More than 90% of cases occur just distal to the ligamentum arteriosum, secondary to acceleration–deceleration injury. Mid-descending thoracic aortic trauma is uncommon, usually caused by compression over the spine.

Immediate death occurs in 80% of victims. Of those who survive, 25% die in the first 24 hours, 40% die in the first 4 days, and the remaining have a 2% per year risk of late rupture secondary to pseudoaneurysm formation.

DIAGNOSIS

Numerous chest x-ray findings have been described but are nonspecific. Computerized tomography (CT) and magnetic resonance imaging (MRI) have now replaced aortography as the diagnostic tests of choice. Echocardiography and intravascular ultrasound may be helpful.

Aortography is able to provide information about intimal tears, dissection, and aneurysm location, greatly aiding operative strategy. The disadvantages include lack of detail about surrounding structures and contrast-induced renal failure or allergic reaction.

CT scan requires radiation exposure and nephrotoxic contrast material, but is more available than MRI. MRI is the imaging method of choice for the descending aorta; it can accurately identify false lumen entries and can distinguish false lumen thrombus from periaortic hematoma.

Transesophageal echocardiography (TEE) allows precise imaging of aortic wall pathology and flow between true lumen and other areas of interest while supplying valuable cardiac information. The disadvantages of TEE are requirement of sedation, limited availability, and operator dependence.

INDICATIONS FOR SURGERY

For patients with aneurysms of a degenerative or chronic nature, elective resection is advised when the diameter is >5.5 cm, or if symptoms are present. Repeated distal embolism from atherosclerosis or thrombus is an uncommon indication.

For acute type B dissections, surgery is indicated for signs of impending rupture (i.e., persisting pain, hypotension, and left-sided hemothorax), malperfusion (i.e., peripheral or visceral ischemia, renal failure, paraparesis, or paraplegia), and failure of medical management.

For chronic dissection, elective surgery is recommended when the diameter is >5.5 cm or when symptoms are present.

PAU and IMH of the descending thoracic aorta are primarily treated with medical therapy. Indications for surgery are identical to those for acute type B dissection or the development of pseudoaneurysm >5.5 cm.

TREATMENT

Medical Management

Patients with acute descending thoracic aortic conditions should be admitted to the intensive care unit (ICU) for invasive blood pressure monitoring and to monitor end-organ function. Pharmacologic therapy aims to minimize shear forces against the aortic wall by lowering systolic blood pressure and by minimizing the rate of rise of aortic pressure. Target systolic blood pressure is 90 to 110 mm Hg. Short-acting intravenous β-adrenergic blockers and sodium nitroprusside are used. β-Blockers should be provided before giving nitroprusside to avoid reflex tachycardia. Patients who do not undergo surgery should have repeat imaging studies periodically.

Surgical Treatment

The principle of surgical management is to excise the diseased segment of the descending aorta and restore flow in the true lumen and relevant branches. Various surgical approaches and methods of circulatory support can be performed. The standard approach is to use partial left heart bypass with moderate systemic hypothermia (30°C). Arterial cannulation is performed in the distal thoracic aorta for operations on the proximal descending aorta or in the femoral artery for operations extending into the abdomen. Venous cannulation is through the left inferior pulmonary vein or the left atrial appendage.

A left posterolateral thoracotomy is performed with single-lung ventilation. The minimal amount of aorta is excised in order to preserve intercostal arterial supply of the spinal cord, to circumvent paraplegia. Paraplegia occurs in 2% to 19% of cases.

After commencing circulatory bypass, the aortic arch is usually clamped between the left common carotid and the left subclavian arteries. If proximal disease precludes cross clamping, deep hypothermic circulatory arrest is required. The aorta is transected distal to the left subclavian arteries and a collagen-impregnated Dacron graft is anastomosed to it. The occluding clamp is then removed and placed on the graft. The distal descending thoracic aorta is opened longitudinally. Back bleeding from branches are controlled and reattached to the aortic graft, if necessary. The clamp is sequentially moved down the graft as each branch is reattached, allowing early spinal perfusion. The distal anastamosis is done last and the cross clamp is then removed.

The incidence of spinal cord ischemia varies with surgical techniques. Left heart bypass with hypothermia provides the lowest incidence of paraplegia (2%). Alternative techniques such as complete bypass, heparinized shunts, and the "clamp and sew" technique are associated with a higher incidence of paraplegia (3%, 11%, and 19%, respectively). The latter technique ("clamp and sew" technique) is most detrimental when ischemic time exceeds 30 minutes. Use of moderate hypothermia, drainage of cerebrospinal fluid, regional spinal cooling by epidural, preoperative identification of the anterior spinal artery, and pharmacologic agents such as steroids may also lower the risk of spinal cord injury.

Endovascular Therapy

Patients who are unfit for surgery, owing to comorbidity and age, are candidates for endovascular therapy. Intraluminal stenting minimizes surgical trauma and physiologic stress in such patients.

PAU is ideal for endovascular stenting because the tissue is often poor quality for suturing, and surgical manipulation carries high risk of distal embolic events. Stenting may also be used for type B aortic dissection because of decreased incidence of malperfusion and improved recovery. Stenting is not indicated for IMH because there is no primary intimal defect.

Technical limitations for stenting include the requirement of radiographic guidance, a minimum of 2 cm of normal proximal and distal aorta for adequate fixation, and a large peripheral vessel for insertion. Their most common complication is stent leak.

OUTCOMES

Descending Thoracic Aortic Aneurysm

Long-term survival in an untreated descending TAA is 80% at 1 year and 40% at 5 years. Survival after elective surgical repair is 90% at 30 days and 60% at 5 years. Major morbidity consists of paraplegia, paraparesis, and acute renal failure. Hemodialysis is required in 5% of previously healthy individuals and 17% of patients with preoperative renal dysfunction.

Descending Thoracic Aortic Dissection

Actuarial survival for all patients with type B dissections is 65% at 1 year and 50% at 5 years. Medically managed patients have a survival of 73% at 1 year and 58% at 5 years. Patients requiring surgery for failed medical management have survival rates of 47% at 1 year and 28% at 5 years.

Penetrating Atherosclerotic Ulcer and Intramural Hematoma

Evidence in the literature on long-term survival with or without surgery is lacking for descending thoracic aorta PAU and IMH.

Traumatic Injury of the Descending Thoracic Aorta

These patients have high complication rates such as paraplegia, sepsis, renal failure, hemorrhage, and acute respiratory distress syndrome. If patients survive the *initial* events, their long-term outcomes are favorable.

SUGGESTED READINGS

Cohn LH, Edmunds LH Jr, eds. *Cardiac surgery in the adult.* New York: McGraw-Hill; 2003.
Kouchoukos NT, Dugenis D. Surgery of the thoracic aorta. *N Engl J Med.* 1997;336:1876–1887.
Tatou E, Steinmetz E, Jazveri S, et al. Surgical outcomes of traumatic rupture of the thoracic aorta. *Ann Thorac Surg.* 2000;69:70–73.
Vignon P, Gueret P, Vedrinne J, et al. Role of transesophageal echocardiography in the diagnosis and management of traumatic aortic disruption. *Circulation.* 1995;92:2959–2968.

Combined Cardiac and Vascular Surgery

Michael A. Borger

COMBINED CARDIAC AND CAROTID ARTERY SURGERY

Patients may present for surgery with both major cerebrovascular and cardiac disease. The incidence of major coronary disease in patients with symptomatic carotid stenosis is 25% to 30%. The incidence of major carotid stenosis in patients undergoing coronary artery bypass grafting (CABG) is 6% to 10%. Only when the indications for both procedures are present should a combined procedure be considered. The primary reason for simultaneous procedures is to prevent a perioperative stroke and/or perioperative myocardial infarction (MI). The surgical approaches for patients undergoing CABG and carotid endarterectomy (CEA) include the combined technique (both procedures performed under one anesthetic), the staged approach (CEA before CABG under separate anesthetics), and the reverse-staged technique (CABG before CEA under separate anesthetics). The coronary bypass portion of the procedure may also be performed using off-pump techniques, but hypotension secondary to heart positioning should be aggressively avoided. Another option that may become increasingly common in the future is CABG plus carotid stenting with filters.

Diagnosis of Carotid Disease

- Symptoms: transient ischemic attack (TIA), reversible ischemic neurologic deficit (RIND), previous stroke.
- Physical examination: neck bruit.

- Noninvasive testing:
  - Duplex scanning combines Doppler scanning and ultrasonography, and is the preferred method.
  - Magnetic resonance angiography (MRA).
  - Computerized tomography (CT) angiography.
  - CT scan or magnetic resonance imaging (MRI) of the brain should be performed if there is a history of stroke.
- Invasive testing:
  - Carotid angiography should be performed when there is concern about the distal vessels or disease in the aortic arch.

Indications for Carotid Endarterectomy

- Symptomatic carotid stenosis—previous TIA or stroke with severe (70% to 99%) stenosis of the ipsilateral internal carotid artery; symptomatic moderate (50% to 69%) stenosis in very low risk patients.
- Asymptomatic carotid stenosis—very controversial. The Asymptomatic Carotid Artherosclerosis Study (ACAS) and the Asymptomatic Carotid Surgery Trial (ACST) revealed that patients with severe asymptomatic carotid stenosis receive a modest benefit from CEA. However, these trials excluded patients with significant cardiac disease, and the benefit of CEA was lost when perioperative stroke and/or mortality rates exceeded 3%. Such a low perioperative stroke and mortality rate is difficult to achieve in patients undergoing combined CEA and CABG. Our practice has therefore been to perform a combined procedure only in patients with severe bilateral asymptomatic disease (e.g., complete occlusion of one carotid artery and >80% stenosis of the other carotid artery).

Operative Techniques

- Simultaneous exposure of the heart and carotid artery.
- Performance of CEA while harvesting the saphenous vein.
- Optional use of carotid shunt while performing CEA.
- Saphenous vein patch of the endarterectomized carotid artery, particularly if it is not large in caliber.
- Proceeding with CABG.
- Maintenance of elevated perfusion pressures (>70 mm Hg) during cardiopulmonary bypass (CPB), with mild to moderate hypothermia (28°C to 34°C).
- Avoidance of close neck incision until patient has received protamine.

The CEA can also be performed during CPB, but this has not been our practice. Moderate or deep hypothermia during CEA may provide additional cerebral protection but will increase the length of the procedure, CPB times, and the risk of coagulopathy.

Intraoperative Concerns

Most strokes that occur during CABG are secondary to ascending aortic atherosclerosis and not to carotid vascular disease. Patients with carotid disease are at particularly high risk for ascending aortic atherosclerosis, and, therefore, epiaortic scanning should be performed in such patients. If major disease is present, consider cannulation of the aortic arch beyond the origin of the carotid artery to minimize cerebral embolization or cannulation of the innominate artery if it is free of disease. Also consider off-pump coronary bypass with *in situ* arterial grafts or with automated proximal anastomotic devices.

Postoperative Care

Maintain adequate perfusion pressure, oxygenation, and cardiac output. Watch for bleeding/hematoma in the neck incision. Reintubate the patient immediately if an expanding neck hematoma is present.

Attempt to wake the patient early after arrival in the intensive care unit (ICU) to assess neurologic status. After awakening with or without extubation the patient may be:

1. Awake and oriented: routine postoperative management.
2. Confused without localizing signs: rule out other causes for confusion and consider imaging with Doppler if concerned about patency of carotid artery.
3. Hemiplegic or hemiparetic: return to the operating room (OR) urgently for angiogram and possible re-exploration of the carotid artery.

Outcomes

The morbidity and mortality rates for combined CABG and CEA are much higher than that for isolated CABG. A meta-analysis revealed that the incidence of stroke during combined surgery is 6%, the incidence of MI is 5%, and the mortality rate is 5%. Outcomes were better in patients who underwent staged CABG/CEA, and we therefore attempt staged procedures whenever possible.

Long-term outcomes are also considerably worse than for isolated CABG. Ten-year survival is 50% to 60%, and freedom from any adverse event (e.g., death, stroke, or cardiac event) is approximately 40%.

COMBINED CARDIAC AND ABDOMINAL AORTIC SURGERY

Patients with symptomatic coronary disease may have a large (>5 cm) abdominal aortic aneurysm (AAA), which is usually asymptomatic. The incidence of AAA in routine patients with CABG is <5%, but increases to 10% to 20% in patients with aneurysms of the ascending aorta. Patients with symptomatic abdominal aneurysm disease often have subclinical coronary disease, with an incidence of approximately 50%. However, symptomatic AAAs (i.e., rupture or threatened rupture) usually require emergent treatment before coronary anatomy can be delineated. Simultaneous CABG and AAA repair is therefore an uncommon procedure but may be considered in select patients.

A potential advantage of combined CABG/AAA is the ability to scavenge shed blood while the aneurysm is being repaired. It is also possible to put the abdominal aortic clamp in place with very little pressure on the aorta simply by temporarily decreasing CPB flow. Performing the aortic procedure during CPB support also avoids the increases in left ventricular afterload caused by aortic clamping. Although combined CABG/AAA procedures have been described in the literature over many years, percutaneous stent-graft treatment is becoming increasingly common in such high-risk patients.

Diagnosis of Abdominal Aortic Aneurysm

- Symptoms: usually asymptomatic, but patients may have back or abdominal pain.
- Physical examination: palpation of a pulsatile abdominal mass, signs of peripheral ischemia if aortoiliac occlusive disease is present.
- Imaging: ultrasonography, CT scan, or MR angiography, or conventional angiography. CT angiography is becoming the method of choice because it demonstrates the size and location of the aneurysm (e.g., infrarenal versus suprarenal) and the status of major branches (e.g., inferior mesenteric artery). Conventional angiography is considered when CT angiography is inconclusive.

Indications for Combined Abdominal Aortic Aneurysm Repair and Coronary Artery Bypass Graft

- Otherwise healthy patient with a low perioperative risk.
- AAA >5 cm, which can be repaired with either a straight tube graft or an aorto-bi-iliac replacement.
- Major coronary artery disease requiring surgical intervention (e.g., severe left main stenosis).

Operative Techniques

- Use an antifibrinolytic agent and consider Trasylol to minimize postoperative bleeding.
- Perform CABG first. Maintain high perfusion pressures (>70 mm Hg) during CPB to minimize end-organ ischemia.
- With the patient on CPB and with the heart beating, the abdomen is opened and the aneurysm is repaired.

Postoperative Care

- Maintain blood pressure between 100 and 120 mm Hg for the first 6 hours. Consider higher pressures if there is evidence of renal hypoperfusion.
- Leave nasogastric tube in place for 2 or 3 days or until there is evidence of normal gastrointestinal peristalsis.
- Optimize fluid administration as significant intra-abdominal third spacing occurs.
- Observe respiratory function closely after extubation because there may be more compromise because of intra-abdominal swelling.
- Maintain adequate urine output.
- Be careful about excessive fluid requirements or falling hematocrit, suggestive of occult intra-abdominal or retroperitoneal bleeding.

Outcomes

Combined CABG and AAA resection is an uncommon procedure, and therefore most studies in the literature contain a small number of patients. Operative mortality is significantly elevated at approximately 10%. Causes of mortality include MI, low cardiac output syndrome, and coagulopathy. Prolonged ventilatory support (>48 hours) is also very common, occurring in one third of patients. Four-year survival is acceptable at 75%.

SUGGESTED READINGS

Borger MA, Fremes SE. Management of patients with concomitant coronary and carotid vascular disease. *Semin Thorac Cardiovasc Surg*. 2001;13:192–198.

Borger MA, Fremes SE, Weisel RD, et al. Coronary bypass and carotid endarterectomy: does combined approach increase risk? A meta-analysis. *Ann Thorac Surg*. 1999;68:14–21.

Borger MA, Ivanov J, Weisel RD, et al. Stroke during coronary bypass surgery: principal role of cerebral macroemboli. *Eur J Cardiothorac Surg*. 2001;19:627–632.

El-Sabrout RA, Reul GJ, Cooley DA. Outcome after simultaneous abdominal aortic aneurysm repair and aortocoronary bypass. *Ann Vasc Surg*. 2002;16:321–330.

Halliday A, Mansfield A, Marro J, et al. for the MRC Asymptomatic Carotid Surgery Trial (ACST) Collaborative Group. Prevention of disabling and fatal strokes by successful carotid endarterectomy in patients without recent neurological symptoms: randomised controlled trial. *Lancet*. 2004;363:1491–1502.

Yadav JS, Wholey MH, Kuntz RE, et al. Protected carotid-artery stenting versus endarterectomy in high-risk patients. *N Engl J Med*. 2004;351:1493–1501.

Chapter 33

Surgery for Mechanical Complications of Myocardial Infarction

Tirone E. David

Rupture of the Free Wall of the Ventricle *285*

Postinfarction Ventricular Septal Defect *286*

Cardiac rupture, mitral valve regurgitation, and ventricular aneurysm are mechanical complications of myocardial infarction. The natural history of acute myocardial infarction has changed considerably in hospitalized patients over the last several decades because of pharmacologic manipulations and interventional procedures. Cardiac rupture and left ventricular aneurysm were common problems in the early days of cardiac surgery, but they are now rare complications of acute transmural myocardial infarction. Left ventricular aneurysms and ischemic mitral regurgitation are discussed in Chapters 38 and 26, respectively.

RUPTURE OF THE FREE WALL OF THE VENTRICLE

The free wall of the left ventricle is the most common site of cardiac rupture following acute transmural myocardial infarction. It usually occurs 4 to 5 days after the infarct, but it ranges from hours to several weeks. The lateral ventricular wall is the most common site of rupture, and it is more likely to occur in women than in men and in older than in younger patients.

The pathogenesis of cardiac ruptures remains unclear. The problem likely begins with infarct expansion, which increases wall tension with further dilation and ultimately rupture. The outcome is determined by the rapidity with which the tear extends through the necrotic muscle and by the size of the rupture. Large and acute ruptures of the free wall of the left ventricle cause sudden hemodynamic collapse, profound hypotension, electromechanical dissociation, and death within minutes. Small and subacute ruptures may be temporarily sealed by clot or fibrinous pericardial adhesions and may be compatible with life for several hours, days, or even longer. On a rare occasion a false aneurysm develops.

Acute rupture of the free wall is invariably fatal. Subacute rupture causes hemo-pericardium, and symptoms and signs of acute tamponade. Unless surgically treated, patients with subacute rupture die within hours or days.

Surgical treatment consists of patching the necrotic area with Dacron fabric or bovine or autologous pericardium. Chronic false aneurysm may be treated like true aneurysms if the margins of the infarcted muscle are scarred, but often they also require a patch to restore left ventricular geometry.

Most reports on myocardial rupture involve a few cases to determine the real oper-ative mortality with these operations. We reported 12 patients with false aneurysms who underwent surgical repair, and of them three died. Most patients had a posterior false aneurysm, and four patients required concomitant mitral valve replacement because of severe mitral regurgitation preoperatively.

POSTINFARCTION VENTRICULAR SEPTAL DEFECT

Rupture of the interventricular septum is the second most common site of cardiac rup-ture. It causes a ventricular septal defect (VSD). The infarct is always transmural and can be anterior or posterior. The rupture usually occurs 2 and 4 days after the infarct. Anterior VSD is caused by occlusion of the left anterior descending artery, and it is located in the distal half of the septum. Posterior VSD results from occlusion of the dominant right coronary artery, and the rupture usually occurs in the proximal half of the posterior part of the septum. Posterior VSD is often associated with extensive right ventricular infarction.

Most patients who develop postinfarction VSD progress into heart failure and/or cardiogenic shock. For this reason, the best approach is emergency surgery. Patients in cardiogenic shock should be stabilized with intra-aortic balloon pumps, vasodilators, inotropes, and assisted ventilation, if necessary. Coronary angiography should be per-formed immediately after hemodynamic stabilization, and surgery should follow soon after. Patients who are hemodynamically stable should have surgery on an urgent basis because they can deteriorate anytime, and once multiorgan failure ensues, mortality rises radically.

Surgery consists of myocardial revascularization and repair of the VSD. The original techniques of repair of the ruptured septum consisted of infarctectomy and recon-struction of the septum with Dacron patches, as illustrated in Figures 33-1 and 33-2. The operative technique of infarct exclusion (see Figs. 33-3 and 33-4) was introduced in the mid-1980s, and, in our hands, made a major difference in survival, particularly in patients with posterior VSD who historically had a higher operative mortality than anterior VSD.

The operative mortality largely depends on the patient's clinical presentation before surgery. Therefore, repair of postinfarction VSD in patients who are hemodynamically stable is associated with an operative mortality of 10% to 20%, but it is as high as 40% to 50% in patients in cardiogenic shock. Operative survivors have good long-term sur-vival, particularly if ventricular function is not severely impaired, and complete revas-cularization is performed at the time of the septal repair.

Transcatheter closure of postinfarction VSD using various types of devices has been successful only in a few patients, but it certainly is a promising technique.

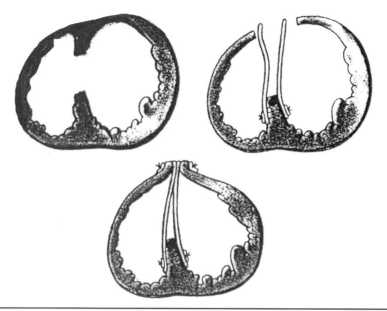

FIGURE 33-1. Infarctectomy and patch repair of anterior ventricular septal defect (VSD).

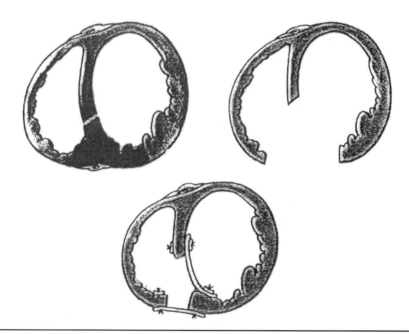

FIGURE 33-2. Infarctectomy and patch repair of posterior ventricular septal defect (VSD).

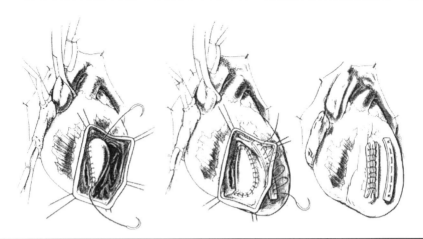

FIGURE 33-3. Infarct exclusion of anterior ventricular septal defect (VSD).

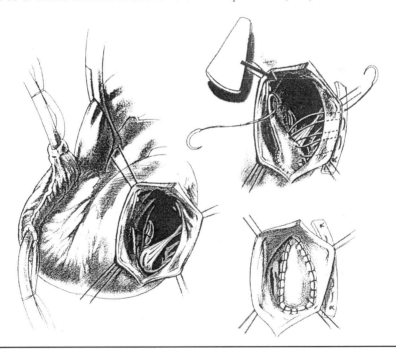

FIGURE 33-4. Infarct exclusion of posterior ventricular septal defect (VSD).

SUGGESTED READINGS

David TE, Dale L, Sun Z. Postinfarction ventricular septal rupture: repair by endocardial patch with infarction exclusion. *J Thorac Cardiovasc Surg*. 1995;110:1315–1322.

Holzer E, Balzer D, Amin Z, et al. Transcatheter closure of postinfarction ventricular septal defects using the new amplatzer muscular VSD occluder. Results of a U.S. registry. *Catheter Cardiovasc Interv*. 2004;61:196–201.

Radford MJ, Johnson RA, Daggett WM Jr, et al. Ventricular septal rupture: a review of clinical and physiologic features and an analysis of survival. *Circulation*. 1981;64:545–553.

Surgery for End-stage Heart Disease and Heart Transplantation

Vivek Rao and Christopher M. Feindel

Congestive heart failure remains the only cardiovascular diagnosis that is increasing in prevalence in the developed world. The gold standard for the treatment of end-stage heart disease not amenable to any other form of conventional therapy is cardiac transplantation. Unfortunately, limited organ availability precludes heart transplantation for many patients who would otherwise benefit from this therapy. Therefore, several centers have re-evaluated the role of high-risk surgical alternatives to transplantation. Although few of these procedures have been evaluated formally for long-term durability, the potential to delay the need for transplantation for even a few years is appealing. For centers with the resources to provide mechanical circulatory support (see Chapter 36), high-risk interventions can be performed in patients with ventricular assist device backup.

Ischemic cardiomyopathy occurs in most patients in this population, and they may potentially benefit from one or more of the following "conventional" procedures: coronary artery bypass graft (CABG), mitral valve repair/replacement, and left ventricular reconstruction.

DIAGNOSIS

The role of ischemia in patients with end stage cardiomyopathy remains controversial. The Surgical Therapy for Ischemic Congestive Heart Failure (STICH) trial is a large, multicenter, international trial designed specifically to address the benefits of revascularization ± left ventricular reconstruction in patients with ischemic cardiomyopathy. Despite the unproven benefits of revascularization for patients with heart failure, most centers continue to advocate diagnostic angiography to rule out potentially treatable coronary artery disease (CAD). Often, the disease is diffuse and widespread and not amenable to conventional revascularization. In these instances, transmyocardial revascularization (TMR), gene therapy with angiogenic factors, or cell transplantation may be the only remaining options.

When CAD is amenable to surgical revascularization, most centers advocate risk stratification with viability testing. The most reliable tests for viability are positron emission tomography (PET), employing radioactive carbohydrates (fluorodeoxyglucose [FDG]) or magnetic resonance imaging (MRI) with gadolinium infusion. Delayed enhancement with gadolinium implies fixed, nonviable tissue. In addition to the viability assessments, MRI provides intricate details about cardiac structure and function, and can differentiate between ischemic dyskinetic segments of viable myocardium and true aneurysmal formation.

Transthoracic echocardiography provides invaluable information with respect to global and regional ventricular function, valvular morphology and function, and transverse/descending aortic atheroma. Transesophageal echocardiography (TEE) should be a routine intraoperative adjunct for all surgical procedures in patients with end-stage heart failure.

For transplant eligibility, several screening tests are performed to identify significant comorbidities, which may preclude successful transplantation. Table 34-1 lists the most commonly performed screening evaluations. Although each transplant program may have its own criteria for transplant eligibility, there are a few standard contraindications:

- Fixed pulmonary hypertension, defined arbitrarily as >4 Woods units, a mean transpulmonary gradient (mean pulmonary arterial pressure minus pulmonary capillary wedge pressure) >14 mm Hg, or a systolic pulmonary to systemic artery pressure ratio >0.5.
- Recent (<5 years) malignancy.
- Active systemic infection.
- Major systemic illness (i.e., diabetes, amyloidosis, hemochromatosis).
- Other end-organ failure.

Relative contraindications include peripheral vascular disease, age more than 65 years, emotional stability, and demonstrated lack of compliance to medical regimens. It is important to realize that most patients would still benefit from cardiac transplantation, but the chronic shortage of suitable donor organs forces transplant programs to rationalize care to those patients who are most likely to derive long-term benefits. Potential candidates are assessed by a multidisciplinary committee to allow for the equitable distribution of these scarce resources.

Donor selection varies amongst transplant centers, but in general, the criteria for acceptable organs continues to evolve as all programs struggle with the chronic shortage of organs to meet increased demand. After matching for ABO blood type and body size (usually within 20% of recipient weight), several factors contribute to the decision-making process when evaluating a potential cardiac donor. The presence of standard cardiac risk factors (including age >50) mandates coronary angiography to rule out occult CAD. Transthoracic echocardiography is also important to evaluate ventricular function in addition to valvular structure and function. It is important to note that a single echocardiogram does not completely rule out a potential donor organ and

▶ **TABLE 34-1 Commonly Performed Screening Investigations to Assess Candidacy for Heart Transplantation**

Routine	Additional
Consultations	
Cardiology	Dental surgery
Cardiovascular surgery	Gynecology
Psychiatry	Respirology
Social work	Transplant immunology
Transplant coordinator	Transplant ID
Anesthesia	Hepatology
	Neurology
	Hematology/Oncology
	Gastroenterology
Investigations	
Right and left heart catheterization	Liver biopsy
Transthoracic echocardiogram	Nerve conduction study
Electrocardiogram	GI endoscopy
Pulmonary function tests	Bone marrow examination
Arterial blood gases	Chest CT scan
Chest x-ray	Mammogram
Abdominal ultrasound or CT scan	Pap smear
Laboratory Tests	
ABO blood type and screen	Protein electrophoresis
CBC, ESR, smear, reticulate	Stool for parasites, C and S, blood
PT, PTT, INR, bleeding time	Prostate specific antigen
Electrolytes, creatinine	
Urinalysis, 24 h creatinine clearance	
Thyroid function tests	
Liver function tests	
Blood glucose (fasting, 2 h PC)	
Cholesterol, triglycerides	
Antibody screen (HBV, HCV, HIV)	
HLA typing	
Anti-HLA antibodies (PRA)	
Antibody titers (CMV, EBV, HSV, Toxo)	

ID, infectious disease; GI, gastrointestinal; CT, computerized tomography; Pap, Papanicolaou; CBC, complete blood count; ESR, erythrocyte sedimentation rate; C and S, culture and sensitivity; PT, prothrombin time; PTT, partial thromboplastin time; INR, international normalized ratio; HBV, hepatitis B virus; HCV, hepatitis C virus; HIV, human immunodeficiency virus; HLA, human leukocyte antigen; PRA, panel reactive antibody; CMV, cytomegalovirus; EBV, Epstein-Barr virus; HSV, herpes simplex virus.

an initially poor evaluation may be considerably improved after hormonal resuscitation (e.g., T4, vasopressin, insulin) and appropriate management of preload and afterload. Unfortunately, due to time constraints, prospective human leukocyte antigen (HLA) matching is not routinely performed for cardiac transplants.

SURGICAL TECHNIQUES

Coronary Artery Bypass Graft

Although the role of revascularization remains controversial in patients with isolated heart failure symptoms without angina, most centers will offer high-risk CABG to those patients with graftable targets and evidence of reversible ischemia. Often, the left anterior descending artery (LAD) is completely occluded and, even if graftable, supplies infarct territory. Therefore, the authors prefer to employ the left internal thoracic artery to graft an important lateral wall target. Similarly, the right coronary artery (RCA) is often found to be diffusely diseased or chronically occluded with no discernible targets. In these instances, an acute marginal branch can often be found that supplies important perfusion to the right ventricular free wall and intraventricular septum.

Meticulous delivery of cardioplegia is extremely important in these cases as patients have little reserve for inadequate myocardial protection. Retrograde cardioplegia may be beneficial, especially in cases where the LAD is chronically occluded. The use of special induction or reperfusion strategies, such as terminal hot shots or amino-acid enriched reperfusates, may also be of benefit (see Chapter 21).

Mitral Valve Repair

Patients with congestive heart failure often have evidence of significant mitral insufficiency. The mitral valve leaflets are normal or, at most, mildly thickened in most patients. The mechanism leading to mitral insufficiency is usually annular dilatation and/or leaflet tethering. Recently, we have treated these patients with an undersized annuloplasty band (≤28 mm) in addition to division of the secondary and tertiary chordae.

Badhwar and Bolling have reported encouraging results with mitral valve repair in patients with poor ejection fraction due to a variety of etiologies. However, the durability of these procedures remains uncertain as the 2-year survival is only 70% and the rate of recurrent mitral regurgitation (MR) is unknown.

In patients with coexisting renal insufficiency, a common comorbidity in this patient population, the benefits of mitral valve repair must be weighed against the risk of a prolonged and complex operation. Certainly, if there is evidence of myxomatous disease in one or both leaflets suggesting the need for a complex repair, one may elect to proceed with formal mitral valve replacement with preservation of all subvalvular structures.

Left Ventricular Reconstruction

The role of left ventricular reconstruction for patients with true or false aneurysms of the left ventricle is clearly established. However, for patients with akinetic areas comprising a mixture of muscle and scar tissue, the role of left ventricular repair is not well defined. The second major hypothesis of the STICH trial is to determine the role of left ventricular reconstruction for patients with ischemic cardiomyopathy.

The Dor procedure was initially described in 1984 and referred to as an endoventricular circular patchplasty of an akinetic or dyskinetic segment of myocardium. Most surgeons now employ a modification of the originally described technique in which the left ventricular defect is plicated with a purse-string suture before closure of the patch. Mickleborough et al. have also reported excellent clinical results using a modified linear closure.

Heart Transplantation

The development of experimental organ transplantation began in 1905 when Drs. Carrel and Guthrie performed an extrathoracic heterotopic canine transplant. However, until the development of cardiopulmonary bypass in 1958, the technique for orthotopic cardiac transplantation could not be perfected. Critical research by Dr. Norman Shumway at Stanford University paved the way for the first human transplant performed by Dr. Christian Barnard in 1967. After an initial flurry of activity, the procedure became virtually abandoned due to recalcitrant rejection and infection. The introduction of cyclosporine in the 1970s revolutionized all solid organ transplants and ushered in the second era of heart transplantation.

The initial technique, described by Shumway, consisted of a biatrial anastomosis employing a cuff of recipient left and right atria. Advances in suture technology and surgical technique have led to the adoption of the cava–cava technique and, in some centers, complete orthotopic transplantation is done with cuffs of left and right pulmonary veins sewn to the donor left atrium.

PERIOPERATIVE CONSIDERATIONS

Irrespective of the surgical intervention involved, patients with end-stage heart disease require careful attention to perioperative fluid and blood product administration. In patients presenting florid heart failure with gross volume overload, consideration should be made to delay operative intervention until renal, pulmonary, and cardiac function is optimized. When emergency surgery is required, it is often useful to incorporate hemodialysis or ultrafiltration in the cardiopulmonary bypass circuit to achieve significant hemoconcentration and avoid the detrimental effects of perioperative anemia. For potential transplant candidates, consideration must be made of the immunologic costs of blood product utilization. Platelet transfusions, in particular, can lead to HLA sensitization and greatly increase the risk of rejection episodes.

Although most patients present with evidence of left ventricular dysfunction, right ventricular failure is a devastating and highly fatal complication. Meticulous detail to hemostasis will minimize blood product utilization. The cytokine release associated with transfusion has been directly correlated to right ventricular failure. Inadequate myocardial protection may also lead to significant right ventricular dysfunction (especially in situations where the RCA territory is incompletely revascularized). The authors prefer a strategy of preventing right ventricular failure as opposed to treating a patient who is hemodynamically labile. The prophylactic use of milrinone, a phosphodiesterase inhibitor, has proven to be a useful adjunct in these critically ill patients. A loading dose of 3 to 5 mg is delivered directly into the pump circuit at the onset of reperfusion. The hypotension associated with this loading dose is usually manageable with increased pump flow rates or intermittent vasoconstrictor support.

If needed, a continuous infusion can be initiated during the attempt to wean from cardiopulmonary bypass.

Persistent right ventricular dysfunction is now managed by early introduction of inhaled nitric oxide, intravenous prostacyclin, or, in some centers, inhaled prostacyclins. Often, rate control with Isoproterenol or temporary atrial overdrive pacing can improve right ventricular function and lead to better left ventricular filling. An early sign of impending right ventricular failure is oliguria. Prompt institution of renal replacement therapy will avoid considerable volume overload, which will only worsen right ventricular function.

As mentioned previously, renal insufficiency is a common comorbid condition in this patient population. To date, there have been no successful renal protective strategies validated in prospective, randomized clinical trials. Nevertheless, many institutions including our own tend to administer low-dose dopamine (2 to 4 μg/kg/minute) throughout cardiopulmonary bypass and in the early postoperative period. Other strategies currently under investigation include N-acetylcysteine and vasopressin infusions, pulsatile cardiopulmonary bypass flows, and the B-type natriuretic peptide (BNP) analogue, neseritide.

OUTCOMES

The morbidity and mortality associated with each of the high-risk alternatives to transplant procedures discussed earlier is extremely surgeon-dependent and can vary from 3% to more than 20%. The current operative mortality associated with heart transplantation is reported to be 10% with an additional attrition of 5% to 10% over the first year due to recalcitrant rejection or infection. Long-term survival following heart transplantation now approaches 80% at 5 years, with an average life expectancy of 9 years. Long-term survival is limited by malignancy or transplant vasculopathy.

SUGGESTED READINGS

Badhwar V, Bolling S. Mitral valve surgery in the patient with left ventricular dysfunction. *Semin Thorac Cardiovasc Surg*. 2002;14:133–136.

Doenst T, Velasquez E, Beyersdorf F, et al. To STICH or not to STICH? *J Thorac Cardiovasc Surg*. 2005;129:246–249 *(in press)*.

Mickleborough LLM, Merchant N, Ivanov J, et al. Left ventricular reconstruction: early and late results. *J Thorac Cardiovasc Surg*. 2004;128:27–37.

Ross HJ, Hendry PJ, Dipchand AI, et al. The 2003 Canadian Cardiovascular Society consensus guideline update for the diagnosis and management of heart failure. *Can J Cardiol*. 2003;19:347–356.

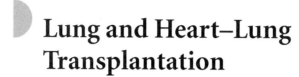

Lung and Heart–Lung Transplantation

Shaf Keshavjee and Stefan Fischer

The surgical options for the treatment of end-stage cardiopulmonary failure have evolved considerably since the initial success of heart–lung and lung transplantation. The first successful single lung transplant and the first successful bilateral lung transplant were performed in Toronto in 1983 and 1986, respectively. The first successful heart–lung transplant was performed at Stanford in 1981. Essentially, given the scarce supply of donor organs and the complications associated with thoracic organ transplantation, transplantation should be performed when no other treatment modality is available. Furthermore, only the organs that need to be replaced should be transplanted. Therefore, lung transplantation is performed for end-stage lung failure, heart transplantation for end-stage heart failure, and combined heart–lung transplantation is reserved for combined irreversible cardiac and pulmonary failure. Lung volume reduction (LVR) is a procedure that may be used in select cases of end-stage emphysema, as an alternative to transplantation, as a bridge to transplantation, or in combination with transplantation.

SURGICAL TECHNIQUE
Donor Procedure

The donor lung retrieval procedure is detailed elsewhere. A brief description of the technique of lung preservation is given in Table 35-1. For technique of cardiac transplant, see Chapter 34.

Recipient Procedure

The lung transplant operation requires cooperation and precise communication between the surgeon and the anesthetist. A single lung transplant is performed through a

▶ **TABLE 35-1** Technique of Lung Preservation

Donor lung protection
- Methylprednisolone 2 g IV to donor
- Pulmonary artery flush with Perfadex (low potassium dextran [LPD]) solution (3), 50 mL/kg, 4°C
- PGE_1 500 μg direct injection into pulmonary artery
- PGE_1 500 μg in flush solution
- Lungs are stored at 4°C in the inflated state ($FIO_2 > 0.5$) for transport

Intraoperative lung protection
- Keep lung cool using a cooling jacket during implantation
- Clear blood and secretions and *gently* reinflate (25 cm H_2O) before reperfusion
- Gradually release pulmonary artery clamp over 10 min (modified reperfusion technique)
- Wash out flush solution and de-air through atrial anastomosis

---

IV, intravenously; PGE_1, prostaglandin E_1; FIO_2, fraction of inspired oxygen.

standard posterolateral thoracotomy, and a bilateral lung transplant is performed through a transverse fourth intercostal space thoracosternotomy or bilateral anterior thoracotomies without dividing the sternum.

Bilateral Lung Transplant Procedure

A pneumonectomy is performed on the side receiving the least blood flow (as determined by a preoperative quantitative V/Q scan). The bronchus, pulmonary artery (PA), and left atrium/pulmonary veins are prepared for anastomosis. The donor lung is trimmed on the back table and then placed in the recipient's chest on a cooling jacket. The patient is given methylprednisolone (Solumedrol), 500 mg intravenously (IV).

The bronchial anastomosis is performed first, with a running 4-0 polydioxane surgical (PDS) suture on the membranous wall and interrupted mattress 4-0 polypropylene sutures on the cartilaginous wall. The bronchus is intussuscepted for one ring. The anastomosis is further buttressed with sutures through peribronchial tissues. The bronchial tree is then suctioned clear by the anesthetist.

A vascular clamp is placed on the proximal PA and the vessel is appropriately trimmed. The pulmonary arterial anastomosis is performed in an end-to-end fashion using a running 5-0 polypropylene suture interrupted in two places.

The pericardium surrounding the pulmonary vein stumps is incised and an atrial clamp is placed on the lateral wall of the left atrium. The vein stumps are opened and their orifices are joined to form a common atrial cuff. The atrial anastomosis is then performed using a running 4-0 polypropylene suture that is interrupted in two places. This is done with a horizontal mattress suture in a completely everting technique so that there is perfect endothelium-to-endothelium apposition. The atrial anastomosis is left untied at this point for later de-airing.

The cooling jacket is removed and the lung is gently reinflated to a maximum pressure of 25 cm H_2O. Once the lung is inflated, ventilation is initiated with a fraction of inspired oxygen (FIO_2) of 0.5, a maximum peak pressure of 15 to 25 cm, and a positive end expiratory pressure (PEEP) of 2 to 5 cm. The PA clamp is gradually removed over a period of 10 minutes to provide gradual reflow (rewarming and distention) of the pulmonary vasculature. The flush solution and blood are allowed to drain out of the atrial anastomosis, and once the lung is de-aired, the atrial clamp is removed and the atrial suture is secured.

The patient is allowed to stabilize for a period of 10 to 15 minutes. The pneumonectomy and implantation procedure are then similarly performed on the contralateral side in the case of a bilateral lung transplant. The patient is supported by the native lung while the first lung is implanted and by the newly transplanted lung while the second lung is implanted. Cardiopulmonary bypass (CPB), therefore, is not routinely used for lung transplantation. In approximately 30% of cases, CPB is necessary. This is usually for cases where CPB is clearly needed such as heart–lung transplant, combined lung transplant and cardiac repair, and severe pulmonary hypertension, or in cases where oxygenation or ventilation become impossible or when the patient becomes hemodynamically unstable. The indications for CPB are listed in Table 35-2.

Heart–Lung Transplant Procedure

The heart–lung transplant procedure is also performed through a transverse thoracotomy incision. The exposure of the posterior mediastinum and pleural spaces that is

▌ **TABLE 35-2 Cardiopulmonary Bypass for Lung Transplantation**

Indications
- SLT   Pulmonary hypertension (primary or secondary)
  Inadequate gas exchange
  Hemodynamic instability
- BLT   Pulmonary hypertension
  Dysfunction of first graft
  Progressive increase in PAP/hypotension
  – Pulmonary edema/hypoxia
- Separate lung ventilation impossible
  Children
  – Copious thick secretions (CF)
- Need for cardiac repair, heart–lung transplant

Cannulation
- Standard: Aortic root and right atrium (two-stage venous cannula)
- Right SLT: right femoral artery and right atrium
- Left SLT: descending aorta or femoral artery, femoral vein or proximal PA

Special considerations
- Do not persist unduly before resorting to CPB if problems with hypoxia or hypotension
- Decrease to 1/2 to 3/4 full PA flow at reperfusion—to gently reperfuse at low pressure
- Maintain ventilation of first lung implanted once reperfused
- Maintain low pressure reperfusion (ejection) of first lung (3/4 full flow) to prevent warm ischemia (note: the transplanted lung has no bronchial blood flow)

SLT, single lung transplant; BLT, bilateral lung transplant; PAP, pulmonary artery pressure; CF, cystic fibrosis; PA, pulmonary artery; CPB, cardiopulmonary bypass.

afforded by this approach has considerably decreased the incidence of postoperative hemorrhage (compared to a median sternotomy). The technique for heart–lung transplantation, which is briefly described subsequently, is adapted from the original description of the procedure by the Stanford group.

The patient is cannulated for CPB in the standard fashion (aorta/bi-caval). The aorta is cross clamped and the heart is excised by transecting the aorta and PA and incising the right and left atria. The pericardium is incised anterior and parallel to the phrenic nerves bilaterally. The posterior wall of the left atrium is divided in the midline and the pulmonary vein/left atrial mobilization is completed extrapericardially, posterior to the phrenic nerve pedicles. The PA is divided at the bifurcation and a button of tissue is left on the ductus arteriosus to preserve the recurrent nerve. The PAs are dissected laterally. Both main bronchi are divided in standard fashion. The carina is then excised, taking care to minimally disrupt the blood supply to the distal trachea.

The heart–lung graft is then placed in the chest. The right lung is passed under the right atrium and the right phrenic nerve pedicle, and the left lung is passed under the left nerve pedicle. The trachea is anastomosed in an end-to-end manner using a running 4-0 PDS suture on the membranous wall and is interrupted with 4-0 Prolene sutures on the cartilaginous wall. The anterior pretracheal donor and recipient tissues are approximated to buttress the anastomosis. Gentle low-volume ventilation with an Fio_2 of 0.5 is then initiated.

The donor right atrium is opened from the inferior vena cava (IVC) to the base of the atrial appendage, and the right atrial anastomosis is performed using a running 3-0 polypropylene suture. A bicaval anastomotic technique may also be used. The aortic anastomosis is then performed using a running 4-0 polypropylene suture. The heart is then carefully de-aired and the cross clamp is released.

POSTOPERATIVE CARE

The postoperative care of patients with a lung (LTx) or heart–lung (HLTx) transplantation begins in the operating room. After the completion of the implantation procedure, meticulous attention must be paid to the hemodynamic optimization of the patient. Cardiac output, filling pressures, and systemic vascular resistance (SVR) should be measured. These patients often have a low SVR syndrome, which requires institution of an infusion of an α-agent (e.g., norephinephrine) and judicious volume replacement. Although volume overload is not desirable, volume depletion is also undesirable in that it contributes to hemodynamic instability; essentially one should aim for a euvolemic state.

After the completion of the operation, the double-lumen endotracheal tube is exchanged for a single-lumen tube, and a bronchoscopic examination is performed to inspect the bronchial anastomosis and to clear the airway of blood and secretions.

The patient is transferred to the intensive care unit (ICU). The central venous pressure (CVP) and pulmonary capillary wedge pressure (PCWP) are kept at the lowest possible values to maintain a mean blood pressure (BP) >65 mm Hg with adequate urine output. Often the low SVR state persists for 12 to 24 hours and a continuous infusion of norepinephrine, with or without dopamine, is required. Patients with elevated PA pressures preoperatively tend to be more hemodynamically labile and more difficult to manage.

Ventilatory Support

A baseline arterial blood gas is obtained on an F_{IO_2} of 1.0, PEEP 5 cm, on arrival in the ICU. Conventional ventilation techniques are used with PEEP; the plateau pressure must be kept at <35 cm H_2O. In approximately 20% of cases, reperfusion injury is severe and life threatening. If conventional ventilation is inadequate, in cases of severe ischemia-reperfusion injury, nitric oxide is used to improve oxygenation and to decrease PA pressure. A low-dose prostaglandin E_1 (PGE_1) infusion can also be beneficial in reperfusion injury. In severe cases, extracorporeal membrane oxygenation (ECMO) is used to support the patient until the acute lung dysfunction recovers. In general, at least 50% of patients will be extubated within 24 to 48 hours of surgery.

Immunosuppression

- Solumedrol 500 mg IV before reperfusion.
- Solumedrol 0.5 mg/kg/day for 3 days.
- Prednisone 0.5 mg/kg/day from day 4 to 14, then taper to 5 mg/week to 20 mg/day.
- Cyclosporine (Neoral) 5 mg/kg PO b.i.d. (target level 250 to 350 mg until 6 months).
- Azathioprine 1.5 mg/kg/day IV/PO.

Anticoagulation

Anticoagulation is desirable because bronchial anastomotic healing depends on microcirculatory blood flow through pulmonary–bronchial collaterals, and deep vein thrombosis (DVT)/pulmonary embolism prophylaxis is also necessary.

Start immediately postoperatively (hold if bleeding is a concern):

- Heparin 100 units/hour IV for 7 days, then 5,000 units sc q12h until discharge.
- Rheomacrodex (5% dextran 40) 500 mL IV over 24 hours for 7 days.

Infection Prophylaxis

- Perioperative antibiotic prophylaxis against bacterial infection: Cefuroxime 1.5 g IV 30 minutes preoperatively, and q8h for 48 hours. Adjust according to culture results of donor and recipient.
- Cystic fibrosis patients: Ceftazidime 2 g IV+tobramycin 5 mg/kg IV (or according to known organisms/sensitivities/synergistic antibiotic testing in the patient).
- Cytomegalovirus (CMV) infection: All patients who are CMV positive (donor, recipient or both)—Gancyclovir 5 mg/kg b.i.d. for 14 days, then qMWF (every Monday, Wednesday, Friday) for 12 weeks.
  - Negative donor and recipient—Acyclovir, 400 mg, PO t.i.d. for 3 months (herpes prophylaxis).
  - Positive donor and negative recipient—CMV hyperimmune globulin immediately and q2wk for 16 weeks.
- *Pneumocystis carinii:* Septra o.d. qMWF, starting on day 14.

SUMMARY

Lung and heart–lung transplantation are potentially lifesaving procedures for patients with end-stage pulmonary and/or cardiac failure. Optimal results depend on careful patient selection and attention to the many details of these complex procedures in patients who are extremely ill. Further information on indications, patient selection, complications, and outcomes are found in Suggested Readings.

SUGGESTED READINGS

DePerrot M, Chaparro C, McRae K, et al. Twenty year experience of lung transplantation at a single center: influence of recipient diagnosis on long-term survival. *J Thorac Cardiovasc Surg*. 2004; 127(5):1493–1501.

DePerrot M, Keshavjee S. Lung transplantation: lung preservation. *Chest Surg Clin N Am*. 2003;13(3): 443–462.

DePerrot M, Liu M, Waddell T, et al. Ischemia- reperfusion injury–state of the art. *Am J Respir Crit Care Med*. 2003;167:490–511.

DePerrot M, Weder W, Patterson GA, et al. Strategies to increase limited donor resources. *Eur Respir J*. 2004;23(3):477–482.

Keshavjee SH, Todd TR. Selection of the donor: excision and storage of the lungs. In: Cooper DKC, Miller LW, Patterson GA, eds. *The transplantation and replacement of thoracic organs*. 2nd ed. Hingham, MA: Kluwer Academic Publishers; 1996.

Keshavjee SH, Yamazaki F, Cardoso P, et al. A method for safe 12 hour pulmonary preservation. *J Thorac Cardiovasc Surg*. 1989;98:529–534.

Pearson FG, Deslauriers J, Ginsberg RJ, et al., eds. *Thoracic surgery*. New York: Churchill Livingstone; 1995.

Smith JA, McCarthy PM, Sarris GE, et al., eds. *The Stanford manual of cardiopulmonary transplantation*. New York: Futura Publishing; 1996.

Todd TR, Perron J, Winton T, et al. Simultaneous single lung transplant and lung volume reduction. *Ann Thorac Surg*. 1997;63:1468–1470.

Urschel HC, Cooper JD. *Atlas of thoracic surgery*. New York: Churchill Livingstone; 1995.

Ventricular Assist Devices

Vivek Rao

Congestive heart failure remains the only cardiovascular diagnosis that is prevalent in the developed world. The gold standard for the treatment of end-stage heart disease, not amenable to any other form of conventional therapy, is cardiac transplantation. Unfortunately, limited organ availability precludes heart transplantation for many patients who would otherwise benefit from this therapy. Ventricular assist devices (VADs) were introduced to provide mechanical circulatory support to patients who are critically ill until a suitable donor organ can be found. Several short-term (days to weeks) and long-term (months to years) devices are now in use with acceptable, although not ideal, clinical outcomes.

The successful use of mechanical circulatory support as a "bridge" to transplantation has led to the consideration of "destination" therapy whereby VAD implantation represents the definitive treatment of patients with refractory heart failure who are not eligible for transplantation. In addition, experience with prolonged (>3 months) circulatory support has revealed that some patients recover native left ventricular function after a period of cardiac decompression and reverse remodeling. Therefore, the use of VADs as a bridge to recovery is a concept that will likely transform the current management strategy for patients with end-stage heart disease.

Regardless of the type of VAD system employed, there are several pre-, peri-, and postoperative considerations when managing a patient who is critically ill and who is dependent on mechanical circulatory support. Careful patient selection remains the predominant key to clinical success.

INDICATIONS FOR MECHANICAL CIRCULATORY SUPPORT

Mechanical circulatory support is now considered a standard of care for certain patients with acute or chronic heart failure. Device selection depends on several factors including presenting illness, likelihood of short-term recovery, neurologic status, and body size. The overriding indication in all patients, however, remains inadequate cardiac function to provide end-organ perfusion. Classic hemodynamic criteria include pulmonary

▶ TABLE 36-1 Commonly Available Ventricular Assist Devices

Name	Type	Mechanism	Duration	Position
ABIOMED BVS5000	BIVAD	Pneumatic	Days-Weeks	Paracorporeal
Thoratec	BIVAD	Pneumatic	Months	Paracorporeal
HeartMate	LVAD	Electrical	Months	Implantable
Novacor	LVAD	Electrical	Months	Implantable
CardioWest TAH	BIVAD	Pneumatic	Months	Paracorporeal
DeBakey	LVAD	Axial flow	Months	Implantable
Jarvik 2000	LVAD	Axial flow	Months	Implantable
HeartMate II	LVAD	Axial flow	Months	Implantable
ABIOMED BIVAD	BIVAD	Pneumatic	Months	Paracorporeal

BIVAD, biventricular assist device; LVAD, left ventriclular assist device; TAH, total artificial heart.

capillary wedge pressure >20 mm Hg, systolic blood pressure <80 mm Hg, and a cardiac index <2.1 L/minute/m², despite optimal fluid and inotropic management. In patients with chronic heart failure awaiting heart transplantation, other factors may also favor earlier consideration of VAD insertion in an otherwise stable patient. These include blood type O and body weight >100 kg (suggesting prolonged wait for donor organ), oliguria or azotemia, inotrope dependency, refractory pulmonary hypertension, or onset of malignant arrhythmias.

Table 36-1 lists the currently available and most commonly employed VADs. Key considerations include eligibility for transplantation (see Chapter 34), likelihood for recovery, and potential need for biventricular support. Extracorporeal membrane oxygenation (ECMO) has been deliberately excluded from this list because any patient who requires pulmonary support, in addition to circulatory assistance, should likely receive ECMO until lung function improves to the point that isolated cardiac support is feasible.

PREOPERATIVE CONSIDERATIONS

As mentioned previously, patient selection is paramount to clinical success following VAD insertion. Many authors have derived risk factor screening scores using multivariable logistic regression analyses to assist in patient selection. Table 36-2 depicts the

▶ TABLE 36-2 Preoperative Risk Factor Screening Scale. Patients with a Combined Score >5 Face a >50% Risk of Operative Mortality after Left Ventricular Assist Device (LVAD) Insertion Compared to <15% in Patients with Scores <5

	Ventilated Patient	4 points
	Previous LVAD *in situ*	2 points
	Postcardiotomy shock	2 points
	CVP >16 mm Hg	1 point
	PT >16 seconds	1 point

CVP, central venous pressure; PT, prothrombin time.

Columbia University screening scale, which is also employed in our institution. For patients with a summation score >5, the estimated operative mortality exceeds 50% compared to <15% for those patients with scores <5. Note that even "low-risk" patients face an operative mortality considerably higher than that of most conventional cardiac surgical procedures, reflecting the burden of their critical illness. In addition to these comorbidities, careful anesthetic and surgical evaluation of the potential VAD candidate should include the following:

- Assessment of coagulation profile, including sickle cell status in appropriate patients. The blood bank should be notified and blood products should be reserved (usually 4 units packed red blood cells [PRBC], 4 units fresh frozen plasma [FFP], and 10 units of platelets for *uncomplicated* VAD cases).
- The presence of any coexisting infection, which may lead to device endocarditis, should be determined. Often, line sepsis precipitates hemodynamic collapse, leading to VAD consideration. If an infection is identified and appropriately treated, VAD insertion can usually proceed safely. However, in patients with sepsis with no clear source of infection, VAD insertion is associated with high mortality.
- Transesophageal echocardiography (TEE) should be done to rule out intracardiac shunts. Even minor atrial septal defects should be closed at the time of left ventricular assist device (LVAD) insertion because they can lead to considerable right to left shunts and hypoxia postoperatively.
- TEE should be done to evaluate cardiac valves. Considerable aortic insufficiency *must* be addressed at the time of LVAD insertion because it can lead to a blind loop phenomenon with poor "real" cardiac output. Aortic stenosis is usually irrelevant unless recovery is anticipated, in which case bioprosthetic replacement is preferred because mechanical valves are prone to thrombose, even with therapeutic anticoagulation (due to lack of normal transvalvular flows). The treatment of mitral insufficiency remains controversial because most devices that completely unload the left ventricle eliminate residual mitral insufficiency. However, for axial flow devices and in situations where recovery is anticipated, several authors recommend repair or replacement of the mitral valve. Owing to the normal transmitral flow, mechanical valves can be employed with appropriate postoperative anticoagulation. Mitral stenosis can lead to poor VAD filling and should be addressed with mitral valve replacement. Secondary tricuspid insufficiency is common in patients with biventricular failure and may complicate management in patients with isolated left-sided support. However, in most cases as the pulmonary vascular resistance decreases with mechanical support, the tricuspid regurgitation abates.
- Surgically amenable coronary artery disease is common in patients with ischemic cardiomyopathy. In patients receiving isolated left ventricular support, care must be taken to optimize right ventricular performance. Therefore, any right coronary artery (RCA) lesions should be revascularized at the time of LVAD insertion, or conversion to biventricular support may be necessary.
- Ventricular arrhythmias are common and are usually eliminated by cardiac decompression following institution of mechanical support. However, in patients with isolated left-sided support, a failing right ventricle can produce hemodynamically significant arrhythmias. Although arrhythmias (both atrial and ventricular)

are usually well tolerated, they often lead to decreased LVAD flows and a loss of normal physiologic responses to increased workload. Persistent atrial fibrillation may also lead to thrombus formation and should therefore be treated with early pharmacologic or electrical cardioversion.

PERIOPERATIVE CONSIDERATIONS

Antibiotic prophylaxis is usually dependent on institutional colonization but commonly includes protection against gram-positive organisms and fungi. Aprotonin is the preferred antifibrinolytic agent, and its use at the time of LVAD insertion does not necessarily preclude repeat administration at the time of LVAD explant and transplantation. Most devices can be inserted by a standard median sternotomy, but some authors have reported lateral thoracotomy approaches to VAD insertion in patients with multiple previous sternotomies. In patients who are critically ill, cardiopulmonary bypass (CPB) is initiated early to stabilize hemodynamics, but, in more stable patients, VAD insertion can often be performed without CPB. Once on CPB, inotropic support is usually halved (not discontinued) and vasopressin infusions should be started (2 to 6 units/hour depending upon the degree of vasoplegia).

Although most of the long-term devices are designed for left ventricular (LV) apical cannulation, the short-term devices can be configured to provide inflow through the right (for right ventricle assist devices [RVADs]) or left atrium. However, even with short-term devices (such as the ABIOMED), ventricular cannulation is preferred to improve decompression (and likelihood of recovery), optimize flow, and prevent potential thrombus formation across the atrioventricular valves.

Placement of the pump housing (in the case of the HeartMate and Novacor devices) remains controversial. Intraperitoneal placement lowers the risk of driveline and/or pocket infections but is associated with significant morbidity at the time of LVAD explant and transplant secondary to intra-abdominal adhesions. Preperitoneal placement facilitates pump exchange and/or explant but does increase the risk of device-related infections.

Intraoperative TEE is also useful to reassess valvular function, rule out right–left intracardiac shunts, and aid in de-airing following device implantation. Weaning from CPB is a coordinated effort involving perfusion, anesthesia, surgery, and the VAD controller. Devices should never be activated if CPB flows are >2 L/minute for risk of air entrainment and subsequent cerebral embolus. Heparin anticoagulation is fully reversed with protamine (even in devices that subsequently require anticoagulation). Blood product administration is common at this point because of inherent coagulation abnormalities present in patients with heart failure.

POSTOPERATIVE CONSIDERATIONS

In the early postoperative period, normal hemodynamic monitoring is employed in addition to continuous evaluation of VAD function. Coagulopathy is common, but persistent chest tube drainage should prompt early surgical exploration. The aortic anastomosis is the most common site of postoperative bleeding. When VAD output is below desired limits (i.e., 2 L/minute/m^2), the differential diagnosis includes hypovolemia, tamponade, and right ventricular (RV) failure (in cases of isolated LVAD support). If volume status is adequate (i.e., central venous pressure [CVP] >15 mm Hg) and tamponade had been ruled out (by TEE or re-exploration), then RV failure is the likely cause of poor LVAD output. Milrinone, dobutamine, and nitric oxide are all useful pharmacologic adjuncts to the management of postoperative RV failure. In approximately 15% of cases, temporary right-sided VAD support may be required. Usually, RV function recovers with LVAD support due to improvements in pulmonary vascular resistance. Therefore, in most cases temporary RVAD support can be withdrawn after 3 to 5 days.

CLINICAL OUTCOMES

The overall operative mortality associated with VAD insertion remains approximately 25%. Most programs now routinely discharge their patients with LVAD and maintain outpatient therapy while the patients are awaiting heart transplantation. Fatal or transplant-precluding complications (stroke) before transplant occur in a very small number of these patients. Owing to the improved physiology secondary to VAD support, outcomes following transplantation are better in this population compared to patients undergoing transplantation without VAD support.

Late complications while on VAD support are often device-specific but include driveline infections, pocket infections, thromboembolic events, and human leukocyte antigen (HLA) sensitization. The latter complication can considerably increase the risk of acute rejection following cardiac transplantation.

To facilitate potential myocardial recovery, most programs now reinstitute antifailure therapy (β-blockade, angiotensin converting enzyme [ACE] inhibition, etc.). The Harefield group has also reported promising results with clenbuterol, a β-agonist that promotes myocyte hypertrophy. Unfortunately, predicting which patients will recover native cardiac function (and maintain it for a prolonged duration) remains a mystery, and therefore, most patients eventually proceed to transplantation.

SUMMARY

Mechanical circulatory support has now become established as a standard of care for the treatment of acute and chronic heart failure. The next generation of devices will be smaller and less morbid, and will be designed to have greater durability than the currently available VADs. As the technology continues to improve, it is likely that mechanical circulatory support will one day provide a real alternative to conventional transplantation.

SUGGESTED READINGS

Delgado DH, Rao V, Ross HJ, et al. Mechanical circulatory assistance: state of art. *Circulation.* 2002;106:2046 2050.

Hon JK, Yacoub MH. Bridge to recovery with the use of left ventricular assist device and clenbuterol. *Ann Thorac Surg.* 2003;75:S36–S41.

Rao V, Oz MC. Mechanical circulatory assistance. In: Yang SC, Cameron DE, eds. *Current therapy in thoracic and cardiovascular surgery*. Philadephia, PA: Mosby; 2004.

Rao V, Oz MC, Flannery MA, et al. Revised screening scale to predict survival after insertion of a left ventricular assist device. *J Thorac Cardiovasc Surg.* 2003;125:855–862.

Rose EA, Gelijns AG, Moskowitz AJ, et al. Randomized evaluation of mechanical assistance for the treatment of congestive heart failure (REMATCH) study group. Long term mechanical left ventricular assistance for end-stage heart failure. *N Engl J Med.* 2001;345:1435–1443.

Chapter 37

Adult Congenital Heart Surgery

Glen S. Van Arsdell, Igor E. Konstantinov, and William G. Williams

Therapy for adult congenital heart disease is evolving and developing as children whose heart disease was repaired 20 years earlier develop secondary problems now. Complex unrepaired cardiac lesions in the adult are now quite unusual for North American–born patients. Most primary disease seen today is a late diagnosis of some type of atrial defect or small ventricular septal defect (VSD). The practice is increasingly

▶ **TABLE 37-1** **Toronto Congenital Cardiac Center for Adults (TCCCA) Surgical Procedures 1973–2003**

Pathology	Percentage
Hypertrophic obstruction cardiomyopathy	25
Atrial septal defect	23 (now substantially declining)
Tetralogy of Fallot	11
Ventricular septal defect	8
Single ventricle	5
Congenitally corrected transposition of great arteries	3
Ebstein anomaly	3
Other	22

shifting to (a) repeat operations for valves or conduits, (b) arrhythmia surgery related to long-standing valve disease or progressive ventricular failure, (c) and revision of Fontan circulation pathways. Table 37-1 lists the various procedures performed in adults with congenital heart defects at the Toronto General Hospital during the last three decades.

Twenty years ago, the Fontan procedure was increasingly becoming utilized for single ventricle disease. Not surprisingly, single ventricle surgery is now becoming a central part of adult congenital surgical practice.

This chapter describes the primary congenital lesions that are frequently or occasionally still seen; it also discusses the current strategy that is being adopted in the late management of single ventricle disease.

LEFT TO RIGHT SHUNTS

The major concern in left to right shunts in the adult is whether there has been development of irreversible pulmonary vascular resistance (PVR). Eisenmenger syndrome would be expected to be present in an adult with a nonrestrictive VSD, but only rarely in one with a large atrial septal defect (ASD). Irrespective of this, the status of pulmonary artery pressures must be evaluated and, if near systemic, a formal PVR study should be performed.

Other consequences of chronic volume loading are right or left heart dilation, or failure for ASD and VSD, respectively. Both initially cause volume overloading. Long-standing volume overload is associated with atrial dilation and subsequent atrial arrhythmias including atrial fibrillation. In a study looking at adult repair of ASDs, it was noted that patients >40 years whose cardiac lesions were repaired had a persistence of atrial arrhythmia. The implication is that associated arrhythmia in adults with ASD or VSD may well need arrhythmia surgery in addition to defect closure. ASD closed before 24 years of age was associated with normal life expectancy.

ATRIAL SEPTAL DEFECTS

Anatomy

ASD occurs as a defect in the fossa ovalis or persistence of the patent foramen ovale. These defects are known as *secundum defects*. Septum primum defects are a defect of the endocardial cushion and are associated with abnormal atrioventricular valve alignment and a cleft in the left-sided valve. Sinus venosus defects occur adjacent to the lateral atrial wall—most commonly close to the superior vena cava (SVC), but they can also occur close to the inferior vena cava (IVC). Sinus venosus defects are usually associated with partial anomalous pulmonary venous drainage. Coronary sinus defects are rare; they are most commonly seen in patients with a single ventricle.

Occasionally, patients will have associated pulmonary valve stenosis that might need to be addressed. In most instances, however, apparent pulmonary stenosis is simply flow acceleration across the pulmonary valve attributable to the volume load from the left to right shunt. The pulmonary valve should be inspected visually if the preoperative gradient is >30 mm Hg.

Operative and Perioperative Issues

ASDs continue to be an important part of adult congenital surgery, but for various reasons, most secundum ASDs in our institution are now treated with device occlusion in the interventional suite; however, some large defects (3 to 4 cm or more), or those without a good rim, continue to need surgical intervention. Surgical indications can also extend to those having significant atrial arrhythmia where concomitant atrial arrhythmia surgery is indicated—usually for those treated at an age >40 years.

Intervention Options

There is continued debate about surgical versus device closure of ASDs. Device closure is only an option for patent foramen ovale or secundum ASDs and not the other type of atrial defects. The advantage of device closure is that it is an outpatient procedure. With the newest nitinol device (Amplatzer) there has been little problem with migration, infection, or significant residual lesions—for appropriately selected cases. Devices have been particularly useful for the treatment of patent foramen ovale associated with paradoxic emboli. The two major downsides to devices are the rare but definable device erosion that can cause death and the lack of long-term assessment of effectiveness or complications. Erosion has been reported rarely, but it can occur in surrounding structures such as the aorta or even outside of the heart.

Surgical repair is more invasive—even using minimally invasive techniques. There are neurologic consequences to even a short run of cardiopulmonary bypass (CPB) that have been identified as significant when compared to neurologic outcomes associated with device closure. There is also a small but definable incidence of death—substantially <1%—that is most frequently associated with undiagnosed postpericardiotomy syndrome. Postrepair patients who are not well and who may live far away from the hospital where the surgery was performed will sometimes receive follow-up care in hospitals or clinics that are not completely aware of the implications of postpericardiotomy syndrome and effusions. This issue has been associated with death following repair—within the first 6 weeks after surgery.

Indications for Surgery

- ASD of hemodynamic significance.
  - Right ventricular (RV) volume and/or pressure overload.
  - RV failure.
  - Decreasing exercise tolerance.
  - Atrial arrhythmia.
  - Paradoxic emboli—manifested as a transient ischemic attack or stroke.
- Asymptomatic with a Qp:Qs >2:1 (usually will have one of the above criteria).

Surgical contraindications to intervention.

- Significant or irreversible pulmonary vascular disease (see Table 37-2).
- Biventricular end stage heart failure.

Procedures

Secundum Atrial Septal Defect

- Device closure of defects <40 mm that have a circumferential rim.
- Sternotomy, partial sternotomy, mini-incision, or anterolateral fourth interspace thoracotomy; most large defects require patch closure—autologous pericardium is useful.

Sinus Venosus

Associated partial anomalous pulmonary veins are tunneled through the defect. The SVC may need to be augmented to prevent SVC obstruction. The sinus defect may also need to be enlarged before the baffle creation to prevent pulmonary venous obstruction. Frequently, a two-patch system is most useful.

Ostium Primum Defect

The left atrioventricular valve cleft is closed. Standard annuloplasty techniques are used only if necessary. Occasionally, late-presenting patients have unrepairable regurgitation, requiring valve replacement.

The primum defect is patched with autologous pericardium. The conduction tissue is at risk and is avoided by leaving the coronary sinus on the left side or sewing the patch to the left atrioventricular valve in the region of the conduction tissue.

> **▶ TABLE 37-2 Relative Contraindications to Surgery Due to Pulmonary Vascular Disease**
>
> - Pulmonary artery pressure >2/3 systemic arterial pressure
> - PVR >2/3 systemic vascular resistance without pulmonary reactivity to O_2 or NO
> - Qp:Qs <1.5:1
> - Lung biopsy with Heath Edwards ≥II

PVR, pulmonary vascular resistance; O_2, oxygen; NO, nitric oxide.

Right-Sided Maze

Those patients who have preoperative documented atrial flutter may benefit from a right-sided maze procedure. We would recommend an electrophysiology mapping procedure to determine the source of arrhythmia. Arrhythmias that have a left-sided component may benefit from a biatrial maze procedure. The right-sided maze alone adds very little time to the operation.

Intraoperative Transesophageal Echocardiography

Intraoperative transesophageal echocardiography (TEE) is used to assess residual lesions and ventricular function. Correctable residual lesions should be corrected. Intraoperative TEE combined with the intraoperative hemodynamic profile assists in determining a treatment strategy in the intensive care unit (ICU)—should the patient be managed as a "well patient" or a "sick patient."

Postoperative Management

Most standard risk patients require only a central line and central venous pressure (CVP) monitoring both intraoperatively and postoperatively. A Swan-Ganz catheter is used for those with significant right ventricular failure or elevated PVR.

For those with major right ventricular failure, right heart assistance is achieved with milrinone, elevating the pH to 7.45 to 7.50, and with nitric oxide. These maneuvers are only necessary for patients who are very sick (see Table 37-3).

Standard risk patients can be extubated in the operating room or soon after their arrival in the ICU.

Early mobilization is useful. Discharge is typically on the third or fourth postoperative day. Atrial arrhythmias can prolong the stay, and standard arrhythmia management is used.

Follow-up

Atrial arrhythmias can occur late in upto one third of patients. Meticulous postoperative follow-up for effusions is required. The patient should be seen within 1 week of

▶ **TABLE 37-3** **Treatment of Right Ventricular Dysfunction and/or Pulmonary Hypertension**

- Adequate sedation and paralysis
- pH >7.45: hyperventilation for target Pco_2 = 25 to 30 mm Hg, bicarbonate IV
- Arterial O_2 saturation approximately 100%
- Adequate RV volume loading with CVP = 15 to 18 mm Hg
- Prevent and treat lung disease/lesions: atelectasis, pneumonia, pulmonary edema
- Pulmonary vasodilators: nitroprusside, nitroglycerin, amrinone/milrinone, PGE_1, NO
- Inotropic support: dobutamine, amrinone/milrinone

RV, right ventricular; CVP, central venous pressure; PGE_1, prostaglandin E_1; NO, nitric oxide.

discharge. One could argue for routine echocardiographic postoperative pericardial effusion surveillance at 2 to 3 weeks and perhaps at 6 weeks.

Pericardial effusions and pericarditis are treated with acetylsalicylic acid (ASA) 325 to 650 mg PO q6h. If the patient is refractory, prednisone 50 to 100 mg PO daily can be added. Frequent echocardiographic surveillance for effusion size is required if the presence of an effusion is identified or if there are pericardial symptoms.

Symptomatic effusions are drained—they should be drained with the patient awake. Sedation or intubation (in order to drain the effusion) can be associated with cardiovascular collapse and death.

Endocarditis prophylaxis is used for 6 months after surgery.

VENTRICULAR SEPTAL DEFECTS

Anatomy

Perimembranous is the most common VSD, although they also occur as muscular, inlet, outlet, or multiple. The presence of a VSD should lead one to look for other lesions such as malposition of the great vessels, coarctation, or hypoplastic ventricles.

Pathophysiology

Patients with VSDs are more likely to develop Eisenmenger syndrome and must therefore be carefully evaluated for suitability of operative therapy. Those patients having small hearts and those who give a history of cyanosis or a history of appearing to improve physiologically in early childhood are likely suffering from irreversible pulmonary vascular disease.

Surgical Indications

- Endocarditis—two episodes of endocarditis are used although even one bout of endocarditis would be an appropriate indication.
- RV outflow obstruction from RV muscle bundles associated with a VSD.
- Ruptured sinus of Valsalva aneurysm—usually associated with an outlet VSD but can also be seen with a perimembranous VSD.
- Associated substantial subaortic stenosis.
- Associated aortic insufficiency (AI)—from leaflet prolapse into the VSD.
- VSDs associated with left heart failure—usually a restrictive VSD that has, over a period, caused left-sided heart dilation. Only a few patients would have Qp:Qs of >2:1.

Interventions

Muscular and small perimembranous defects can now be closed using interventional occluders—usually the Amplatzer nitinol device. Larger defects, inlet defects, and outlet defects must still be closed surgically.

Surgical closure is performed through the right atrium for most lesions. For perimembranous and inlet defects, the conduction tissue leaves the triangle of Koch and runs close to the VSD rim on the rightward side of the defect. Care must be taken to stay away from the edge of the VSD in this region. Closure of outlet defects is best performed through a pulmonary arteriotomy just above the pulmonary valve. Most defects are best repaired employing a patch. Dacron is our material of choice.

Postoperative Management

Intraoperative TEE is performed to ensure there is no significant residual lesion. Specific evaluation sites are the tricuspid valve, the aortic valve, the RV outflow, and the VSD itself looking for residual lesions. Tiny residual lesions are not a problem—usually just a few pixels width on the TEE. Repair of residual lesions with a shunt of >1.2:1.0 is indicated. Shunt fraction is calculated by measuring aortic, right atrial (RA), and pulmonary artery (PA) saturations. An assumption is made that aortic and pulmonary vein saturations are equal. An example calculation is as follows:

$$\text{Aorta} = 100\%$$
$$\text{RA} = 60\%$$
$$\text{PA} = 80\%$$
$$(100 - 60)/(100 - 80) = 2:1. \tag{37.1}$$

For those patients with hemodynamic indications for surgery, a Swan-Ganz catheter would be placed to monitor pulmonary artery pressures and cardiac output. Standard heart failure therapies are used for low cardiac output. Other monitors of cardiac output can also be used, such as pulmonary artery or SVC saturations. Serum lactate level is also useful as a marker of cardiac output.

Poor cardiac output can be caused from poor filling of the left side of the heart—a potential consequence of elevated PVR. This is dealt with by manipulating PVR. Medical maneuvers for lowering PVR are to hyperventilate and raise the pH to around 7.5. Milrinone and nitric oxide can also be useful. For severe problems with filling of the left side of the heart, it may be necessary to create an atrial fenestration as a "pop-off" for left-sided heart filling. In rare cases, the patient may benefit from a VSD fenestration.

Approximately 1% of patients will develop a heart block. Temporary pacing is used until it is determined whether the heart block is permanent. Conduction that does not normalize in 72 hours should be treated as a permanent heart block. A transvenous pacemaker system is then implanted.

PATENT DUCTUS ARTERIOSUS

Indications for Intervention

The indications for intervention are the presence of a patent ductus arteriosus (PDA) and absence of Eisenmenger syndrome. These lesions are closed because of the high risk of endocarditis, volume loading of the left ventricle, and prevention of Eisenmenger syndrome. Most lesions can be closed by catheter occlusion. Large lesions warrant a full pulmonary hypertension study.

Operative Repair

Although the concept is simple, closure can be hazardous because of calcification of the duct. For patients <40 years, who have no evidence of calcification, a standard posterolateral thoracotomy approach is utilized. Division between clamps or triple ligation is used. A calcified duct in a patient is repaired using CPB by a sternotomy approach. Control of the PAs is required at the initiation of bypass so there is not a steal phenomenon. The PA is opened and the duct is occluded by compression or a balloon catheter. If this is not possible, circulatory arrest can be utilized for adequate visualization. The duct is repaired by sewing on a patch from within the pulmonary artery—just as one would do for a VSD.

Postoperative Management

Postoperative management is similar to managing pulmonary hypertension associated with a VSD. Recurrent nerve palsy may occur.

RIGHT TO LEFT SHUNTS

Pathophysiology

Right to left shunts caused by pulmonary stenosis or pulmonary atresia protect the pulmonary vasculature so that pulmonary hypertension is not an issue. Patients are affected by profound cyanosis, which can cause death. Extreme polycythemia can cause strokes. Cerebral abscess may also occur.

Anatomy

The most common anatomic cause of cyanosis in the adult patient is untreated tetralogy of Fallot (TOF). These patients have anterocephalad deviation of the infundibular septum with an associated VSD. The deviation of the infundibular septum causes varying degrees of pulmonary stenosis or atresia. Cyanosis can also be caused by a VSD associated with RV muscle bundle obstruction (a double-chambered RV). Other cyanotic lesions (other than Eisenmenger) presenting in adulthood would most commonly be a form of single ventricle physiology or Ebstein anomaly.

Surgical Indications

Unrepaired TOF should be repaired. Investigation for pulmonary artery size, presence or absence of aortopulmonary collaterals, and coronary anatomy for a left anterior descending (LAD) artery arising from the right coronary artery and crossing the RV outflow should be performed.

Surgical Repair

Repair of "simple" TOF consists of release of RV muscle bundles, VSD closure, pulmonary arterioplasty, and decision making about the management of the pulmonary valve. Valves that can achieve close to normal size with a valvotomy are preserved. If one elects to preserve the valve, RV pressures need to be measured following termination of bypass. RV pressure of less than two thirds that of the systemic is acceptable. If the pressures are greater than two thirds that of the systemic, bypass should be reinstituted and a transannular patch inserted.

Patients who have pulmonary atresia and who survive into adulthood most likely will have multiple aortopulmonary collaterals (MAPCAs). Repair consists of what is know as a unifocalization procedure—connecting all the MAPCAs together to achieve one connected central source of a pulmonary arterial tree so that an RV to new PA connection can be achieved. These procedures may be performed as a single stage by a sternotomy or through staged thoracotomies with staged systemic to pulmonary artery shunts. Approximately two thirds of the segments need to be present and unobstructed in order to achieve complete closure of the VSD. Even with complete unifocalization of all segments, there can be very high pulmonary artery pressure, thereby necessitating a fenestrated VSD.

Perioperative Care

An intraoperative TEE is performed to ensure appropriate residual lesions. Inappropriate residual lesions are corrected before leaving the operating room (OR).

The most common postoperative issue is poor RV function—usually diastolic dysfunction manifested by antegrade flow in the pulmonary arteries with atrial contraction. Management consists of volume loading, minimization of inotropes, and minimization of ventilation pressures. Early extubation is beneficial because negative-pressure ventilation assists pulmonary blood flow. For severe cases of restrictive physiology, draining both pleural spaces and the peritoneum is beneficial. This allows for the lowest airway pressures and best cardiac filling. In patients for whom severe restriction is anticipated, a 4- to 6-mm atrial fenestration can be left in place. This fenestration can be made so that it is adjustable. Those patients with poor cardiac output despite all other maneuvers will likely benefit from an open chest surgery.

Most patients have little trouble following surgery. Routine fluid management with mild volume loading is beneficial. A Swan-Ganz catheter may be quite beneficial. CVP may need to be pushed as high as 15 to 20 mm Hg for severe cases of restriction.

Occasionally, full perfusion of the pulmonary vasculature will result in pulmonary edema. Expectant ventilation and diuretics usually resolve the problem with time.

Pulmonary Valve Implantation for Repaired Tetralogy of Fallot

Up to 10% to 15% of patients having previous repair of TOF develop RV failure manifest by atrial arrhythmias, ventricular tachycardia, QRS complex width of >160 ms, and a dilated poorly functioning RV. These patients require replacement of the pulmonary valve. We have chosen the bioprosthesis method where the valve is implanted, ventricular mapping is sometimes performed, and then arrhythmia pathways are cryoablated, if appropriate. Concomitant tricuspid valve repair is frequently necessary. Atrial arrhythmia surgery may also be needed but is less common. Perioperative care is standard care with early extubation and management of arrhythmias. It is important to operate earlier rather than later on these patients; otherwise the ventricles do not improve but merely stabilize.

Data is now emerging that repair is appropriate when the ventricular volume reaches 160 mL/m^2 by magnetic resonance imaging (MRI) measurement.

COARCTATION OF THE AORTA

Classic coarctation occurs at the site of the ductus arteriosus insertion into the aorta— just distal to the left subclavian artery. There is frequently an associated VSD or a bicuspid aortic valve. Many single ventricle lesions are also associated with coarctation but survival into adulthood would be unusual. Some coarctation is also associated with an abnormally small arch.

Pathophysiology

Adult presentation of coarctation is usually discovered because of hypertension. The consequences of long-standing coarctation include ventricular hypertrophy, vascular aneurysms in the brain or intercostals arteries, endocarditis, and aortic dissection. There can be premature coronary artery disease and the development of end-stage heart disease.

Interventional Indications

Interventional indications are the presence of greater than a 50% narrowing and/or upper to lower limb blood pressure gradient of 20 to 30 mm Hg or more. Exercise gradients are usually substantially higher.

Interventional Approaches

Most adults presenting with discrete coarctation are currently managed by interventional stent implantation. If there is associated arch narrowing or a failed interventional attempt, surgical repair through a left posterolateral thoracotomy is performed. Patients with good distal pulses have well developed collaterals. Repair can be performed at 34°C, and the occurrence of paraplegia is less likely. Arterial pressure proximal to the coarctation should be maintained normotensive or somewhat hypertensive (100 to 140 mm Hg). Patients with poor distal pulses or distal pressures of <70 mm Hg may benefit from femorally based CPB whereby distal perfusion can be maintained above 70 mm Hg and the patient can have controlled cooling to 34°C.

Repair is achieved by resection and an end-to-end anastomosis. Where mobility is insufficient, a Dacron or Gore-Tex tube graft can be inserted.

Those patients needing repair of recoarctation or those who have an associated hypoplastic arch are treated using a median sternotomy approach—usually along with circulatory arrest.

Postoperative Care

Bleeding from enlarged intercostals or chest wall collaterals may be problematic. Reexploration may need to be performed. Insertion of tube thoracostomies may be complicated by further chest wall arterial bleeding.

- Paraplegia occurs in approximately 1%—usually associated with poor collateral development. Intraoperative strategies are important in preventing paraplegia. Good distal perfusion pressures are maintained during recovery. Mild hypertension is better than mild hypotension. CVP approximately 10 mm Hg or less is maintained—to maintain cerebral spinal fluid (CSF) pressure <10 cm Hg. Some have advocated CSF drainage to keep CSF pressure low. Nipride is relatively contraindicated because it may cause "steal" from the spinal cord.
- Postoperative hypertension can cause bleeding, rupture of the suture line, and aortic dissection. Blood pressure is kept under control with esmolol.
- Postcoarctation syndrome: Up to 5% of patients develop abdominal pain, ileus, possible perforation, and pancreatitis caused by mesenteric arteritis. Hypertension should be controlled. The bowel should be rested and observations for an acute abdomen should be done. A nasogastric (NG) tube may be helpful until gut function returns.
- Other complications: Phrenic nerve palsy, chylothorax, and recurrent nerve injury may occur.

EBSTEIN ANOMALY

Anatomy

Ebstein anomaly contains three major components: displacement of the posterior and septal leaflet of the tricuspid valve deep into the ventricular cavity, abnormally thin and poorly functional ventricular muscle, and an ASD. Accessory conduction pathways may coexist. The heart is typically giant on a chest x-ray (CXR)—mostly from right atrial enlargement.

Pathophysiology

Symptoms vary on the basis of the degree of tricuspid insufficiency and or RV outflow obstruction. Patients with little tricuspid insufficiency and no obstruction to RV outflow can be fully saturated and reasonably asymptomatic. Patients with poor functional capacity of the right ventricle may have marked cyanosis and right ventricular failure. Biventricular failure may develop.

Surgical Treatment

Surgery is indicated for major cyanosis or heart failure related to tricuspid insufficiency. Valve repair is achieved by narrowing the annulus so that the large anterior leaflet works as a monocusp. Alternatively, a sliding leaflet plasty along with a ventricular plication and annuloplasty can be performed. The atrial defect is closed. Repair is achieved in 50% to 90% of patients. For those having valve replacement, a tissue valve is used. Mechanical valves are thought to be contraindicated because of problems with valve thrombosis even in the face of adequate anticoagulation. Heart block is avoided by placing the sutures cephalad to Koch triangle and the coronary sinus.

Some patients benefit from volume unloading of the right heart. This allows a tighter annuloplasty and may decrease wall tension on the poorly functioning RV. Volume unloading of approximately 25% can be achieved by performing a concomitant bidirectional cavopulmonary shunt (BCPS). This type of repair is known as a $1\frac{1}{2}$ *ventricle repair*. A BCPS can only be performed if left atrial pressures are low— <10 mm Hg, and if pulmonary artery pressures are less than approximately 15 to 18 mm Hg mean.

Postoperative Management

A Swan-Ganz catheter is utilized. Right ventricular failure is treated by decreasing PVR (pH 7.45–7.50, milrinone, nitric oxide, and minimal mean airway pressure) and by lowering left atrial pressure. All effusions should be drained if the patient is struggling postoperatively. The enlarged right heart can cause compression of the left ventricular outflow tract (LVOT); this can be exacerbated with excessive inotropic use. Increasing systemic vascular resistance with Neosynephrine or vasopressin may be useful in this scenario. In general, these patients can act much like patients with single ventricles— their poor right ventricles function as a weakly pulsatile Fontan.

SINGLE VENTRICLE SURGERY (FONTAN OPERATION)

The Fontan procedure consists of routing all systemic venous blood directly to the pulmonary arteries. The functional single ventricle is the systemic ventricle, it may be either a morphologic right or a left ventricle. The ventricle must not have outlet obstruction, and ventricular function needs to be good as does atrioventricular valve function. See Table 37-4 for relative risks and indications.

Options for managing single ventricles excluding the Fontan procedure include systemic to pulmonary artery shunts and a classic Glenn shunt. The classic Glenn shunt is an SVC to isolated right pulmonary artery (RPA) connection and has considerable long-term consequences of pulmonary arteriovenous fistulas. The systemic to pulmonary

▌ **TABLE 37-4** **Single Ventricle Patient Classification and Procedure Selection for a Fontan**

Parameter	Surgical Risk		
	Low	Intermediate	High
Pulmonary vascular resistance (Woods)	<2	2–3	>3
Mean pulmonary artery pressure (mm Hg)	<15	15–20	>20
Transpulmonary pressure (mm Hg)	<7	7–12	>12
Ventricular end-diastolic pressure (mm Hg)	<6	6–12	>12
Ventricular ejection fraction	>50	40–50	<40
Ventricular outflow tract gradient (mm Hg)	<20	20–30	>30
A-V valve regurgitation	None	Mild	>mod
Surgical option	Fontan	BCPS-SPS ± late Fontan	BCPS-SPS + correct anomalies

BCPS-SPS, bicavopulmonary shunt associated with a systemicopulmonary shunt if arterial saturation is inadequate.

artery shunt causes volume loading of the heart and eventual heart failure. The Fontan circulation volume unloads the heart (although not completely because of collateral formation) and allows full saturation; it, however, requires the single ventricle to work through two capillary resistance beds (systemic and pulmonary). Consequently, over a period, heart failure and arrhythmia may develop.

Fontan Revisions

The early Fontan operations for tricuspid atresia were performed with an atriopulmonary connection and ASD closure. Those patients now have an enlarged right atrium and poor fluid energetics. Many have atrial arrhythmias, which, when left with an uncontrolled rate, can result in poor ventricular function. Additionally, enlarged atria can hold thrombi that may cause pulmonary emboli.

Patients with good ventricular function but declining exercise capacity, and those who have significant problems with atrial flutter and/or fibrillation, are candidates for an atrial arrhythmia surgery (maze) and conversion to a more energy-efficient lateral tunnel or extracardiac Fontan. These patients should have a preoperative electrophysiology study to determine the value and the type of arrhythmia surgery needed.

Those patients having complex previous palliative procedures, including the classic Glenn, associated with pulmonary arteriovenous malformations, may also benefit from conversion to a modern type of Fontan connection. See Table 37-4 for selection criteria.

Operative Issues

Standard redo sternotomy techniques are used. Bicaval cannulation is performed. An aortic cross clamp is used for the intracardiac portion of the revision. Once the maze is completed the cross clamp is removed. A 22 to 24 mm Gore-Tex connection is created between the IVC and the undersurface of the RPA. The SVC is transected and a BCPS is performed. Permanent biventricular epicardial pacing wires may need to be placed. Pulmonary artery obstructions are resolved.

Any valve repair or replacement that might need to be performed is also achieved.

Postoperative Care

The postoperative care operations are long and tedious. Bleeding can be very excessive. A great deal of patience and perseverance needs to be applied to stop the bleeding with various blood products. A rule of thumb that is more often correct than not is the following: For each hour of pump time an hour should be allocated to stop the bleeding. Aprotinin may be helpful, but mostly it is the meticulous mechanical hemostasis along with the generous use of blood products that achieves control of bleeding. It is imperative that there is good hemostasis—tamponade will be very poorly tolerated. Even mild compression from mediastinal clots may be devastating to hemodynamics.

It is not possible to achieve measurement of cardiac output. We use a TEE to assess function and then monitor right-sided filling pressures with a central line. The CVP usually needs to be 15 to 20 mm Hg for the first 12 to 48 hours. SVC saturations are a useful marker of systemic blood flow. We prefer to see SVC saturation levels of 60 or above, assuming arterial saturation levels of 90% and more.

Inotropic support is usually needed. Milrinone is our first choice followed by dopamine up to 10 mics/kg/minute. Epinephrine and norepinephrine may also be indicated. We prefer to start the dosage at 1.0 mics/kg/minute. Occasionally, these patients become hyperdynamic and have too low a systemic vasodilator response (SVR). In that situation, we use vasopressin starting at 0.0001 mics/kg/minute.

Management of ventilations is, as previously described, to minimize PVR. Drainage of both pleural spaces and even the peritoneum is useful. Early extubation may increase cardiac output because of the respiratory assist to pulmonary blood flow and subsequently left heart filling.

Those patients with poor hemodynamics should have an atrial fenestration created at the time of repair. It should be adjustable but measuring up to 5 to 7 mm in size, which allows direct filling of the left heart at the expense of mild cyanosis. The fenestration can be closed at a later time.

Intermediate Postoperative Care

We fully anticoagulate our patients undergoing Fontan until the fenestration is closed. Thereafter, it is not clear whether there should be antiplatelet therapy, full anticoagulation, or no anticoagulation at all. Our choice is at least for some anticoagulation.

Patients need to be followed for heart failure, arrhythmia, and the formation of clots in the Fontan circuit.

HYPERTROPHIC OBSTRUCTIVE CARDIOMYOPATHY

Anatomy/Histology

Abnormal unexplained segmental myocardial hypertrophy is usually marked at the septum, immediately below the aortic valve. There is a large genetic predisposition: 55% of patients have autosomal dominant transmission.

Histologically, the septal myocardium is characterized by disarray of the alignment of the myocytes. This is associated with abnormal intimal and medial thickening of intramyocardial coronaries.

Pathophysiology

Subvalvar dynamic obstruction is due to septal hypertrophy and narrowing of the outflow tract of the left ventricle (LV) (and rarely in the RV) resulting in flow acceleration and a pressure gradient. The flow acceleration pulls the mitral valve (usually the anterior leaflet) toward the septum in late systole (systolic anterior motion [SAM]) thereby aggravating the obstruction and producing mitral regurgitation (MR). MR develops in late systole as the anterior mitral leaflet moves toward the ventricular septum. Following myectomy, the MR is minimal unless there is the presence of concomitant mitral valve disease.

Increases in contractility, reduction in preload, and vasodilation decrease ventricular volume and promote SAM.

There is markedly reduced diastolic compliance with high filling pressures.

LV function is usually supranormal, with an ejection fraction (EF) >80%. LV failure occurs late in the course of the disease and is a result of a myocardial infarction (MI) and/or severe MR.

Surgical Indications

Patients who are intolerant to medical treatment or with incapacitating symptoms, despite optimal treatment with an LVOT gradient >50 mm Hg under resting conditions of >80 mm Hg provoked with amyl nitrate, isoproterenol, or postextrasystolic beat with a septal thickness >18 mm, should undergo myectomy.

Young patients with atrial fibrillation and patients thought to be high risk for sudden death can also benefit from myectomy. Risk factors for sudden death include markedly increased LV wall thickness and mass, "malignant" family history, syncope, ischemia, survivors of a sudden death episode, slow burst of asymptomatic ventricular tachycardia on Holter monitor, and inducible sustained ventricular arrhythmia on electrophysiologic testing.

Surgical Procedure

Preoperative TEE is performed to determine the depth and length of the septal muscle resection needed to alleviate the obstruction completely.

A generous transverse aortotomy and delicate retraction of the aortic valve allows the hypertrophic septum to be visualized beneath the right coronary cusp.

The first incision of the septal myectomy is 2 to 3 mm to the right of the center of the right coronary cusp and directed toward the ventricular apex. The second incision is made 2 mm from the lateral fibrous trigone, below the commissure between the right and left coronary cups, and runs parallel to the first incision. The third incision is placed approximately 2 to 3 mm below the aortic annulus and joins the other two incisions. The depth of the incisions is calculated such that the resulting septal thickness is approximately 8 mm thick.

Postoperative TEE can measure the septal thickness precisely; identify a residual LVOT obstruction, SAM, and MR; or detect iatrogenic AI or VSD.

Postoperative Management

General Recommendations

- Monitoring: Swan-Ganz catheter.
- Maintain preload: diastolic pulmonary artery pressure (PAP) of wedge >18 mm Hg: colloid solution or blood products (targeted Hb = 100 g/L).
- Avoid peripheral vasodilation: (e.g., nitrates).
- Avoid inotropes: if hypotensive despite adequate preload, administer a vasopressor (e.g., phenylephrine).
- Tachycardia and hypertension are treated with β-blockers.

Dysrhythmias

- Postoperative left bundle branch block (LBBB) occurs in 45% of patients; 1% to 2% require a permanent pacemaker.

▌**TABLE 37-5** Postoperative Antiarrhythmic Medications—Hypertrophic Obstructive Cardiomyopathy Patients

Accepted	Controversial/Avoided
β-Blockers	Verapamil
Disopyramide	Digitalis
Amiodarone	

- Rapid atrial fibrillation should be treated with metoprolol 5 mg intravenously (IV) given for 5 to 10 minutes, and repeated twice at 15 minute intervals, if needed. Specific antiarrhythmic medications should be used cautiously (see Table 37-5).
- If unstable, electrical cardioversion should be attempted immediately.
- If atrial fibrillation persists for more than 24 hours, begin a continuous heparin infusion and attempt electrical cardioversion once anticoagulated. If cardioversion is successful, begin sotolol 40 to 80 mg PO b.i.d. If unsuccessful, warfarin is begun.

Prophylaxis

Rapid atrial fibrillation during the immediate postoperative period is common. Therefore, postoperative prophylaxis is recommended, with Sotalol 40 mg PO b.i.d. in the morning following surgery, which may be increased to 80 mg t.i.d. if heart rate (HR) is >80 beats/minute at rest.

SUGGESTED READINGS

Dearani JA, Danielson GK. Congenital heart surgery nomenclature and database project: Ebstein's anomaly and tricuspid valve disease. *Ann Thorac Surg*. 2000;69(Suppl. 4):S106–S117.

Gatzoulis MA, Balaji S, Webber SA, et al. Risk factors for arrhythmia and sudden cardiac death late after repair of tetralogy of Fallot: a multicenter study. *Lancet*. 2000;356:975–981.

Gatzoulis MA, Freeman MA, Siu SC, et al. Atrial arrhythmia after surgical closure of atrial septal defects in adults. *N Engl J Med*. 1999;340:839–846.

Mavroudis C, Deal BJ, Backer CL. The beneficial effects of total cavopulmonary conversion and arrhythmia surgery for the failed Fontan. *Semin Thorac Cardiovasc Surg Pediatr Card Annu*. 2002; 5:12–24.

Chapter 38

Ventricular Reconstruction or Aneurysm Resection for Ischemic Cardiomyopathy

Lynda L. Mickleborough

The treatment of ischemic heart disease continues to be a challenge with an ever-increasing patient population presenting with congestive heart failure. In patients with coronary artery disease and a previous infarct, the necrotic muscle is replaced by a fibrous tissue, and if the infarct is large enough, an area of akinesis or dyskinesis develops. To compensate for loss of contractile function of the infarcted segment the ventricle dilates and undergoes adverse remodeling. Depending on the extent of scarring and other factors, the infarcted area may undergo significant thinning.

We define a ventricular aneurysm as an akinetic or dyskinetic area of the ventricle resulting from previous infarction, with subsequent scarring and some degree of thinning that, in our opinion, makes the area suitable for resection. The scarred area may involve, to a variable extent, the free wall of the left ventricle and/or the septum. The goal of surgical therapy in these patients should be not only to prevent ongoing ischemia but also to minimize the negative effects of the infarct on ventricular structure and function.

DIAGNOSIS

Areas of akinesis or dyskinesis can be identified by echocardiography or on a ventriculogram. At the present time, magnetic resonance imaging (MRI) is the best method to identify areas of significant thinning of the ventricular free wall suitable for reconstruction. Extent of thinning or aneurysmal bulging of the septum can also be reliably assessed with this technique. Coronary angiograms are required to define the coronary anatomy. Echocardiographic assessment for possible mitral regurgitation should be done.

INDICATIONS FOR SURGERY

Surgery may be indicated for control of symptoms due to congestive heart failure, ventricular arrhythmias, ongoing ischemia, or systemic emboli (associated with ventricular thrombus). In addition, surgery may be indicated in asymptomatic patients if there is critical coronary anatomy, or if progressive ventricular dilatation or mitral insufficiency can be demonstrated on serial examinations over time.

OPERATIVE TECHNIQUE

There are several approaches currently recommended for surgical reconstruction of the scarred left ventricle. The following is a brief outline of our approach. Familiarity with normal ventricular size and geometry is essential for obtaining good results with this technique.

The decision whether or not to perform free wall resection or patch exclusion of the septum is made on the basis of preoperative studies. At surgery, with the heart supported on cardiopulmonary bypass, an incision is made in the scarred area parallel to the infarct vessel. If an endocardial clot is present, it is carefully removed before the insertion of a ventricular vent. In the beating heart, regional wall motion and viability can be assessed by finger palpation of the surrounding wall. The extent of resection of the nonfunctioning wall is tailored to restore left ventricular cavity size and shape toward normal as much as possible while ensuring that an adequate diastolic volume remains in the cavity resulting from the modified linear closure. If the septum is thinned or aneurysmal, this part of the ventricle is excluded with a septal patch (glutaraldehyde fixed bovine pericardium), which is incorporated anteriorly into the modified linear closure. The free wall defect is then closed with 2-0 polypropylene mattress sutures buttressed with Teflon felt strips. By taking wide bites on the ventricular wall and narrow bites on the felt, the length of the incision is plicated in the closure, which helps to restore ventricular shape toward normal. A second continuous layer of the same suture is applied to ensure hemostasis. Revascularization of the proximal left anterior descending artery and all other diseased vessels is then carried out under cardioplegic arrest. Mitral valve replacement or repair is performed, if indicated.

CONSIDERATIONS IN PATIENTS WITH VENTRICULAR ARRHYTHMIAS

In patients with clinical or inducible ventricular arrhythmias, additional surgical maneuvers are taken to reduce the risk of arrhythmias or sudden death during follow-up. At surgery, any areas of homogeneous septal scar are excised (2 to 3 mm deep), and overlapping cryolesions are applied at the periphery of the excision. If the septum is significantly thinned, a patch septoplasty is carried out.

POSTOPERATIVE CARE

Most of these patients have congestive heart failure preoperatively and are on a number of medications. All patients require careful perioperative monitoring including use of a Swan-Ganz catheter. In the early postoperative period, patients undergoing ventricular reconstruction require a rapid heart rate and increased filling pressures to maintain an adequate cardiac output. Inotropic or intra-aortic balloon pump support is often needed for 1 or 2 days. Temporary pacing may be required, and atrioventricular sequential pacing is superior to ventricular pacing alone. As the heart adapts to the repair procedure, diuresis can be started to get rid of excess fluid without compromising cardiac output. The aim should be to get the patient as dry as possible without compromising renal function before discharge. Signs of ventricular irritability should be observed, and anything more than unifocal premature ventricular contraction is treated aggressively with intravenous amiodarone. On the second or third postoperative day, angiotensin converting enzyme inhibitors are started and dosage is adjusted while monitoring renal function. A postoperative echocardiogram should be performed (at 1 week) to rule out ventricular thrombus associated with the repair. If thrombus is seen, anticoagulation for 3 months is recommended.

Patients who were on amiodarone before surgery are at increased risk for acute respiratory distress syndrome. To avoid this potentially lethal complication, keep patients on the lowest fraction of inspired oxygen (FIO_2) needed to maintain adequate oxygenation postoperatively; vigorous diuresis is done as soon as possible. Daily chest x-rays are indicated, and if there is any suspicion of pulmonary infection, early and aggressive treatment is recommended.

Upon discharge, these patients should be followed closely in a heart failure clinic to ensure optimal adjustment of medical therapy. Changes in drug dosages are often required, particularly in the first 3 months as the heart and circulation adjust to the reconstruction procedure.

OUTCOMES

We recently reported the results achieved with our approach for left ventricular reconstruction in 285 patients with akinesia or dyskinesia. Preoperatively, 83% were in symptom class III or IV, with congestive heart failure in 61%, angina in 55%, and ventricular tachycardia (VT) in 38%. The average preoperative ejection fraction was 24%. Patch septoplasty was an important part of the reconstruction procedure in 22%. Additional operative procedures included coronary artery bypass graft in 92%, ablation of VT in 41%, and a mitral valve procedure in 2%. Perioperative support included intra-aortic balloon pumping in 17% and inotropic drugs in 54%. Improvement in symptom class was documented in 67% of the survivors. Ventricular reconstruction resulted in a significant increase in ejection fraction and a significant decrease in ventricular volumes (end-diastolic and end-systolic). MRI assessment documents a more normal ventricular shape after the procedure. Survival at 1 and 5 years was 92% and 82% respectively. During follow-up, nine patients needed an automatic implantable cardioverter defibrillator (AICD). Freedom from sudden death at 1 and 5 years was 99% and 97%, respectively.

Our experience demonstrates that in select patients, ventricular reconstruction using a modified linear closure technique combined with patch septoplasty, when indicated, can be done in the beating heart with low mortality. The procedure is associated with objective evidence of improved ventricular function and provides good symptomatic relief and excellent 5-year survival.

SUGGESTED READINGS

Athanasuleas CL, Stanley AW, Buckberg GD, et al. Surgical anterior ventricular endocardial restoration (SAVER) for dilated ischemic cardiomyopathy. *Semin Thorac Cardiovasc Surg.* 2001; 13:448–458.

Dor V, Saab M, Coste P, et al. Left ventricular aneurysm: a new surgical approach. *J Thorac Cardiovasc Surg.* 1989;37:11–19.

Mickleborough LL, Maruyama H, Mohammed S, et al. Are patients receiving amiodarone at increased risk for cardiac operations? *Ann Thorac Surg.* 1994;58:622–629.

Mickleborough LL, Merchant N, Ivanov J, et al. Left ventricular reconstruction: early and late results. *J Thorac Cardiovasc Surg.* 2004;128:27–37.

Implantable Cardioverter Defibrillator and Pacemaker Insertion

Raymond Yee and Jonathan Prychitko

In 1997, an estimated 164,000 new cardiac pacemakers (permanent pacemakers [PPMs]) and 29,000 new implantable cardioverter defibrillators (ICDs) were implanted in patients in North America. Expanding indications have likely increased the number of persons presenting for implantation of these devices since then, and the volume will continue to grow. Therefore, physicians will inevitably encounter these arrhythmia management devices in the course of their work and need to be familiar with the basic principles of their function and about how to treat patients who will receive, or have already received, these devices. This chapter provides the reader with a basic understanding of pacemakers and ICDs, methods for device implantation, and management strategies for patients with devices that are undergoing noncardiac procedures.

PACEMAKER AND IMPLANTABLE CARDIOVERTER DEFIBRILLATOR COMPONENTS

Pacemaker or ICD systems consist of two basic hardware components: generator and lead(s). The generator contains the lithium battery energy source, electronic components, and software that allow the device to perform its programmed functions, components that store information about cardiac events that occurred, and therapies that have been delivered by the device during follow-up. For the generator to deliver therapy to the heart, the generator must be connected to the myocardium by one or more leads. Most leads are designed for implant in the right atrium or ventricle although newer leads have been developed for coronary vein implantation for left ventricular pacing. A lead is covered in polyurethane or silicone insulation except at the distal end where electrodes make contact with the myocardium and the proximal end that plugs into the generator.

Leads possess either passive or active fixation mechanisms that help resist dislodgment of the lead tip until fibrotic tissue envelops the lead–endocardium interface (see Fig. 39-1). Passive fixation leads have short soft barbs that hook onto existing trabeculae or chordae and require no active manipulation to achieve fixation (Fig. 39-1A). Active fixation leads possess a helix (screw) that is driven into the endocardium and holds the lead in position (Fig. 39-1B). Active fixation leads possess a helix or screw at the tip, which requires the physician to actively rotate into the endocardial tissue.

A unipolar lead has a single electrode, and the generator serves as the second electrode to complete the electrical circuit. A bipolar lead has two closely spaced electrodes, and

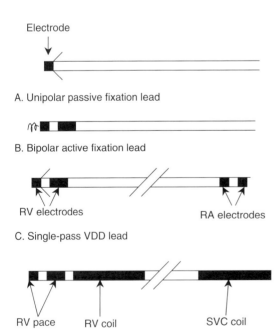

A. Unipolar passive fixation lead

B. Bipolar active fixation lead

RV electrodes
RA electrodes

C. Single-pass VDD lead

RV pace   RV coil   SVC coil

D. ICD quadripolar lead

FIGURE 39-1. Lead types. VDD, ventricular pacing; SVC, superior vena cava; ICD, implantable cardioverter defibrillators.

electricity flows between them. Historically, unipolar leads have a greater risk of skeletal or diaphragmatic muscle stimulation and recording skeletal muscle and electromagnetic noise in the environment than bipolar leads. Bipolar leads are more popular, but some physicians favor unipolar leads because the pacing stimulus artifact is more easily seen on electrocardiogram (ECG) and the minimum energy required to excite (capture) myocardium or "pacing threshold" tends to be slightly lower. Unipolar and bipolar leads can be implanted in the atrium or ventricle. There is also a special quadripolar lead (four electrodes) known as a "single-pass" lead where the two distal electrodes are placed in the right ventricle and the two proximal electrodes rest in the right atrium (Fig. 39-1C). This single lead permits both cardiac chambers to be included in a dual chamber pacemaker system.

ICD leads differ from PPM leads in that they possess one or two additional long coil electrodes used for delivering shocks. When positioned properly, one coil rests in the right ventricle while the second is located in the superior vena cava (Fig. 39-1D).

The device settings of all modern PPM or ICD are set or changed using a computer programmer, which has a wired programmer wand that is placed on the skin overlying the generator and communicates with it by radiofrequency transmissions.

PRINCIPLES OF PERMANENT PACEMAKER AND IMPLANTABLE CARDIOVERTER DEFIBRILLATOR FUNCTION

Pacemakers are used primarily to treat patients with bradycardias and increase the cardiac rate by delivering small amounts of electrical energy (microjoules) to excite myocardial tissue. They are commonly referred to as low-voltage devices. In contrast, ICDs are intended for patients in whom life-threatening ventricular tachyarrhythmias occur or for patients who are at risk for sudden cardiac death from ventricular fibrillation (VF). Modern ICDs contain many of the functions of a PPM but have the added capability to deliver high-energy shocks to cardiovert or defibrillate and are referred to as high-voltage devices. Implantable atrial defibrillators and pacemakers that contain pacing algorithms to prevent and pace-terminate atrial tachycardias or flutter have also been developed, although relatively few patients have received them.

PPMs and ICDs must be able to perform two basic functions: sense the intrinsic cardiac rhythm of the patient and deliver electrical therapy (pacing or shocks) when required. During the patient's spontaneous rhythm, myocardial depolarization generates an electrogram signal that is conducted by the lead to the generator where it is processed and interpreted by the device's software algorithms. The devices measure the electrogram rate in each chamber sensed and withhold or deliver pacing or shock therapies depending on the programmed settings. Newer ICDs are also able to analyze the electrogram morphology to try to differentiate ventricular from supraventricular tachycardias.

PACEMAKER AND IMPLANTABLE CARDIOVERTER DEFIBRILLATOR TYPES

Various types of PPMs exist that can be programmed in a number of different modes. A single chamber device delivers electrical therapy to one cardiac chamber (atrium or ventricle), and only one lead is required. A dual chamber device encompasses the

▶ **TABLE 39-1 NASPE/BPEG Generic (NBG) Pacemaker Code (Revised 2000)**

Chamber Paced	Chamber Sensed	Response to Sensing	Rate Modulation	Multisite Pacing
A—atrium	A—atrium	T—triggered	R—rate modulation	A—atrium
V—ventricle	V—ventricle	I—inhibited	O—none	V—ventricle
D—dual (atrium and ventricle)	D—dual (atrium and ventricle)	D—dual (triggered and inhibited)		D—dual (atrium and ventricle)
O—none	O—none	O—none		O—none

right atrium and right ventricle. Two separate leads are usually necessary, but a single-pass lead may be sufficient in certain patients. Recently, devices were introduced that pace three chambers (atrium and both ventricles); these are called *biventricular* or cardiac resynchronization therapy (CRT) devices. These devices are intended for treatment of specific patients with congestive heart failure.

To convey information about the capabilities of different PPM or ICD types or the programmed operating mode, a standardized device coding system was established and has been modified as technology progressed. Table 39-1 shows the coding scheme for PPMs. The four-letter coding scheme is most commonly used (e.g., DDDR or VVIR), but there is provision for up to five-letter coding. The first and second letters of the code denote the cardiac chamber paced and sensed, respectively. The third letter indicates the device's response to a sensed electrogram, whereas the fourth letter denotes whether the device is capable of pacing rate variation in response to various sensors in the device (rate-responsive or rate-adaptive behavior). For example, a VVIR device paces and senses only the ventricle and, if a spontaneous beat occurs in the ventricle, the device inhibits or withholds pacing therapy. In brief, it is a ventricular-demand pacemaker with rate-response capability. A similar coding system was developed for ICDs but is not commonly used. Currently, ICD types are mostly referred to as single chamber-, dual chamber- or CRT-ICDs (atrial and biventricular), but this simple classification may change with time.

The choice of the device type or pacing mode that is offered to a patient depends upon the bradycardia indication, functional status of the patient, comorbidities, and expected longevity of the patient, but the incremental benefit of a dual chamber pacemaker must be weighed against the greater cost and complexity. Randomized clinical trials (e.g., Canadian Trial of Physiologic Pacing [CTOPP], Mode Selection Trial [MOST], and United Kingdom Pacing and Cardiovascular Events [UKPACE] Trials) have showed no difference in mortality, stroke, or quality of life between DDD and VVI pacemakers in patients with sinus node dysfunction or aortic valve (AV) block. However, DDD pacemakers reduce the incidence of atrial fibrillation in patients with bradycardia after pacemaker implantation.

In general, if the problem is sinus node dysfunction but AV node conduction is intact, AAIR pacing mode may be preferable although the risk of patients developing high-grade AV block on follow-up and requiring upgrade to a DDDR pacemaker is approximately 1% annually. Because of this possibility, some physicians prefer to directly use a DDDR pacemaker. For patients with permanent atrial fibrillation and impaired AV conduction, VVIR pacing is the choice. If a patient has AV block but sinus node function is intact, a VDD pacemaker (senses the atrium and paces the ventricle synchronously) is sufficient because atrial pacing is not required. In a situation where both sinus node and AV conduction are impaired, a DDDR pacemaker is desirable, especially in patients with noncompliant left ventricles or in those who exhibit symptoms and signs of pacemaker syndrome when ventricular paced. In principle, dual chamber pacing to maintain AV synchrony is preferred in all patients, but it is recognized that many patients may not appreciate any benefit compared to VVIR pacing. It must also be noted that recent studies (The Dual Chamber and VVI Implantable Defibrillator [DAVID] Trial DAVID and MOST sub-study) suggest that chronic right ventricular apical pacing may increase mortality and heart failure risk because of abnormal ventricular activation sequence. Therefore, an important principle is to minimize the amount of ventricular pacing the patient experiences when ventricular pacing is not essential.

PACEMAKER AND IMPLANTABLE CARDIOVERTER DEFIBRILLATOR INDICATIONS

Evidence-based professional guidelines governing the clinical indications for pacemaker and ICD implantation have been published, and the reader is advised to consult these publications for a detailed description of various indications (see Suggested Readings). Device indications are divided into three classes (see Table 39-2). Class I are those indications for which there is strong scientific evidence or general agreement in favor of device therapy. Class II indications are those where evidence or opinion is conflicting and is subdivided into A or B subgroups on the basis of the degree of consensus. Class III constitutes those conditions for which there is evidence or agreement that a device is not useful or may be harmful.

Pacemakers are most commonly implanted for documented and symptomatic bradycardia due to sinus node dysfunction and advanced AV block. There are also some conditions where PPM is recommended even though the bradycardia is mild or asymptomatic but progression to severe or symptomatic bradycardia is likely (e.g., second degree Mobitz type 2 AV block). Pacing for hypertrophic cardiomyopathy and medically refractory vasovagal syncope remain controversial. However, an emerging use for pacing therapy is in patients with New York Heart Association (NYHA) class II-III congestive heart failure, left ventricular systolic dysfunction (ejection fraction $\leq 30\%$ to 35%), and who have significant intraventricular conduction delay on the electrocardiogram (ECG) (QRS ≤ 120 msec). Biventricular or CRT pacing in these patients appears to improve symptoms and functional capacity, but there is currently no evidence that CRT pacing alters mortality.

ICDs are intended for patients at risk for sudden cardiac death secondary to ventricular tachyarrhythmias (see Table 39-3). Survivors of cardiac arrest, VF, or hemodynamically unstable ventricular tachycardia episodes without identifiable reversible cause (e.g., acute myocardial ischemia, hypokalemia) have the greatest risk, and ICDs are indicated as secondary prevention (Antiarrythmics Versus Implantable Defibrillator [AVID] Study, Canadian Implantable Defrillator Study [CIDS], and Cardiac Arrest Study Hamburg [CASH] Trials). Randomized clinical trials have also shown that ICDs improve survival in patients with left ventricular (LV) ejection fraction <30%, but without prior

▌TABLE 39-2 **Common Indications for Permanent Pacemaker Implantation**

Class I	*Class IIA*	*Class IIB*
Sinus node dysfunction		
Sinus node disease causing symptomatic bradycardia or chronotropic incompetence	Unexplained recurrent syncope in patients with abnormal sinus node function measurements on electrophysiologic testing	Minimally symptomatic patients with heart rates of <40 bpm while awake
Acquired atrioventricular block		
Third-degree and advanced second-degree AV block in the following settings: • Symptoms OR ≥ 3.0 s asystole OR • Asymptomatic patients with escape rate <40 bpm while awake. • Following catheter ablation of the AV junction. • AV block not expected to resolve after cardiac surgery. • Neuromuscular diseases.	Asymptomatic third-degree block with average awake ventricular rate 40 bpm or greater (especially with LV dysfunction or cardiomegaly)	Marked first degree AV block causing heart failure. Neuromuscular diseases with any degree of AV block, with or without symptoms
Others		
	Markedly symptomatic vasovagal syncope patients with documented spontaneous or head-up tilt test provoked bradycardia Biventricular pacing in NYHA class III or class IV heart failure patients, QRS width ≥55 mm, LV end diastolic dimension	Medically refractory, symptomatic hypertrophic cardiomyopathy with LV outflow tract obstruction

bpm, beats per minute; AV, aortic valve; LV, left ventricle; NYHA, New York Heart Association.

history of ventricular arrhythmias (Multicenter Automatic Defibrillator Implantation Trial [MADIT] II and Sudden Cardiac Death in Heart Failure Trial [SCD-HeFT]). ICD therapy may also be considered as primary prophylaxis in high-risk patients with rare conditions such as hereditary repolarization syndromes (Long QT syndrome, Brugada syndrome) and hypertrophic cardiomyopathy with a family history of sudden death.

PACEMAKERS AND IMPLANTABLE CARDIOVERTER DEFIBRILLATOR IMPLANTATION PROCEDURES

Implant Setting

Devices are commonly implanted in the operating room suite, but there has been a gradual trend in performing the implant procedure in special procedure rooms,

▌TABLE 39-3 Common Indications for Implantable Cardioverter Defibrillators

Class I	Class IIA
Cardiac arrest due to VF or VT without a transient or reversible cause	Patients ≥30 d post-myocardial infarction or >90 d postrevascularization surgery with LVEF <30%
Spontaneous VT associated with structural heart disease	
Syncope of undetermined origin with clinical and hemodynamically significant VF or VT at electrophysiologic study where drug therapy is ineffective or not preferred	
Nonsustained VT in patients with coronary disease, prior MI, LV dysfunction, and inducible VF or VT at electrophysiologic study not suppressible by a Class I antiarrhythmic drug	
Spontaneous VT in patients with structurally normal hearts not amenable to other therapies	

VF, ventricular fibrillation; VT, ventricular tachycardia; LVEF, left ventricular ejection fraction; MI, myocardial infarction.
Adapted from Gregoratos G, Abrams J, Epstein AE, et al. ACC/AHA/NASPE 2002 guideline update for implantation of cardiac pacemakers and antiarrhythmia devices: summary article: a report of the American College of Cardiology/American Heart Association Task Force on Practice Guidelines (ACC/AHA/NASPE Committee to Update the 1998 Pacemaker Guidelines). *Circulation.* 2002;106:2145–2161.

cardiac catheterization or electrophysiology laboratories. This trend coincides with the increasing number of devices being implanted by cardiologists instead of surgeons. Implant rooms must be equipped with fluoroscopic x-ray equipment and an x-ray-lucent table. Patients also need to have ECG and oxygen saturation monitored during the procedure and should be attached to a transthoracic pacing and a defibrillation unit.

Patient Preparation

Like other operative procedures, patients arrive for device implantation in the postabsorptive state. Oral anticoagulants need to be discontinued and high-risk patients should be converted to intravenous heparin or low-molecular-weight heparin before the procedure. An intravenous access line must be *in situ* and is useful for administering sedative drugs and antibiotics but can also be used to infuse contrast dye to assess patency and location of the subclavian or cephalic vein. An intra-arterial line for monitoring blood pressure is often inserted for patients undergoing ICD implantation. Prophylactic intravenous antibiotics should be given to patients where indicated by clinical practice guidelines (e.g., valvular heart disease), but their routine use in all patients is controversial.

Sedation and Anesthesia

Infiltration of the venous access and pocket sites with local anesthetic agents is usually sufficient to keep the patient comfortable during implantation. For mature, cooperative adult patients undergoing PPM implantation, small doses of intravenous sedative and analgesic drugs (e.g., midazolam and fentanyl) may be given to relieve anxiety. Children, adolescents, and uncooperative patients may require larger doses of sedative agents or general anesthesia. ICD implantation is similar to PPM implantation, but deeper sedation (e.g., propafol or larger doses of midazolam combined with fentanyl) is required before testing the ICD where VF is induced and defibrillation is performed.

Implant Site

In infants or small children and patients with mechanical prosthetic tricuspid valves, PPM and ICD systems are usually implanted in the abdominal wall with leads applied directly to the epicardial surface. Virtually all other patients have devices implanted in the left or right infraclavicular region with transvenous leads fixed to the endocardial surface. Devices are typically implanted contralateral to the dominant hand of the patient.

Implant Procedure

Device implantation involves several fundamental steps:

- Securing venous access for the leads.
- Creating the generator pocket.
- Inserting and anchoring the lead(s) in place.
- Connecting the generator and lead(s) before closing the incision.

Venous Access

One commonly used method for accessing the vein is percutaneous needle puncture with the subclavian vein being the most commonly targeted vein. Other veins such as an external jugular, internal jugular, or ileofemoral have been used. The infraclavicular approach is most frequently used to reach the subclavian vein although a supraclavicular technique has also been described. In the infraclavicular technique, the intrathoracic segment of the subclavian vein is usually targeted (see Fig. 39-2). A variant of the infraclavicular approach involves puncturing the extrathoracic segment of the subclavian vein before it passes between the clavicle and first rib; this is called the *axillary vein approach*. Once punctured, a guidewire is inserted to maintain access to the vein. This process can be repeated for each lead to be inserted although some physicians prefer to insert all leads through a single vein puncture. If there is any difficulty finding the subclavian vein, contrast dye can be injected through the intravenous line to visualize it. The other vein-access method involves cutdown onto the cephalic vein, ligating the distal end and introducing the lead through a venotomy. Cephalic veins vary in diameter and small veins may only accommodate a single lead; subclavian vein puncture may be required for any other leads.

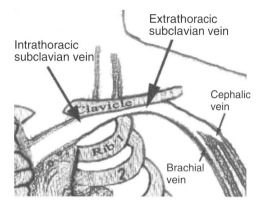

FIGURE 39-2. The course of the subclavian vein as it passes between the clavicle and first rib.

Generator Pocket Creation

After securing venous access, the pacemaker pocket is created proximate to the venous access site. Some physicians prefer to make a horizontal incision inferior to the clavicle (see Fig. 39-3). Others use a more lateral diagonal incision following the delta-pectoral groove, especially when the same incision is also used for the cephalic vein cutdown approach. Rarely, cosmetic considerations require the incision and pocket be made in a more concealed location such as under the breast. This requires the lead to be tunneled subcutaneously to the pocket. The incision is carried down to the prepectoral fascia where a subcutaneous pocket is then created overlying the pectoralis major muscle. The lateral margin of the pocket should not be extended to the anterior axillary line because a more lateral generator pocket can hinder arm movement and cause patient discomfort. A submuscular pocket is preferred where the device size or insufficient subcutaneous tissue over the pocket increases the risk of pocket erosion. The pectoral muscle can be split along the axis of the muscle fibers and a pocket created between the pectoralis major and minor muscles. With the more lateral pocket incision, it is possible to dissect around the lateral margin of the pectoralis major muscle.

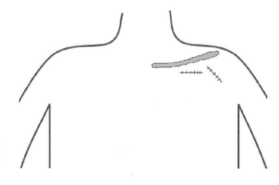

FIGURE 39-3. Potential location of device pocket and incisions.

Lead Implantation

With the percutaneous puncture technique, an introducer sheath is passed over the guidewire and the lead advanced through the sheath lumen. Leads are packaged with wire stylets that can be inserted down the central lead lumen. Stylets can be manually shaped into varying curves to help direct the pacemaker lead tip to the desired site. The pacing leads are guided into position using fluoroscopy and fixated in place. The most common locations for implanting leads are the right atrial appendage and right ventricular apex, but there is currently debate about the optimal pacing sites in the atrial and ventricular chambers. Newer leads have been developed for placement in the coronary veins through the coronary sinus to pace the left ventricle. Once lead fixation is achieved, electrical measurements are taken to confirm adequate and stable contact with the myocardium. The pacing threshold (the minimum amplitude of electrical voltage necessary to excite myocardium) and the electrogram size of the intrinsic myocardial systole are measured. When the right ventricle is paced, it is important to ensure that paced QRS complexes on the surface ECG display left bundle branch block morphology. Once adequate implant locations are achieved, sutures are tied tightly around the anchoring sleeve on the lead and then anchored to the pectoral fascia. The proximal lead ends are connected to the generator and the entire system is inserted into the pocket. For ICDs, defibrillation efficacy is assessed usually by inducing VF and testing the amount of electrical energy required to terminate the episode. The programmer wand placed over the generator directs the ICD to induce VF by rapid ventricular pacing or low energy T-wave shocks. Once induced, defibrillation shocks are delivered by the device. If the device fails to defibrillate, the patient can be rescued by a transthoracic shock. A minimum of two VF episodes is usually induced. Enough time should be allowed between VF inductions to permit stabilization of cerebral, cardiovascular, and hemodynamic functions (minimum of 3 to 5 minutes). If defibrillation efficacy is judged to be inadequate, programming adjustment may be implemented, or additional leads (including a subcutaneous lead on the left chest) might be implanted. Once testing is completed, the generator is anchored to the fascia by a suture to prevent migration, following which the incision is closed.

PROCEDURAL RISKS

Acute complications can be related to the venous access technique, lead placement, or pocket creation. Percutaneous venipuncture has a small risk of pneumothorax, hemothorax, air embolism, and inadvertent subclavian artery puncture that is avoided by using the cephalic vein cutdown approach. Both techniques are associated with a small risk of air embolism and can be minimized by putting the patient in the Trendelenburg position.

During lead placement, extrasystoles from the target chamber are common and atrial fibrillation may be induced by lead manipulation. VF is uncommon but the physician should be aware of this possibility in any patient with structural heart disease, especially patients undergoing ICD implantation. During intraoperative ICD testing, myocardial infarction, systemic emboli, stroke, and cardiogenic shock leading to death are all possible. Myocardial perforation by the lead causing hemopericardium and cardiac tamponade is rare. However, perforation not causing hemodynamic or clinical consequences may occur more frequently than believed or reported. It is more likely to occur in elderly patients. Leads can rarely become entrapped in the tricuspid valve apparatus and can be damaged if excessive traction force is applied to free the lead. Lead dislodgement is often detected before discharge from the hospital, and the most common cause is failure to adequately tie down the lead securely using the anchoring sleeve, allowing traction forces on the lead to pull the lead out. Dislodgement of atrial leads from the atrial appendage has been markedly decreased by development of active fixation leads and leads with preformed J-shaped curves. Finally, care must be taken to connect the lead and generator properly; otherwise, reoperation will be necessary to correct the problem.

Good hemostasis reduces the probability of pocket hematoma, but patients receiving chronic oral anticoagulation, low-molecular-weight heparin, or antiplatelet agents remain at risk. Pressure dressings are often applied in the hope of reducing the amount of bleeding. Opening the pocket to evacuate the hematoma and ligate culprit vessels may be necessary in certain circumstances, but reaccumulation of blood may occur anyway and potentially introduces bacterial organisms into the pocket.

Some late lead complications include late myocardial perforation with diaphragmatic muscle or phrenic nerve stimulation, rise in pacing threshold because of inflammation and fibrosis at the lead–endocardial interface or microdislodgement, and thrombosis of the subclavian vein or, rarely, the superior vena cava. Lead dislodgement usually is seen in the early phase but can occur up to several months postimplantation. Lead failure due to fracture of the conductor wires or breach of the lead insulation can occur years after initial implantation. Lead crush injury at the thoracic inlet is the most common site of lead damage and occurs when percutaneous subclavian puncture is performed too medially.

Device-related complications include pocket infection, erosion, device migration, and chronic pain at the implant site. Device system infection usually necessitates removal of the whole system because eradication of the organism is difficult owing to the presence of foreign body material. Finally, pacemaker syndrome (palpitations, lightheadedness, or hypotension) during VVI pacing mode may occur, alleviated by AV-synchronous modes such as DDD.

PACEMAKERS AND IMPLANTABLE CARDIOVERTER DEFIBRILLATORS IN THE HOSPITAL ENVIRONMENT

Some equipment within the hospital operating room environment emits electromagnetic energy that could interfere with the normal function of a PPM or ICD. If this occurs, these pacemakers and ICDs can respond in several ways. Rapidly oscillating electromagnetic interference (EMI) emitted by the electrocautery units can be mistaken by the device for cardiac electrical activity. Consequently, pacemakers may respond by not delivering pacing output, which could lead to asystole. An ICD might interpret the same rapid EMI as a pathologic tachycardia and deliver shocks in a vain attempt to stop it. Large amplitude EMI such as shocks delivered by a transthoracic defibrillator may damage circuitry within a PPM and ICD or reset these devices to a default "reset" mode that would provide only minimal device therapy. Another source of environmental interference for PPMs and ICDs is strong magnetic fields. Low-strength magnetic fields temporarily switch some PPMs to a fixed-rate pacing mode at a preset rate, thereby ignoring the patient's own intrinsic cardiac rhythm so long as the magnetic field is present. The effect on ICDs is different. Most ICDs will continue to provide back-up bradycardia pacing in the programmed pacing mode, but the detection and delivery of therapies for tachycardias is inhibited so long as the magnetic field is detected. This behavior in the presence of weak magnetic fields may be useful in certain circumstances. If equipment such as electrocautery must be used, applying a magnet over the PPM or ICD generator forces the device to ignore EMI signals and continue to pace the heart.

In strong magnetic fields such as those emitted by magnetic resonance imaging scanners, PPM or ICD leads entering the magnetic field can induce electrical current that can damage the generator or cause burns to the endocardium.

CONCLUSION

The subject of arrhythmia devices and their implantation has matured into a medical field that requires a dedicated period of training for those interested in making this activity a part of their long-term career. This chapter has but briefly brushed the surface of an interesting but complex subject, but it hopefully provides inspiration to newer trainees and to mature practicing physicians to learn more.

SUGGESTED READINGS

Bernstein AD, Parsonnet V. Survey of cardiac pacing and implanted defibrillator practice patterns in the United States in 1997. *Pacing Clin Electrophysiol.* 2001;24:842–855.
Gregoratos G, Abrams J, Epstein AE, et al. ACC/AHA/NASPE 2002 guideline update for implantation of cardiac pacemakers and antiarrhythmia devices: summary article: a report of the American College of Cardiology/American Heart Association Task Force on Practice Guidelines (ACC/AHA/NASPE Committee to Update the 1998 Pacemaker Guidelines). *Circulation.* 2002;106: 2145–2161.
Mond HG. The world survey of cardiac pacing and cardioverter defibrillators: calendar year 1997. *Pacing Clin Electrophysiol.* 2001;24:869–870.

Cardiac Surgical Recovery Unit

Routine Cardiac Surgery Recovery Care: Extubation to Discharge

Daniel Bainbridge and Davy C. H. Cheng

EARLY TRACHEAL EXTUBATION AND PROCESS OF CARE

- The process of postoperative cardiac surgery care must be modified to complement early tracheal extubation for maximum cost efficiency. Fast-track cardiac anesthesia provides the opportunity for the paradigm shift in postoperative care of patients who have undergone cardiac surgery.
- The concept of providing graded levels of care in a cardiovascular intensive care unit (CVICU) can be categorized by patient flow and postoperative recovery:
  - Conventional model: This is the conventional flow of patients from operating room (OR) to ICU, then to a freestanding intermediate care unit, and ward.
  - Parallel model: This is a freestanding intermediate care unit, which directly admits postoperative cardiac patients and operates in parallel to a medical surgical ICU.
  - Integrated model: This is a fully integrated intermediate care unit with ICU. Patients are admitted directly from the OR and recover with a flexible nursing ratio for different acuity level of care.

ADMISSIONS TO CARDIAC SURGERY RECOVERY UNIT

It should be a smooth transition of care from the OR team to the cardiac surgery recovery unit (CSRU).

Anesthesiologist's Report

An anesthesiologist's report includes the following:

- Surgical procedure and brief preoperative history.
- Cardiac risk factors: hypertension, diabetes, renal disorders, and so on.
- Allergies.
- Technical problems: difficult intubation, line insertion.
- Anesthetic regimen: propofol, fentanyl, muscle relaxant.
- Prebypass stability: blood pressure (BP), rhythm, bleeding.
- Cardiopulmonary bypass (CPB) information: duration, circulatory arrest, difficulty in arresting heart.
- Weaning off bypass: number of attempts, pacing, drugs, intra-aortic balloon pump (IABP), hemodynamics (BP, cardiac output [CO], pulmonary artery diastolic pressure [PAD]).
- Transesophageal echocardiography (TEE) findings: left ventricular (LV) function pre- and post-bypass, valvular disease, diastolic disease, and aortic pathology.
- Metabolic: potassium (K^+) level, glucose concentration, urine output, hemoglobin (Hb) (packed red blood cells, [PRBC]), A-a gradient.
- Bleeding: pharmacotherapy (e.g., protamine, tranexamic acid, desmopressin, and ε-aminocaproic acid), blood products.

Surgeon's Report

A surgeon's report includes the following:

- Coronary artery bypass graft (CABG): native circulation (quality of bypasses and distal vessels).
  - Number of bypasses, location, and quality.
  - Current LV function.
  - Endarterectomy, vein patch, radial artery graft, other arterial grafts.
  - Need for nitroglycerin, calcium channel blockers, or antiplatelet agents.
- Valve: repair or replacement, tissue versus mechanical, anticoagulation plan.
- Congenital: Which way does the blood flow? What lines? What hemodynamic goals?
- BP guidelines (low if bleeding friable aorta; high if cerebral or renal disease).

Admission Procedure

Standard admission order sheets and clinical forms (Appendix A and B) are filled out.

- The nurse, respiratory therapist (RT), CSRU staff, surgeon, and anesthesiologist work together to admit and stabilize the patient. This includes the following:
  - Put patient on the ventilator, auscultate lungs, and check endotracheal tube (ETT) placement (assist-controlled ventilation rate [AC] at 10 to 12 breaths/minute [bpm]; tidal volume [TV] 8 to 10 mL/kg; positive end expiratory pressure [PEEP] 5; maintain $ETco_2$ at 35 to 45 mm Hg and oxygen saturation [Sao_2] >95%).
  - 12-lead electrocardiogram (ECG).
  - Transduce and zero the pressure lines (scan quickly for heart rate [HR], rhythm, BP, and filling pressures).

- Check for Swan-Ganz position to be inserted <55 cm and trace to ensure that it is not in the right ventricle or wedged; assess CO.
- Check blood loss from chest tubes, urine output, and general tissue perfusion.
- Ensure pacemaker box is attached and is functioning.
- Check appropriate laboratory data when available including ECG, chest x-ray (CXR) (if indicated), arterial blood gas (ABG), complete blood count (CBC), electrolytes, and prothrombin time (PT)/partial thromboplastin time (PTT).

- Patients who arrive extubated should have an ABG drawn after admission to ensure adequate ventilation and oxygenation: Sao_2 >95%, a fraction of inspired oxygen (Fio_2) of 0.5, and partial pressure of arterial carbondioxide ($Paco_2$) <45 mm Hg. Check to ensure if patient has received intrathecal opioid or thoracic epidural analgesia.
- Protamine: An extra 50 to 100 mg is usually given over 30 minutes.
- Potassium replacement: between 0 and 20 mEq in 2 mEq increments on the basis of intraoperative K^+ and urine output.
- CXR if indicated (Pao_2/Fio_2 ratio <200; peak airway pressure >30 cm H_2O; asymmetric air entry to lung; uncertainty of pulmonary artery catheter position [poor trace, unable to wedge]; hypotension resistant to treatment; excessive bleeding; nasogastric/orogastric tube feeds).
- Continuing operative drugs (e.g., inotropes, dipyridamole) and preoperative bronchodilators, steroids, anticonvulsants, and so on.

ROUTINE POSTOPERATIVE COURSE

- Patients are continuously monitored with bedside ECG, Sao_2, transduced arterial line and central venous pressure (CVP) (or PA pressure), and hourly urine outputs. Cardiac outputs are done every 6 hours or as clinically indicated and the PAD is followed rather than following repeated pulmonary capillary wedge pressure (PCWP). Test results (ABG, K^+, glucose and hematocrit [Hct]) are rapidly available as needed. Additional laboratory tests including CBC, PT/PTT, Cr, Ca^{2+}, and Mg^{2+} are usually done daily. If stable, discontinue sedation when the patient meets the criteria for early extubation.

COMMON MANAGEMENT STRATEGIES

For details on common management strategies see Chapter 41.

- Fluids and hemodynamics: Most patients require additional volume of fluids to maintain optimal filling pressures and adequate urine output. During the first 24 hours, avoid large volumes of crystalloids in favor of colloids intravenously (IV). Maintain systolic blood pressure (SBP) 90 to 130 mm Hg, particularly in the higher range for elderly patients or in patients at risk of cerebral vascular accident (CVA).
- Bleeding: Expect some amount of postoperative bleeding, consider the following abnormal rates of bleeding, and inform the surgeon if the coagulogram is normal:
  - Bleeding >400 mL/hour for first hour.
  - Bleeding >200 mL/hour for first 2 hours.
  - Bleeding >100 mL/hour after first 4 hours (maximum 1,000 mL).
- Glucose and electrolytes: Euglycemia should be maintained in all patients following cardiac surgery. Various regimens of insulin and glucose may be required in patients

who are both diabetic and nondiabetic. Risk factors for postoperative hyperglycemia include: diabetes, administration of steroids before CPB, volume of glucose-containing solutions administered, and use of epinephrine infusions. Electrolyte imbalances should be corrected.

■ Shivering: Shivering tends to increase arterial Pco_2, decrease arterial PO_2, and may interfere with ventilation. Treat with meperidine 25 to 50 mg IV; increase the propofol infusion or pancuronium 2 mg IV if needed. The patient should be warm and not shivering before reversal of neuromuscular blockade.

■ Extubation: Manage early extubation patients according to the CSRU weaning protocol (Appendix F). Patients should be awake and cooperative; hemodynamically stable; no occurrence of active bleeding or coagulopathy; respiratory strength should be assessed by hand grip or head lift to ensure complete reversal of neuromuscular blockade; and temperature should be >35.5°C. Consider T-piecing or an endotracheal ventilation catheter (ETVC) in patients who have known difficult intubation.

■ Postoperative pain: In order to facilitate early extubation, patients receive fewer intraoperative narcotics than in the past. Parasternal block and local anesthetic infiltration of the sternotomy wound and mediastinal tube sites can be a useful analgesic adjunct. Non-selective nonsteroidal anti-inflammatory drugs (NSAIDs) may be used in patients without renal dysfunction and ulcer disease, and in those who are <70 years (diclofenac or indomethacin 50 to 100 mg pr before extubation). Within 24 hours of extubation most patients are managed by oral analgesics such as Tylenol No. 3 or equivalent.

■ Sedation: Patients who are not early extubation candidates are sedated postoperatively with an infusion of narcotics and/or benzodiazepines.

● Narcotic analgesics: morphine 20 mg/100 mL 5% dextrose water (D5W) (2 mg/10 mL) at 1 to 4 mg/hour or fentanyl 1,000 μg/100 mL D5W (10 μg/mL) at 100 to 200 μg/hour.

● Benzodiazepine: midazolam 20 mg/100 mL D5W (2 mg/10 mL) at 1 to 3 mg/hour.

UNSTABLE PATIENTS AND CHEST REOPENINGS

■ Although most patients follow a stable postoperative course and are discharged from the CSRU within 12 to 24 hours, some are critically ill. These patients frequently have an IABP, multiple inotropes, low urine output, unstable hemodynamics, or even an open chest. These patients require continuous intensive management and frequent attention to their clinical status. Strive for 12 to 24 hours of relative stability before gradually weaning inotropes or IABP. Abruptly discontinuing support may lead to an acute deterioration in the patient's condition (see Chapter 41).

■ Chest re-opening for postoperative bleeding is a potentially lifesaving intervention. Indications vary but are usually related to an acute failure to thrive (arrest or pre-arrest), to relieve tamponade, or facilitate open cardiac massage and resuscitation. Patients may require further operative interventions (see Chapter 44).

MEDICAL ROUNDS AND DISCHARGES

■ Multidisciplinary (CSRU consultant, fellow, surgeon, respiratory therapist [RT], and charge nurse) rounds every morning help make discharge decisions. Should a patient's condition change, making him or her not suitable for discharge, he or she will remain in the CSRU and be managed appropriately with medical attention and nursing staff ratio.

■ During morning rounds, the nurse and fellows present the patient's course in CSRU to the consultant in order to make management decisions.
  ● Need for antihypertensives, anticoagulation.
  ● Review of current ECG and laboratory results (i.e., CBC, Cr, ABG).
  ● Urine output, fluid balance, and the need for volume or diuresis.
  ● Chest tube is removed and CXR is checked.
  ● Adequacy of pain control.
  ● Suitability for transfer out of CSRU (order either enteric coated aspirin [ECASA]) or appropriate anticoagulation; reorder the preoperative medications including noncardiac medications; continue anticholesterolemia, antiarrhythmic, and afterload reduction; continue antihypertensives though initial dose may need to be adjusted on the basis of current BP).

■ In complicated patients additional time is spent on:
  ● Review of drugs and hemodynamics.
  ● Ventilation requirements and plan for weaning or extubation.
  ● Further investigations or consultations.

SUGGESTED READINGS

Bainbridge D, Cheng D. Initial perioperative care of the cardiac surgical patient. *Semin Cardiothorac Vasc Anesth*. 2002;6:229–236.

Cheng DCH. Fast track cardiac surgery pathways: early extubation, process of care, and cost containment. *Anesthesiology*. 1998;88:1429–1433.

Cheng DCH, Byrick RJ, Knobel E. Structural models for intermediate care areas. *Crit Care Med*. 1999;27:2266–2271.

Cheng DCH, Karski J, Peniston C, et al. Early tracheal extubation after coronary artery bypass graft surgery reduces costs and improves resources: a prospective, randomized, controlled trial. *Anesthesiology*. 1996;85:1300–1310.

McDonald S, Jacobsohn E, Kopacz D, et al. Parasternal block and local anesthetic infiltration with levobupivacaine after cardiac surgery with desflurane. *Anesth Analg*. 2005;100:25–32.

Westaby S, Pillai R, Parry A, et al. Does modern cardiac surgery require conventional intensive care? *Eur J Cardiothorac Surg*. 1993;7:313–318.

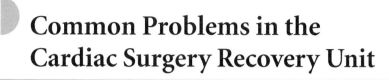

Chapter 41

Common Problems in the Cardiac Surgery Recovery Unit

Annette Vegas

Management of the postoperative cardiac surgery patient in the intensive care unit (ICU) emphasizes ongoing vigilance. Most of these patients experience an uneventful recovery. This chapter reviews the diagnosis and treatment of some of the common problems faced by these patients, including altered hemodynamics, bleeding, and low urine output. In addition, some patients may sustain multiple organ dysfunction requiring meticulous cardiovascular, respiratory, and metabolic support.

HEMATOLOGIC PROBLEMS

- Bleeding: This is a common postoperative complication and surgeons should be informed of ongoing abnormal chest tube losses. Rarely, patients develop unmanageable postoperative coagulopathies (disseminated intravascular coagulation [DIC]). Patients who have undergone cardiac surgery will have received an antifibrinolytic as discussed in Chapter 18. Management of postoperative bleeding in patients who have undergone cardiac surgery includes the following:
  - If generalized, bleeding may reflect coagulopathy; examine for other bleeding sites.
  - Check complete blood count (CBC), prothrombin time (PT), partial thromboplastin time (PTT), fibrinogen level, activated clotting time (ACT), and chest x-ray (CXR).
  - Minimize rises in systolic blood pressure (80 to 100 mm Hg).
  - Warm the patient by using blood warmers, if there is a large volume of fluids, and a warming blanket.
  - Increase positive end expiratory pressure (PEEP) (7.5 to 10 cm H_2O).

- Pharmacotherapy:
  - ▲ Protamine 50 to 100 mg intravenously (IV) (check ACT <150, PTT <23 to 32.5 seconds).
  - ▲ Tranexamic acid (Cyklokapron) 50 mg/kg IV over $\frac{1}{2}$ hour.
  - ▲ Desamino-D-arginine-vasopressin (DDAVP) 16 to 20 μg IV slowly over $\frac{1}{2}$ hour (repeat in 12 hours if needed).
  - ▲ Vitamin K 10 mg IV slowly over $\frac{1}{2}$ hour.
  - ▲ Factor VIIa IV 70 to 90 μg/kg.
- Blood products:
  - ▲ Packed red blood cells (PRBC): maintain Hct 0.24 (Hgb 80 g/L).
  - ▲ Platelets (normal >150,000 to 300,000/μL): consider 5 units of platelets if count is <100,000 or if dysfunction is suspected (aspirin [ASA] or long pump run). Expect each unit of platelets to raise blood platelet count by 5,000 to 10,000/μL.
  - ▲ Fresh frozen plasma (FFP): consider FFP if increased PT (normal 11.5 to 15 seconds) or increased INR (normal 0.8 to 1.2 seconds) and ongoing patient bleeding. Each unit of FFP increases coagulation factors by 5%. For normal hemostasis, maintain factor levels at >50% to 80%. Treatment guidelines are according to international normalized ratio (INR)/PT: 1.5 to 15 seconds (2 units FFP), 2.0 to 30 seconds (4 units FFP), 3 to 30 seconds (6 units FFP). Note that patients who required a high dose of intraoperative heparin may be antithrombin 3 deficient and paradoxically bleed more if FFP is given.
  - ▲ Cryoprecipitate (normal fibrinogen = 1.5 to 3.5 g/L): usually fibrinogen level >1 g/L is adequate for hemostasis. Consider 5 units if there is massive bleeding and demonstrated low fibrinogen level. On an average, 1 unit of cryoprecipitate raises the fibrinogen level to 0.06 to 0.1 g/L.
- Thrombocytopenia: This is a common occurrence postoperatively and is usually self-resolving. Low platelet counts could be related to the presence of an intra-aortic balloon pump (IABP), heparin-induced thrombocytopenia (HIT), or sepsis. If platelet counts decrease by 30% or to <100,000 within 24 hours of using heparin, discontinue heparin and screen for HIT. Transfuse platelets only if the platelet count is <50,000 and a procedure is planned. Avoid platelet transfusions in patients with HIT. If the patient requires anticoagulation use alternatives to heparin.
- Anticoagulation: Postcardiac surgery patients will differ in their anticoagulation requirements depending on their surgical procedure and heart rhythm. Guidelines are provided in Appendix H. Coumadin should be started when the patient can swallow pills. If the patient cannot swallow by 24 hours after surgery, then heparinization is recommended, but the therapeutic level and duration of therapy should be determined by the specific circumstances. All patients should receive deep vein thrombosis prophylaxis until mobilized.

CARDIOVASCULAR PROBLEMS

- Hypertension: The differential diagnosis includes hypothermia, anxiety, pain, hyperdynamic left ventricle, and severe hyperglycemia. There are many drugs available to manage postoperative hypertension; the choice depends in part on treatment goals (see Table 41-1).

▶ **TABLE 41-1**   Classes and Effects of
                   Antihypertensive Drugs

	Pre-load	After-load	HR	Contractility
Vasodilator	↓	↓	↑	↑
Calcium channel	↔	↓	↓	↓
ACE inhibitor	?↓	↓↓	∅	↑
β-Blockers	↑	↑	↓	↓

HR, heart rate; ACE, angiotensin converting enzyme.

In the early postoperative period, use short-acting, easily titratable intravenous drugs to adapt to changing hemodynamic parameters and ensure adequate absorption. If the patient is intubated, consider additional sedation and analgesia. Patients who have pre-existing hypertension should resume their preoperative medications when tolerated in the postoperative period.

- Vasodilators:
  - ▲ Nitroglycerin (NTG) 100 mg/250 mL 5% dextrose water (D5W) at 5 to 50 mL/hour IV infusion.
  - ▲ Sodium nitroprusside (SNP) 50 mg/250 mL D5W at 5 to 50 mL/hour IV infusion.
  - ▲ Hydralazine 5 to 10 mg IV bolus q4h.
- β-Blockers:
  - ▲ Esmolol 10 to 20 mg IV bolus.
  - ▲ Metoprolol 1 to 5 mg IV bolus.
  - ▲ Labetalol 5 to 20 mg IV bolus.
- Calcium channel blockers:
  - ▲ Nifedipine 10 mg sublingual.
  - ▲ Diltiazem 5 to 10 mg IV qh as infusion.
- Hypotension: There is a wide differential in the postoperative setting as outlined in Table 41-2. Before starting any drugs, *examine the patient*; remember to corroborate any numerical data obtained. Ensure that the numbers obtained are accurate and remember that the patient, not the numbers, requires management. If the patient is sinking fast *act quickly* by placing the patient in the Trendelenburg position, stopping sedation and vasodilators, giving volume and calcium chloride 1 g IV: These are useful temporizing measures until a more definitive diagnosis is reached. A simple practical approach to get you started can be seen in Table 41-3.
- Bradycardia: Atrial and/or ventricular epicardial leads are placed intraoperatively. Pace patients in asystole, third-degree heart block or bradycardia, preferably atrial greater than atrioventricular greater than ventricular alone. If the condition persists for more than 48 to 72 hours, the patient may need a permanent pacemaker. Sinus bradycardia may respond to low-dose dopamine, isoproterenol, or epinephrine and the patient usually recovers.
- Tachycardia and dysrhythmias: Treatment depends on atrial or ventricular dysrhythmia, and hemodynamic stability. Hemodynamically unstable rhythms are cardioverted (see Table 41-4).

▶ **TABLE 41-2** Differential Diagnosis in Hypotension

Diagnosis	Treatment
↓ **SVR**	↑ **SVR**
• Vasodilation (drugs, histamine, fever, ↑ CO_2, acidosis, sepsis)	• Eliminate vasodilating factors
• ↓ Blood viscosity	• Administer vasoconstrictor
	• Correct anemia
↓ **Preload (CVP, PA_D)**	↑ **Preload (CVP, PA_D)**
• Hypovolemia, venodilation	• Position patient to ↑ venous return (Trendelenburg)
• ↓ Venous return (IPPV, tamponade)	• Fluids: colloid, blood
	• Relieve tamponade, ↓ airway pressure
• Loss of atrial kick	• Restore atrial kick (AV pacing, cardiovert)
• RV failure (↓ LV preload)	• Rx: RV failure (↑ CVP, ↓ PVR, inotrope)
↑ **Afterload (↑ SVR)**	↓ **Afterload (↓ SVR)**
• Hypertension, pain	• Consider volume
• Vascular obstruction	• Administer vasodilator (Nipride)
• ↑ Airway pressure (affects RV)	• Aonsider inodilator (milrinone)
• Hypovolemia	• IABP
Dysrhythmias	**Dysrhythmia treatment**
• ↑ HR, ↓ HR	• Correct etiology (↑>↓ K^+, ↑Mg^{2+}, ischemia)
• Atrial	• Antiarrhythmics
• Ventricular	• Pacemaker
↓ **Contractility (↓ CO)**	**Systolic (inotrope)**
• Acute hypertension	• Eliminate cardiac depressants
• Ischemia, infarct	• Relieve ischemia
• Ventricular over distention	• Inotropes
• Acute valvular dysfunction	• Avoid ventricular distention
• Myocardial depressants	**Diastolic (lusitropic)**
• ↓ O_2, ↑ CO_2, acidosis	• B1 agonist or phosphodiesterase inhibitor
	↓ **Cardiac work**
	• Treat hypertension
	• IABP, LVAD

SVR, systemic vascular resistance; CVP, central venous pressure; IPPV, intermittent positive pressure ventilation; LV, left ventricular; AV, aortic valve; RV, right ventricular; PVR, pulmonary vascular resistance; IABP, intra-aortic balloon pump; HR, heart rate; LVAD, left ventricular assistive device; CO, carbon monoxide; CO_2, Carbon dioxide; O_2, oxygen; PA_D, pulmonary artery diastolic pressure.

■ Premature ventricular complex (PVC): This may reflect marginal coronary perfusion and ongoing ischemia or a serum electrolyte problem. Check serum electrolytes; repeat the 12 lead electrocardiogram (ECG) and note the patient's hemodynamics. Treat PVCs aggressively if multifocal and frequent.
  ● Check Swan-Ganz catheter position; remove if not required.
  ● Serum K^+ concentration (4 to 5 mEq/L): to optimize give potassium chloride (KCL) 10 to 20 mEq IV: slowly through a central line.
  ● Magnesium sulfate: 1 to 2 g IV, may repeat as poor correlation with serum level.
  ● Lidocaine: 100 mg IV bolus (± repeat 50 mg/kg IV bolus), infusion 1 to 4 mg/minute.

▶ **TABLE 41-3** Management of Hypotension

Check blood pressure by cuff
⇓
Check heart rate, rhythm (90 bpm, atrial kick)
⇓
Check filling pressures (additional volume)
⇓
Check cardiac output

If low, add inotrope	*If high,* add vasopressor
Dopamine	Phenylephrine
Dobutamine	Norepinephrine
Milrinone (+ vasopressor)	Vasopressin
Epinephrine	

Blood pressure (BP) = cardiac output (CO) × systemic vascular resistance (SVR)
Cardiac output (CO) = stroke volume × heart rate (HR)
Stroke volume depends on preload, afterload and myocardial contractility.

- Amiodarone, 50 to 300 mg IV slowly over 15 to 30 minutes, infusion 900 mg/250 mL D5W over 24 hours.
- Overdrive pace rhythm.

■ Cardiac tamponade: This is a lethal, but often difficult to diagnose condition in the postcardiac surgery patient. Suspect the diagnosis if there is (a) sudden absence of bleeding from chest tubes, (b) rising filling pressures (central venous pressure [CVP] = PA_D >20 mm Hg) with fall in blood pressure (BP), (c) fall in cardiac output and poor peripheral perfusion, and (d) falling urine output. Echocardiography (transthoracic or transesophageal echocardiography [TEE]) may help distinguish right ventricular (RV) failure from tamponade. A localized clot may compress the heart and is more likely to compress if the pericardium is closed. Despite equivocal evidence, the surgeon may choose to re-explore the patient to release pericardium or evacuate the clot.

▶ **TABLE 41-4** Postcardiac Surgery Arrhythmia Management

Rhythm	*Treatment*
Sinus bradycardia	Pacing, β1 (dopamine, epinephrine, isoproterenol), atropine
Sinus tachycardia	Underlying cause, β-block
Premature atrial beats (PAC)	Atrial overdrive pacing, $MgSO_4$, digoxin
Atrial fibrillation (AF)	$MgSO_4$, digoxin, β-block, Ca^{2+} channel block, amiodarone
Atrial flutter (AFL)	Rapid atrial pacing, digoxin, amiodarone
Third HB, junctional	Pacing
Premature ventricular (PVC)	See text, page 350
Ventricular tachycardia (VT)	β-block, lidocaine, amiodarone, quinidine
Ventricular fibrillation (VF)	Defibrillation, ACLS protocol

ACLS, advanced cardiac life support.

RESPIRATORY PROBLEMS

- Hypoxia: The differential diagnosis of a wide A-a gradient includes: pre-existing chronic obstructive pulmonary disease (COPD), endotracheal tube misplacement, bronchospasm, pneumothorax, pleural effusion, airspace disease, or post-cardiopulmonary bypass (CPB) (acute respiratory distress syndrome [ARDS]). Examine the chest and check a CXR for correctable causes. Management strategies include:
  - If intubated: add PEEP (7.5 to 10 cm H_2O), increased F_{IO_2}, diurese, bronchoscopy, bronchodilators.
  - If extubated: pain control, chest physiotherapy, diuresis, increased F_{IO_2}, facial continuous positive airway pressure (CPAP), bronchodilators.
  - If pneumonia: sputum culture, Gram stain, bronchoscopy, antibiotics.
- Chest tubes: All postoperative cardiac surgery patients have chest tubes inserted intraoperatively to drain extra fluid in the pleural spaces, mediastinum, and pericardial space. These chest tubes are usually removed 12 to 48 hours postoperatively provided there is minimal drainage, no air leak, and stable respiratory status. A CXR is performed 1 hour after chest tube removal to exclude a pneumothorax.
- Pneumothorax: Suspect the clinical presence of a pneumothorax by auscultation and confirm by CXR. Chest tube insertion is required if the pneumothorax is >50% in size, is a tension pneumothorax, or the patient is symptomatic with poor gas exchange.

RENAL PROBLEMS

- Urine output (low): This is an important reflection of overall patient condition and requires close attention. Management is controversial and may include the following steps:
  - Check volume status (filling pressures) or administer volume bolus.
  - Check hemodynamics (BP and cardiac output [CO]); this may require a vasopressor to maintain adequate perfusion pressure and/or an inotrope to optimize CO.
  - Ensure patency of urinary catheter by flushing with saline.
  - Stop all nephrotoxins (indomethacin, aminoglycosides, angiotensin converting enzyme [ACE] inhibitors).
  - Consider dopamine 1 to 3 μg/kg/hour.
  - Consider adding low-dose vasopressin (0.5 to 2 units/hour).
  - Consider diuretics:
    - ▲ Furosemide 10 to 300 mg IV bolus, ± drip 10 to 20 mg/hour.
    - ▲ Metolazone 5 to 10 mg PO/ng before furosemide bolus.
    - ▲ Ethacrynic acid 50 to 100 mg IV bolus.
- Urine output (high): This may occur because of mannitol in the CPB prime, furosemide given in the operating room (OR), low-dose dopamine infusion, or hyperglycemia. Try to keep the patient volume replete, and if possible stop the dopamine infusion. Consider a single-dose desmopressin (DDAVP) 4 μg IV to treat postoperative diabetes insipidus.
- Dialysis: Renal replacement is started for patients with acute or chronic renal insufficiency and/or volume overload. Indications for dialysis include hypervolemia,

hyperkalemia, acidosis and increased blood urea nitrogen (BUN), and creatinine (Cr). If the patient is hemodynamically stable, intermittent hemodialysis can be done through an Uldall line or pre-existing AV access. Ultrafilteration or hemodialysis may be started using continuous venous-venous hemodialysis (CVVHD) through appropriate line access. This is the preferred technique in the patient who is hemodynamically unstable because it varies with how much fluid removal occurs per hour.

CENTRAL NERVOUS SYSTEM PROBLEMS

- Seizures: Postoperative seizures are infrequent and may be difficult to differentiate from residual muscle relaxant, rigors, or shivering. Document the location and frequency of seizures. Seizures are usually transitory owing to emboli (air, debris), but if persistent may require an electroencephalograph (EEG) and neurology evaluation. Check and normalize serum electrolyte concentration (Ca^{2+}, Mg^{2+}, and Na^+), glucose level, arterial oxygen (Pao_2), and carbon dioxide ($Paco_2$) pressure. Specific anticonvulsant treatment may include:
  - Valium (2 to 5 mg IV bolus), lorazepam (1 to 2 mg IV bolus).
  - Dilantin 10 to 15 mg/kg IV (maximum 1 g) load, maintain 3 to 5 mg/kg/day.
  - Phenobarbital 10 to 15 mg/kg IV (maximum 1 g) load, maintain 2 to 4 mg/kg/day.
- Stroke: The incidence is 1.4% to 6.6% in the postcardiac surgery patient. The clinical presentation is variable and depends on the cause, site, and extent of cerebral damage. Common presentations include transient ischemic attacks (TIA), focal deficits, and coma. Document the neurologic deficit and any progression. A computed tomographic (CT) scan should be done urgently (24 to 48 hours) if there is a need for anticoagulation, otherwise it can be done electively (5 to 7 days). Because of their recent surgery, these patients are not candidates for thrombolytic therapy. The patient must be able to adequately protect his or her airway before extubation and swallow properly before oral feeding. Consider early tracheotomy, feeding jejunostomy, or swallowing studies if the patient requires prolonged care.
- Coma: It is unusual for patients to be comatose after cardiac surgery. Exclude metabolic, drug, or primary central nervous system (CNS) events. An early CT scan, if the patient is hemodynamically stable, will help document structural brain damage. Consider CNS protection by normalizing Pao_2, $Paco_2$, and serum glucose level, and maintain an adequate cerebral perfusion pressure. There is currently no role for mannitol, steroids, or calcium channel blockers in this setting.
- Agitation/delirium: Agitation or delirium is a common occurrence in the postoperative elderly patient. Risk factors include preoperative organic brain disease, severe cardiac disease, multiple medical problems, and complex and prolonged surgical procedures. It is necessary to exclude and correct metabolic problems (decreased glucose level, increased $Paco_2$, extremely decreased Pao_2), reassess drugs, or consider alcohol withdrawal. Sedation options may include narcotic analgesics, benzodiazepines, or Haloperidol.

METABOLIC PROBLEMS

- Diabetes: Hyperglycemia is often present after CPB because of impaired insulin production and peripheral insulin resistance. Strict glucose control is currently advocated to improve wound healing and reduce perioperative complications. Patients on multiple inotropes may need a more generous insulin dose. A sliding insulin scale is followed as outlined in Appendix I.

- Potassium (K^+): Total body potassium (K^+) concentration is 3,500 mEq (50 mEq/kg lean body weight) but only 2% is extracellular (<70 mEq). There is a nonlinear relation between total body K^+ and serum K^+ (see Fig. 41-1).

  Hypokalemia (<3.5 mEq/L) results in muscle weakness, CNS changes, AV block, ECG changes (ST segment depression, "u" wave, T wave flat), and potentiates digoxin toxic arrhythmias. Administer KCl, 10 to 20 mEq, through a central line to replenish deficits. Hyperkalemia (>5.5 mEq/L) is uncommon but can cause skeletal muscle weakness, diarrhea, widened QRS, bradycardia, and asystole. Treat if serum K^+ >6 mEq/L or in the presence of any ECG changes. Treatment options include: calcium chloride 1 g IV, Humulin R 10 units IV bolus with D50W in case of low glucose level, furosemide 10 to 20 mg IV, Kayexalate 20 to 50 g in 50 mL of 20% sorbitol PO or PR q3h or dialysis.

- Phosphate (Po_4^{3-}): Only 2% of phosphorus is located in the extracellular space. Normal serum levels show a diurnal change (normal range 3 to 4.5 mg/dL or 0.8 to 1.45 mmol/L). Hypophosphatemia is uncommon but can be related to the following conditions: dextrose infusion, refeeding, phosphate binding antacids, alcohol withdrawal, respiratory alkalosis, sepsis and total parenteral nutrition (TPN). The consequences of severe hypophosphatemia (serum Po_4 <1.0 mg/dL) may involve muscle weakness including myocardial and respiratory contractility. Intravenous replacement is recommended even if there is no clinical sequela. Administer potassium phosphate 15 to 30 mmol in 100 mL D5W over 4 hours, and follow serum phosphate levels; repeat if needed.

- Calcium (Ca^{2+}): Hypoalbuminemia decreases the protein bound fraction and, therefore, the total serum calcium level (n = 2.1 to 2.5 mmol/L), but does not affect

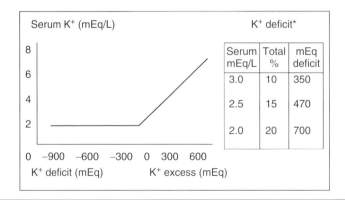

FIGURE 41-1. Relationship of serum K^+ to total body K^+ excess or deficit.

the serum ionized Ca^{2+} level (n = 1.1 to 1.3 mmol/L). The differential of ionized hypocalcemia (<1.1 mmol/L) includes sepsis, alkalosis, acute pancreatitis, renal insufficiency, blood transfusion, CPB, and drugs. Findings associated with severe hypocalcemia include neuromuscular excitability, hypotension, left ventricular failure, and prolonged QT interval. Administer intravenous calcium in the form of calcium gluconate 10% (90 mg [4.5 mEq] Ca^{2+}/10 mL) or calcium chloride 10% (272 mg [13.6 mEq] Ca^{2+}/10 mL).

■ Magnesium (Mg^{2+}): This is the second most abundant intracellular cation, though with uneven distribution in the body. The body contains a total of 1,000 mmol of Mg^{2+} that is distributed as serum Mg^{2+}, 2.6 mmol (0.3%), and bone Mg^{2+}, 530 mmol (53%). Serum levels of Mg^{2+} (normal = 0.70 to 1.10 mmol/L) have a poor correlation with total body levels. Urinary Mg^{2+} is likely a better indicator of total body stores. Measured low serum levels are treated with magnesium sulfate 2 to 4 g IV. This is also of therapeutic value for patients with atrial or ventricular arrhythmias and normal serum magnesium levels.

■ Metabolic acidosis: The most common differential diagnosis in postcardiac surgery patients relates to hypoperfusion (increased lactate level), renal failure (increased Cr level), and diabetes (increased ketone concentration). The anion gap can be calculated and helps differentiate different types of metabolic acidosis:

● Normal anion gap = 10 to 12 mEq/L, calculated as $Na^+ - (Cl^- + HCO_3^-)$.

● Normal anion gap acidosis (increased Cl^-) results from HCO_3^- loss typically from the gut, pancreas, or kidney (renal tubular acidosis).

● Elevated anion gap acidosis (normal Cl^-) results from H^+ gain related to ketoacidosis (starvation, diabetes), lactate, or acute intoxication (salicylate). Acidosis adversely affects myocardial contractility and attenuates the positive inotropic effects of catecholamines. Treatment depends on the underlying cause and hemodynamic profile. Ensure that the patient can eliminate the additional CO_2 produced before administering sodium bicarbonate ($NaHCO_3$).

● The physiologic correction for metabolic acidosis is a compensatory respiratory alkalosis; a decrease of 1 mEq/L HCO_3^- should cause a decrease of 1.1 mm Hg $PaCO_2$. The $PaCO_2$ cannot be <10 mm Hg.

● Replace half of the calculated total base deficit with $NaHCO_3$ (1 ampule [50 mL] = 44 mEq HCO_3^-).

▲ Base deficit = normal HCO_3^- (24 mmol/L) – measured base deficit.

▲ Calculate total mEq deficit = HCO_3^- deficit (base deficit) × 0.3 × weight (kg).

INFECTIOUS DISEASE PROBLEMS

■ Antibiotic prophylaxis: To be effective, administer perioperative prophylactic antibiotics for cardiac surgery in the OR before skin incision. Common antibiotic choices are cefazolin, 1 g IV, or vancomycin, 1 g IV, for patients who are allergic to penicillin. The regimen is continued for the recommended number of doses and then discontinued (see Table 41-5).

■ Fever: In the first postoperative 24 hours, it is reasonable to treat fever symptomatically with an antipyretic drug. If the patient is febrile beyond 24 hours, culture urine, blood, and sputum and check white blood cell count. Consider early antibiotic treatment if the patient has prosthetic material (valve or graft). If the patient has

▶ **TABLE 41-5** Cardiac Surgery Antibiotic Recommendations

Coronary Bypass Graft	Prosthetic Valve Surgery
Cefazolin 1 g IV preoperative, then 1 g IV q8h for 24 h postoperative (total of 3 doses)	**Cefazolin** 1 g IV preoperative, then 1 g IV q8h for 24 h postoperative (total of 6 doses)
IF PENICILLIN ALLERGY **Vancomycin** 1 g IV preoperative, then vancomycin 1 g IV q12h for 24 h postoperative (total of 2 doses)	**Vancomycin** 1 g IV preoperative, then vancomycin 1 g IV q12h for 24 h postoperative (total of 3 doses)

a pre-existing infection (bacterial endocarditis), then continue preoperative antibiotics on the basis of the final tissue culture results from the OR.

■ Line changes: Intravenous lines are routinely changed to minimize nosocomial line infections. Change arterial lines only if the site is inflamed or infected, or if the site is in a position that interferes with mobilization. Change central lines prophylactically every 7 to 10 days depending on patient condition and alternate access sites. Remove unused lines and catheters as soon as possible to minimize infections.

GASTROINTESTINAL PROBLEMS

■ Gastritis prophylaxis: Patients who do not undergo mechanical ventilation for >48 hours and who have no coagulopathy are at extremely low risk (0.1% versus 6.0%) of clinically important gastric bleeding and therefore do not require prophylaxis. The optimal drug (sucralfate, H2 blockers, proton pump inhibitors) for stress ulcer prophylaxis is debatable. Treat patients with active ulcer disease with intravenous proton pump inhibitors (omeprazole).

■ Nutrition: Enteral feeds should start early if patient recovery is anticipated to take a long time. Irrespective of bowel sounds, begin full strength formula at 10 mL/hour and increase slowly. Consider metoclopramide 10 mg IV q8h if there is delayed gastric emptying. Use regular nasogastric (ng) or Silastic feeding tube, but there is absolutely a need for CXR to confirm tube position before feeds commence. TPN is started only after enteral feeds have failed or are contraindicated.

■ Diarrhea: The most common causes in postcardiac surgery patients are enteral feeds, intestinal ischemia, or pseudomembranous colitis. Management includes checking stool for clostridium difficile toxin, a reassessment of medication, and ruling out systemic hypoperfusion. Stop any gastric prokinetic agents and enteral feeds. A rectal tube may be inserted and loperamide (Imodium), 4 mg PO initially and then 2 mg PO after each bowel movement (maximum 16 mg/day), should be administered.

■ Liver and pancreatic dysfunction: Liver dysfunction is unusual but may occur in patients with a past history of liver disease (pre-existing right heart failure), an episode of hypoperfusion, or use of high-dose vasopressors. Watch for very high cardiac output, low systemic vascular resistance (SVR), low blood sugar, persisting acidosis, and elevations in liver enzyme levels. There is no specific treatment except supportive measures by minimizing hepatic congestion and avoiding hepatotoxins. Postoperative patients may have an elevated amylase suggesting perioperative pancreatic injury. These patients may have an elevated glucose level and be critically ill on multiple inotropes. Most often, the amylase level falls within 24 hours without specific treatment; consider discontinuing the propofol infusion, if present.

SUGGESTED READINGS

Aronson S, Blumenthal R. Perioperative renal dysfunction and cardiovascular anesthesia: concerns and controversies. *J Cardiothorac Vasc Anesth.* 1998;12:567–586.

Arrowsmith JE, Grocott HP, Newman M. Neurologic risk assessment, monitoring and outcome in cardiac surgery. *J Cardiothorac Vasc Anesth.* 1999;13:736–743.

Despotis GJ, Skubas NJ, Goodnough TG. Optimal management of bleeding and transfusion in patients undergoing cardiac surgery. *Semin Thorac Cardiovasc Surg.* 1999;11:84–104.

Gomez M. Magnesium and cardiovascular disease. *Anesthesiology.* 1998;89(1):222–240.

Kollef MH, Sharpless L, Vlasnik J, et al. The impact of nosocomial infections on patient outcomes following cardiac surgery. *Chest.* 1997;112:666–675.

Pires LA, Wagshal AB, Lancey R, et al. Arrhythmias and conduction disturbances after coronary artery bypass graft surgery: epidemiology, management and prognosis. *Am Heart J.* 1995; 129:799–808.

Chapter 42

Atrial and Ventricular Arrhythmia Management

Christopher A. Palin and Charles W. Hogue, Jr.

A broad spectrum of cardiac arrhythmias can occur after cardiac surgery including supraventricular tachycardias and immediate life-threatening ventricular fibrillation (VF) or ventricular tachycardias (VTs). Clinicians caring for patients who have undergone cardiac surgery, therefore, must be familiar with the emergency management of cardiac rhythm disturbances. This chapter reviews the management of atrial and ventricular arrhythmias in the patient who has undergone cardiac surgery including the current Advanced Cardiac Life Support (ACLS) guidelines (2000) for the treatment of these arrhythmias.

ATRIAL ARRHYTHMIAS

All subtypes of atrial arrhythmias are possible after cardiac surgery including atrial fibrillation (AF) and flutter, atrial tachycardia (ectopic or re-entrant), atrioventricular (AV) nodal re-entry tachycardia, and multifocal or accessory pathway tachycardias. By far, the most common is AF, which occurs in >30% of patients after coronary artery bypass grafting (CABG) surgery, and in even more patients after cardiac valvular surgery. The high prevalence of AF has not been eliminated with "off-pump" procedures. The most consistent risk factor for AF is increased patient age. AF after cardiac surgery is associated with increased risk for stroke, longer duration of hospital stay, and increased hospital costs.

Treatment of Atrial Arrhythmias

The goals for treatment of AF are heart-rate control, restoration of sinus rhythm, and prevention of thromboembolic complications. There is a high rate of spontaneous conversion to sinus rhythm in those patients who have AF after cardiac surgery. Correction of oxygen desaturations and treatment of hypokalemia and hypomagnesemia may be all that is needed in some patients. Electrical cardioversion is mandatory in the presence of hypotension, evidence of myocardial ischemia, congestive heart failure (CHF), or when improvement in diastolic ventricular filling might be improved with restoration of the "atrial kick" (e.g., patients with left ventricular [LV] hypertrophy or other forms of marked diastolic dysfunction). Overdrive atrial pacing may effectively convert some forms of atrial flutter (type I, flutter rate <340/minute). Determination of atrial rate and rhythm may be facilitated with atrial electrocardiograms (ECGs) obtained by the connection of temporary atrial pacing wires to an ECG lead. In noncardiac surgical populations, prospective randomized trials suggest that patient outcome with AF is no different for patients managed with anticoagulation and heart-rate control compared with those given antiarrhythmic drugs for pharmacologic cardioversion.

Direct Current Cardioversion

Energy levels for *synchronous* direct current (DC) cardioversion of atrial flutter are typically 50 to 100 J and for AF 100 to 200 J. Effectiveness is enhanced by placement of electrodes (preferably self-adhesive) over the anterior aspect of the heart and posteriorly below the left scapula. Compared with the prior standard monophasic waveform current, biphasic waveform energy delivery is associated with a higher rate of cardioversion, lower energy requirement, and less dermal injury. Energy settings for a biphasic cardioversion are substantially less and may be initially 50 to 100 J for transthoracic cardioversion of AF. Sedation is required for patient comfort. Potential complications include ventricular or bradycardia arrhythmias, and thromboembolism. Elective cardioversion is often considered after the first episode of AF or in symptomatic patients.

Anticoagulation

In nonsurgical populations, cardioversion within 48 hours of arrhythmia onset is generally recommended to avoid thromboembolism. It is apparent that mural thrombus may form in a shorter interval. Anticoagulation of the surgical patient must consider the added risk of pericardial bleeding and pericardial tamponade after mediastinotomy. The lack of safety and efficacy data for anticoagulation of the cardiac surgical patient requires an individual assessment of risk versus benefit of this therapy. Patients with low cardiac output and AF are particularly at a high risk for stroke. Antiplatelet drugs are often started soon after surgery. Aspirin reduces the incidence of thrombosis for noncardiac surgery patients in AF, for patients with no structural heart disease, and few risk factors for stroke.

A target international normalized ratio (INR) of 2 to 3 for 3 weeks is recommended before attempting elective cardioversion for patients with AF >48 hours duration. A strategy of heparin anticoagulation along with transesophageal echocardiography exclusion of left atrial thrombus is equally effective for preventing thromboembolization. Anticoagulation is continued for 3 to 4 weeks after restoration of sinus rhythm because both AF and cardioversion may lead to atrial stunning and continued risk for thrombus formation.

▶ **TABLE 42-1** Drugs for Heart Rate Control in Postoperative Atrial Fibrillation with Examples of Adult Doses and Common Side Effects

Drug	Dose	Side Effects/Comments
β-blockers		Bronchospasm, hypotension, worsening heart failure, rapid onset
Atenolol	1–5 mg IV over 5 min, then 50–100 mg b.i.d. PO	
Metoprolol	1–5 mg IV over 2 min, then 25–100 mg t.i.d. PO	
Esmolol	0.5 mg/kg IV over 1 min, then 0.05–0.20 mg/kg/min	Short acting
Calcium channel blockers		Hypotension, worsening heart failure, rapid onset
Diltiazem	0.25–0.35 mg/kg over 10 min, then 5–15 mg/h IV	
Verapamil	2.5–10 mg IV over 2 min, then 80–120 mg PO t.i.d.	More negatively inotropic
Digoxin	0.25–1 mg IV (slowly), 0.125–0.500 mg/d PO	Heart block, anorexia, and nausea

IV, intravenous; PO, by mouth; b.i.d., twice a day; t.i.d., three times a day.

Heart Rate Control

Many patients with postoperative AF may be managed simply with heart rate control. β-adrenergic receptor blockers or calcium channel blockers are the primary agents for this purpose (see Table 42-1). Digoxin is considered when there are contraindications for these drugs or for patients with left ventricular dysfunction. Digoxin slows the heart rate by enhancing the parasympathetic tone. Decades of experience has shown that heart rate slowing effects of digoxin are attenuated in states of high sympathetic tone such as exercise. For similar reasons, it is less effective perioperatively in the setting of heightened sympathetic drive than β-blockers or calcium channel antagonist. The slow onset of digoxin is another consideration. Target ventricular response rates of 60 to 90 bpm at rest are often used for nonsurgical patients with AF and may be applied in the postoperative setting. Patients with accessory AV conduction pathways (e.g., Wolf-Parkinson-White syndrome) deserve special consideration. Because conduction through the accessory pathway is not slowed as is conduction through the AV node, drugs that slow heart rate by the latter mechanisms may actually promote accessory conduction of fibrillatory waves. In patients with accessory pathway, AF may rapidly degenerate to VF. Treatment must be aggressive and is aimed at slowing accessory pathway conduction with antiarrhythmic drugs.

Antiarrhythmic Drug Therapy

Antiarrhythmic drugs are indicated for pharmacologic cardioversion of AF and for maintenance of sinus rhythm after electrical cardioversion. A similar consideration of risk for thromboembolism as for electrical cardioversion is necessary before attempts

▶ **TABLE 42-2** Drugs for Arrhythmia Control in Postoperative Atrial Fibrillation with Examples of Adult Doses and Common Side Effects

Drug	Dose	Side Effects/Comments
Amiodarone	2.5–5 mg/kg IV over 20 min, then 15 mg/kg or 1.2 g over 24 h	Hypotension, bradycardia pulmonary fibrosis, phlebitis, photosensitivity, thyroid and hepatic dysfunction, Torsade de pointes, polyneuropathy
Sotalol	1 mg/kg IV or 80–160 mg PO, then 160–320 mg/d	Bradycardia, hypotension, CCF, Torsade de pointes
Procainamide	Up to 1 g IV at 25–50 mg/min	Fever, lupuslike syndrome, accumulates in renal failure, drug level monitoring
Disopyramide	2 mg/kg IV, then 0.4 mg/kg/h	Urinary retention, dry mouth, glaucoma
Ibutilide	1 mg IV over 10 min and can repeat after 10 min	Torsade de pointes
Dofetilide	4–8 μg/kg IV	Dose adjusted in renal failure, Torsade de pointes
Propafenone	2 mg/kg IV over 10–20 min or 450–600 mg PO	Avoid with LV dysfunction, hypotension
Flecainide	1–2 mg/kg over 10–30 min	Avoid in coronary artery disease and LV dysfunction

IV, intravenous; PO, by mouth; LV, left ventricular; CCF, congestive cardiac failure.

for pharmacologic cardioversion. Antiarrhythmic drugs from Vaughan-Williams classes IA, IC, and III are all effective for converting AF to sinus rhythm (see Table 42-2). Guidelines have been produced by a joint committee from the American College of Cardiology, American Heart Association, and the European Society of Cardiology. Although these guidelines mainly concern the nonsurgical patient, they can be applied equally to patients after cardiac surgery.

Of particular importance is the proarrhythmic potential of antiarrhythmic drugs, particularly in Torsade de pointes. Risk factors for the latter include prior proarrhythmia, long-QT interval, coronary artery disease, hypertrophy, and LV dysfunction. Recent research suggests a genetic susceptibility to prolongation of the QT interval on exposure to certain drugs. This "double-hit" phenomenon results in a normal QT interval in the absence of offending drugs, but there is QT prolongation upon exposure. However, continuous ECG monitoring with particular attention to the heart rate–adjusted QT interval is advised when antiarrhythmic drug treatment is initiated.

The risk of proarrhythmia is highest with class I antiarrhythmic drugs (e.g., procainamide, quinidine, flecainide), less with sotalol, and least with amiodarone. Amiodarone is the agent of choice in the presence of left ventricular dysfunction or other risk for proarrhythmia.

Procainamide is a class IA antiarrhythmic with efficacy for both atrial and ventricular arrhythmias, but its use can result in significant hypotension, a lupuslike syndrome, and gastrointestinal (GI) upset. Monitoring of plasma levels of its major metabolite (*n*-acetyl procainamide or NAPA) is necessary to avoid accumulation of this active compound. Procainamide possesses anticholinergic properties that may lead to increased heart rate if heart rate slowing drugs are not first initiated. Both flecainide and propafenone are class IC agents with significant negative inotropic effects and should be avoided in patients with LV dysfunction or coronary artery disease. Neither agent is available in parental form in the United States.

Sotalol is a nonselective β-blocker with class III properties similar to amiodarone. Sotalol also lacks an approved intravenous (IV) formulation in the United States. Its use can be associated with bradycardia, hypotension, and the risk of proarrhythmia effects. Newer class III drugs such as ibutilide and dofetilide are available for the acute pharmacologic conversion of AF. Ibutilide has few hemodynamic side effects but it is associated with a high rate of Torsade de pointes. Dofetilide is better tolerated but its dose is carefully adjusted to creatinine level. Dofetilide is not a primary agent for conversion of AF.

Prevention of Atrial Fibrillation

Postoperative β-blockers can be recommended for the prevention of postoperative AF after cardiac surgery on the basis of multiple trials. Although both amiodarone and sotalol have also been shown to be effective prophylactic agents, in some studies there are conflicting data and the findings have not been universally accepted. Further, the lack of safety data about the widespread use of these drugs warrants careful consideration. Therefore, amiodarone or sotalol are not first-line drugs for postoperative AF prevention, and their use for this purpose is individualized. Magnesium supplementation after cardiac surgery, although of low risk, has not been shown to have a consistent benefit. Thoracic epidural analgesia has also produced conflicting results. The trials of postoperative atrial pacing have been inconsistent; however, biatrial pacing may be of more benefit.

VENTRICULAR ARRHYTHMIAS

Ventricular ectopy and nonsustained VT are common after cardiac surgery with a reported frequency as high as 50% in studies using Holter monitoring. In the absence of left ventricular dysfunction or structural heart disease, these arrhythmias are self-limited. Addressing precipitating factors such as electrolyte abnormalities, hypoxemia, acidosis, or direct mechanical irritation from intravascular catheters or chest tubes may be all that is necessary for treatment. Ongoing myocardial ischemia even after CABG surgery must be considered and aggressively treated. Careful assessment of other precipitants such as catecholamine infusions, proarrhythmic drug effects, or even rare causes such as electrical microshock should be considered. Suppression of ventricular ectopy with lidocaine has not been demonstrated to be associated with improved patient outcomes, and prophylactic use of lidocaine has not been convincingly shown to prevent more malignant ventricular arrhythmias after cardiac surgery. In contrast to ventricular ectopy and nonsustained VT, sustained VT and VF are less common, occurring in <1% of patients. The occurrence of nonsustained VT in the setting of ventricular impairment, sustained VT, or VF requires careful assessment as they identify patients at high risk for subsequent sudden death. Consultation with an electrophysiology cardiologist is prudent. Implantation of an internal cardiovertor/defibrillator device may be considered if reversible causes of an arrhythmia are identified.

Advanced Cardiac Life Support Guidelines (2000)

New recommendations for the emergency treatment of ventricular arrhythmias are based on a careful critique of existing data using an evidence-based approach (See ACLS Guidelines, 2000). These guidelines reinforce that the most important treatment of hemodynamically significant VT or VF is prompt electrical counter shock beginning at 200 J followed by shocks of 300 J and 360 J. At the time of their publication, there was insufficient data for recommendation of energy settings for biphasic waveform current delivery. Biphasic waveform requires less energy and is more effective than cardioversion/defibrillation with monophasic delivery. Beginning with 200 J with transthoracic biphasic waveform cardioversion/defibrillation or 5 to 10 J direct epicardial cardioversion/defibrillation is prudent.

The algorithms for treating narrow-complex tachycardia, stable VT, and pulseless VT or VF are included here for reference (see Figs. 42-1, 42-2, and 42-3). Drug therapy for life-threatening ventricular arrhythmias is considered as secondary treatment. Of note, intravenous amiodarone is often recommended when drug therapy is indicated for atrial and ventricular arrhythmias. In contrast, lidocaine is recommended as a secondary drug for hemodynamically stable VT and is rated "class indeterminate" for hemodynamically significant VT or VF based on insufficient evidence to support its recommendation. Vasopressin (40 U) may also be considered now in place of epinephrine during cardiac arrest to increase coronary and cerebral perfusion pressure.

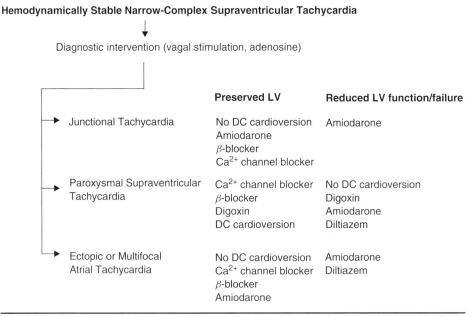

FIGURE 42-1. Treatment protocol for hemodynamically stable narrow-complex tachycardia. LV, left ventricular; DC, direct current. (Adapted from ACLS Guidelines [2000]. *Circulation.* 2000;102(8):1–384.)

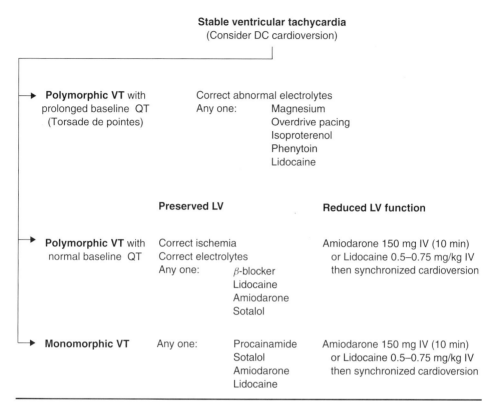

FIGURE 42-2. Treatment protocol for hemodynamically stable ventricular tachycardia. VT, ventricular tachycardia; LV, left ventricular; IV, intravenous. (Adapted from ACLS Guidelines [2000]. *Circulation.* 2000;102(8):1–384.)

In patients with confirmed supraventricular tachycardia with aberrancy, treatment can be given as outlined in the ACLS narrow-complex tachycardia algorithm (Fig. 42-1). Agents that block the AV node (calcium channel blockers, β-blockers, and adenosine) are potentially dangerous in patients with VT and therefore should not be used when the diagnosis of wide-complex tachycardia is uncertain. Empiric treatment of wide-complex tachycardia of unknown origin should be limited to DC cardioversion, amiodarone, or procainamide.

Sustained Ventricular Tachycardia

On the basis of the QRS morphology, VT can be divided into monomorphic or polymorphic subtypes. The QRS complexes in monomorphic VT are similar or repetitive. This arrhythmia is associated with previous myocardial infarction, dilated cardiomyopathy, and right ventricular dysplasia. Monomorphic VT can be either hemodynamically stable or unstable. Hemodynamically unstable VT requires immediate termination with synchronized cardioversion. IV lidocaine was recommended for the treatment of hemodynamically stable VT. However it is now considered second

Basic CPR and Defibrillation
Activate emergency team and call for defibrillator
Start basic CPR: airway, breathing, chest compressions
Defibrillate: Shock VF or pulseless VT up to three times (200J, 300J, 360J or biphasic 200J)

↓

Persistent or recurrent VF/VT?

↓

ADVANCED TREATMENT
Secure airway and ventilate to assure oxygenation
Establish intravenous access
Monitor and identify cardiac rhythm
Consider differential diagnosis

↓

Epinephrine 1 mg IV and repeat every 3 to 5 minutes
Or
Vasopressin 40 U IV once only

↓

Resume attempts to defibrillate without a delay of more than 60 seconds

↓

Consider amiodarone, lidocaine, magnesium, procainamide, and buffers

↓

Resume attempts to defibrillate

FIGURE 42-3. Treatment protocol for ventricular fibrillation or pulseless ventricular tachycardia. CPR, cardiopulmonary resuscitation; VF, ventricular fibrillation; VT, ventricular tachycardia; IV, intravenous. (Adapted from ACLS Guidelines [2000]. *Circulation.* 2000;102(8):1–384.)

line to IV procainamide, IV sotalol, IV amiodarone, or other IV β-blockers. Patients with CHF and/or reduced LV function are particularly susceptible to the negative inotropic effects of antiarrhythmic agents. Amiodarone is the least negative inotropic agent and is currently the recommended drug for this clinical situation.

Polymorphic VT is a condition where the QRS morphology constantly varies. In the setting of pre-existing prolongation of the QT interval, polymorphic VT is termed Torsade de pointes. This distinction is important in guiding treatment. Polymorphic VT not associated with prior QT interval prolongation (i.e., not Torsade de pointes) is usually associated with hypotension, although stable hemodynamics might be present at the start of the arrhythmia. Importantly, polymorphic VT may rapidly degenerate into VF, necessitating prompt and aggressive treatment. Polymorphic VT is commonly associated with ongoing myocardial ischemia particularly in the setting of myocardial infarction.

Hemodynamically Stable Wide-Complex Tachycardias

Both monomorphic VT and supraventricular tachycardias (with aberrant conduction) can present with a hemodynamically stable tachycardia patient with an ECG showing a wide QRS complex (>0.12 ms). Acutely differentiating supraventricular versus ventricular origin of the arrhythmia is challenging, and existing algorithms are insensitive. A history of structural heart disease suggests VT as the most likely etiology. Previous aberrant conduction problems or accessory pathway problems suggest a supraventricular tachycardia with aberrant conduction. Careful examination of the ECG may help to identify the loss of AV relation and other changes in QRS morphology in VT, although misdiagnosis is common (>50%).

Ventricular Fibrillation or Pulseless Ventricular Tachycardias

The ACLS guidelines highlight the proven efficacy of early defibrillation for VF/pulseless VT. Antiarrhythmic therapy is considered after the first series of three precordial shocks. Lidocaine has no proven efficacy as a treatment in cardiac arrest and has been superseded by IV amiodarone, which has improved early survival in out-of-hospital arrest. Antiarrhythmics are of particular value where an appropriate cardiac rhythm can be restored but not maintained by defibrillation.

Torsade de Pointes

Torsade de pointes is a form of polymorphic VT in the setting of pre-existing prolonged QT interval. Prolongation of the QT interval can be congenital or acquired. The acquired form of QT interval prolongation can occur with a variety of antiarrhythmic drugs, antihistamines, phenothiazines, antifungal drugs, butyrophenones, and many more. A careful search for precipitating agents is necessary whenever Torsade de pointes occurs because discontinuing the offending drug is necessary. Internet Websites are helpful and can be easily accessed using the search term Torsade de pointes. Electrolyte disturbances are also associated with the arrhythmia, and proper replenishment can be curative. Cardioversion is necessary when Torsade de pointes is associated with hemodynamic instability. In addition to removing/correcting reversible precipitating conditions, treatment of drug-associated Torsade de pointes often includes administration of 1 to 2 g IV of magnesium. There is insufficient evidence, though, on the effectiveness of this therapy, but it is generally associated with few risks in the absence of renal insufficiency. Increasing the heart rate to >90 beats per minute (bpm) with a catecholamine infusion or pacemaker is often used when bradycardia precedes episodes of Torsade de pointes, but there is insufficient data to judge the effectiveness of this strategy. Because antiarrhythmic drugs can precipitate Torsade de pointes, they are avoided, particularly in Class I and newer Class III drugs.

SUGGESTED READINGS

ACLS Guidelines (2000). *Circulation*. 2000;102(8):1–384.
DiMarco JP. Medical progress—implantable cardioverter-defibrillators. *N Eng J Med*. 2003;349: 1836–1847.
Fuster V, Ryden LE, Asinger RW, et al. American College of Cardiology/American Heart Association/ European Society of Cardiology Board. ACC/AHA/ESC guidelines for the management of patients with atrial fibrillation: executive summary. *J Am Coll Cardiol*. 2001;38:1231–1266.

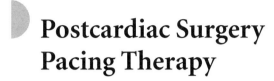

Chapter 43

Postcardiac Surgery Pacing Therapy

Douglas A. Cameron

Temporary epicardial cardiac pacing has emerged as an important nonpharmacologic tool in the early management of arrhythmias following cardiac surgery. Applications vary from standard bradycardia indications to hemodynamic support and tachyarrhythmia diagnosis and management. Knowledge of the indications, techniques, various applications, and complications of temporary pacing is essential in the postoperative cardiac care setting.

TEMPORARY ELECTRODES

Pairs of teflon-insulated stainless steel unipolar myocardial electrodes spaced 0.5 to 1 cm apart are used for temporary cardiac pacing. By convention, atrial leads are exposed to the right of the sternum, and ventricular leads are exposed to the left of the sternum.

All temporary pacing requires electrode pairs. Bipolar pacing uses paired intramyocardial electrodes; unipolar stimulation is achieved by one intramyocardial electrode (cathode), with a second myocardial electrode passed through the skin to function as the subcutaneous anode.

LEAD USES

Bradycardia Support

- Relative bradycardia: Immediate postoperative inappropriate sinus bradycardia (<80 bpm) associated with low output and/or atrial/ventricular ectopy. Atrial pacing or atrioventricular (AV) pacing is preferred.

- Pathologic bradycardia: AV block, tachycardia/bradycardia, sinus dysfunction, antiarrhythmic drug-provoked bradycardia.

Overdrive Pacing

- Hemodynamic: Atrial or AV overdrive of accelerated junctional or idioventricular rhythm (restore AV synchrony), rate augmentation for relative sinus bradycardia.
- Arrhythmia: Suppression of atrial or ventricular ectopy, suppression of *torsade de pointes* ventricular tachycardia (VT), prevention of atrial fibrillation (AF).
- Rate control: Acceleration of atrial flutter to AF with improved rate control (concealed conduction).
- Pace termination, supraventricular tachycardias (SVTs), and atrial flutter.

Arrhythmia Diagnosis

- Atrial intracardiac electrogram (IEGM): Intracardiac atrial electrogram recording that evaluates AV relationship during undefined tachycardias.

Prognostic Testing

- Bradycardia: AV conduction and sinus node recovery time testing.
- Tachycardia: Electrical physiology (EP)-programmed ventricular stimulation study.

EXTERNAL PULSE GENERATORS

The different features of the external pulse generator are shown in Table 43-1.

Typical temporary pacing modes use a standard three-position code as summarized in Table 43-2.

Temporary pacing may be complicated by the failure of sensing with potential proarrhythmia or failure to capture. Table 43-3 provides a guideline to troubleshooting common temporary pacemaker malfunctions.

▶ **TABLE 43-1 Features of External Pulse Generators**

Single chamber:	• Constant current outputs programmable up to 20 mA
	• Variable rates 30–180 bpm
	• Variable sensitivity 0.5 mV—asynchronous
High output:	• Constant current single chamber output up to 50 mA
	• Asynchronous: pacing will compete with intrinsic rhythm
	• Used in high pacing threshold situations
	• These units no longer are commercially available
Dual chamber:	• Rate, output AV interval programmable
DVI mode	• Adds atrial sensitivity settings, atrial high rate overdrive up to
DDD mode	• 800 bpm

NOTE: No mode switching is available in DDD mode during atrial tachycardias and therefore may inappropriately pace at upper tracking limit.
AV, atrioventricular.

▶ **TABLE 43-2** **Typical Temporary Pacing Modes: Three Position Code**

	Chamber Paced	*Chamber Sensed*	*Response Mode*
AAI	A	A	I
AOO	A	0	0
VVI	V	V	I
DVI	D	V	I
DDD	D	D	D

AAI: Indications: sinus dysfunction, excitable atrium, stable atrioventricular (AV) conduction
Contraindications: atrial fib/flutter, AV block
AOO: Indications: avoid atrial oversensing, pace termination supraventricular tachycardia (SVT)
Contraindications: AV block, atrial fibrillation
VVI: Indications: AV block, bradycardia, inexcitable atrium (atrial fibrillation)
DVI: Indications: sinus bradycardia with AV block; no atrial sensing, therefore, loss of AV synchrony during sinus accelerations with AV block
DDD: Indications: variable sinus rates with unstable AV conduction
Contraindications: atrial fibrillation (recall no mode switching)
A, atrium; V, ventricle; D, dual; I, inhibited; 0, off; DVI, sequential pacemaker based on ventricular activity only; DDD, pacemaker based on both atrial and ventricular activity.

▶ **TABLE 43-3** **Temporary Pacing Troubleshooting Guide**

Pattern	*Checks*	*Etiology*
Loss of capture **Pacer spike absent:**	**Visible LED output signal** • Check cable connectors • Trace/inspect leads • Unipolarize	**Open circuit** • Faulty contact • R/O fracture • Single lead fracture
	No LED output signal • Confirm power on • Reduce sensitivity • Change battery • Change pulse generator	**Power failure** • Oversensing • Battery depletion • Generator failure
Loss of capture **Pacer spike present:**	• Increase output • Check cable connections • Unipolarize electrodes • Change battery	• Threshold rise • Poor/wrong contact • Exit block/fracture • Battery depletion
Undersensing:	• Increase sensitivity • Increase sensitivity/overdrive • Unipolarize	• Rising threshold • VPB • Exit block/fracture
Oversensing:	• Reduce sensitivity • Unipolarize • Secure connectors • Adjust permanent pacemaker • Check grounding/patient isolation	• Farfield • Lead fracture • Poor contact • Crosstalk • EM interference

LED, light emitting diode; R/O, rule out; VPB, ventricular premature beat; EM, electromagnetic.

Overdrive Pacing

AF remains the most common postoperative complication following cardiac surgery occurring in approximately one third of patients typically on the second or third postoperative day. Growing evidence supports the role of atrial overdrive pacing, to prevent AF, with relative risk reductions of 2.5. The role of alternate site atrial overdrive pacing through the interventricular septum or left atrium is under investigation and is not yet proved to be superior to conventional right atrial overdrive pacing. Evidence so far is conflicting on the benefits of biatrial pacing. Exit block, phrenic nerve stimulation, and subtle loss of left atrial capture may complicate this modality of temporary pacing. It is important to remember that atrial overdrive pacing may potentially be proarrhythmic if loss of atrial sensing or capture is present, causing unintentional initiation of AF. Future application of newer AF prevention pacing algorithms, as well as improving techniques for alternate site pacing, may lead to greater efficacy of acute pacing interventions in the prevention of postoperative AF. Successful awake low energy internal atrial defibrillation using custom removable temporary atrial electrodes placed intraoperatively has been reported. Despite this, cardioversion is not typically recommended early postoperatively owing to the high propensity for early recurrence of AF.

Pace termination is most frequently used for atrial flutter. Classic atrial flutter (atrial rates 230 to 340 bpm with an inverted saw-tooth pattern in the inferior leads) is most amenable to pace termination. Atrial electrograms can be displayed on the V_1 electrocardiogram (ECG) lead by using an alligator clip attached between the V_1 lead and the atrial electrode. This allows confirmation of the diagnosis and measurement of the atrial cycle length. Before attempting to pace terminate, one should initially pace atrially at maximal output and low rates to exclude unintentional ventricular stimulation. Subsequently initiate asynchronous atrial burst pacing, starting just below the flutter rate, and sequentially increase the rates until evidence of capture is observed on ECG or is inferred through change in ventricular response. Pace 10 to 30 seconds at each rate, followed by abrupt termination before the next attempt. Typical termination rates are 120% to 140% of the atrial cycle length. If unsuccessful, faster overdrive rates may trigger AF with slower ventricular response (concealed conduction). AF itself, however, is not amenable to pace termination.

Management of Patients with Automatic Implantable Cardioversion Defibrillator

Patients with an automatic implantable cardioversion defibrillator (AICD) pose unique difficulties postcardiac surgery. There is the possibility of lead dislodgement and/or damage intraoperatively, which could lead to inappropriate or failed bradycardia or tachycardia therapy. The tachyarrhythmia features on the device should be routinely disabled perioperatively and only re-enabled following complete reassessment to ensure proper sensing and pacing behavior. External temporary pacing may result in inappropriate shocks owing to inappropriate oversensing by the AICD and should not be deployed while the antitachycardia and shock features are armed. If temporary pacing is required with the device enabled or with unknown status, the application of a pacemaker magnet over the device will temporarily disable the antitachycardia and shock therapies while applied, thereby preventing inappropriate shocks. Magnet application will also prevent inappropriate shocks caused by cautery, or secondary to rapid tachycardia responses to atrial arrhythmias. Unlike permanent pacemakers, the magnet does not influence the normal pacemaker behavior. This response is intentional to avoid inappropriate pacing that could lead to unprotected arrhythmia inductions. The application of a magnet in a patient with a cardiac resynchronization therapy (CRT) AICD, in addition to disabling the shock therapies, will suspend resynchronization pacing, with only single-site right ventricular (RV) pacing present during the magnet application. Knowledge of this behavior is important because loss of biventricular pacing may adversely affect hemodynamics.

PERMANENT CARDIAC PACING

Postoperative conduction abnormalities result from multiple causes including pre-existing conduction disease, direct surgical trauma, mechanical injury (annular calcification), ischemic injury, drugs, and/or metabolic factors. Permanent cardiac pacing is needed in 0.8% to 4.0% of patients following cardiac surgery. Risk factors predisposing to permanent pacemaker insertion include valve surgery, right ventricular outflow tract (RVOT) and ventricular septal surgery, age >75 years, and preoperative conduction disorders.

Permanent epicardial pacing electrodes should be prophylactically inserted intraoperatively in high-risk patients with conditions precluding standard transvenous pacing including tricuspid valve replacement, vascular obstruction, and intracardiac shunts. Consider intraoperative permanent epicardial left ventricular (LV) electrode placement in patients with severe LV dysfunction where postoperative resynchronization pacing is strongly considered.

Active fixation atrial leads should be routinely used postoperatively because passive fixation is often unstable or difficult owing to the atrial scarring and/or amputation of atrial appendage.

Indications for permanent pacemaker are as per the American College of Cardiology (ACC)/American Heart Association (AHA) guidelines. Timelines before committing to permanent pacing are not standardized. Recovery may be delayed and premature pacemaker insertion may result in unnecessary pacemaker usage. In this era of shorter hospital stays, delaying pacemaker insertion may result in prolonging monitoring time and in potentially longer hospital stays. A risk/benefit assessment for optimal timing for permanent pacemaker insertion must be done on each postoperative temporary-paced patient.

Biventricular CRT utilizing RV and LV leads is now an approved therapy option in patients with symptomatic heart failure associated with moderately severe LV dysfunction, with wide QRS on maximal medical management. CRT has been proven to improve hemodynamics acutely, and increase dp/dt_{max} and increase cardiac index, without a concomitant increase in myoenergetics. This benefit is achieved through improved LV mechanical synchrony and improved optimization of AV interval timing. The role of acute temporary LV epicardial pacing or biventricular pacing is under investigation. To date, results are conflicting and routine attempts to provide acute biventricular pacing postoperatively are not recommended. It should be considered in patients who are at high risk for poor LV function and who have difficulty coming off bypass.

SUGGESTED READINGS

Daoud EG, Snow R, Hummel JD, et al. Temporary atrial epicardial pacing as prophylaxis against atrial fibrillation after heart surgery: a meta-analysis. *J Cardiovasc Electrophysiol.* 2003;14(2): 127–132.

Ellenbogen KA, Kay GN, Wilkoff BL. *Clinical Cardiac Pacing.* Philadelphia, PA: WB Saunders; 1995.

Furman S, Hayes DL, Holmes DR. *A practice of cardiac pacing.* New York: Futura Publishing; 1993.

Glikson M, Dearani JA, Hyberger LK, et al. Indications, effectiveness, and long–term dependency in permanent pacing after cardiac surgery. *Am J Cardiol.* 1997;80:1309–1313.

Gregoratos G, Abrams J, Epstein AE, et al. ACC/AHA/NASPE 2002 guideline update for implantation of cardiac pacemakers and antiarrhythmia devices-summary article. *J Am Coll Cardiol.* 2002;40:1703–1719.

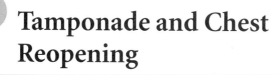

Tamponade and Chest Reopening

Terrence M. Yau

Chest reopening after cardiac surgery may be indicated for the diagnosis and/or therapy of postoperative hemorrhage, tamponade, shock, or cardiac arrest. Patients with suspected sternal osteomyelitis or mediastinitis may require resternotomy, and those with sternal dehiscence may require repeat sternal closure. In addition, early reoperation for failure of a coronary bypass graft, valve repair, or prosthetic valve dysfunction may, on rare occasions, be necessary.

INCIDENCE

The incidence of chest reopening in 2003 at the Toronto General Hospital is listed, by procedure and indication, in Table 44-1.

The independent preoperative predictors of sternal reopening included urgent or emergent surgery, active endocarditis, and decreasing body surface area. Not surprisingly, when intraoperative factors were included in the modeling, the duration of cardiopulmonary bypass was also a significant independent predictor of reopening.

▶ **TABLE 44-1   The Incidence of Chest Reopening in 2003 at the Toronto General Hospital**

Incidence by procedure		
	CABG (*N = 1,097*)	5.8%
	Valvular ± CABG (*N = 432*)	6.3%
	Other (*N = 329*)	9.7%
Incidence by indication		
	Hemorrhage	4.6%
	Tamponade	0.5%
	Shock/cardiac arrest	0.2%
	Sternal osteomyelitis/ mediastinitis	0.3%
	Sternal dehiscence	0.1%
	Redo surgery	0.5%
	Other	0.4%

CABG, coronary artery bypass graft.
Other: procedures such as cardiac transplantation, thoracic aortic surgery, repair of adult congenital heart defects, etc.

INDICATIONS

Postoperative Hemorrhage

Progressive refinements in blood conservation strategies have resulted in considerably reduced shed blood volume and transfusion requirements compared to the decade of the 1990s. However, increasing use of antiplatelet agents and glycoprotein IIb/IIIa inhibitors has increased transfusion requirements, particularly of platelets, in a subset of patients undergoing urgent or emergent surgery.

Our approach to postoperative hemorrhage is biased toward early reopening and minimization of blood product usage. In the absence of a significant coagulopathy, or if adequate clot formation is noted in the chest drains, re-exploration is indicated for drainage of 200 mL of blood in 1 hour, or sustained drainage of 100 mL/hour for 3 to 4 hours.

Clinical suspicion of a surgical site of bleeding, hemodynamic instability, or restricted access to blood products because of patient objection or rare blood types should prompt earlier reintervention.

The objectives of re-exploration are to establish hemostasis and to evacuate the hemopericardium and/or hemothorax, thereby preventing further fibrinolysis, coagulopathy, and exacerbation of mediastinal adhesions.

Tamponade

Cardiac tamponade remains a clinical diagnosis. In the early postoperative period, this diagnosis is often based on decreasing cardiac indices in the presence of increasing pulmonary artery pressures, equalization of central venous and diastolic pulmonary artery pressures, oliguria, and signs of systemic hypoperfusion. Patients may have had moderate hemorrhage initially, that has significantly abated.

Immediate resternotomy in the cardiovascular intensive care unit (CVICU) or in the ward is indicated for critical hemodynamic instability or collapse with a clinical picture suggestive of tamponade. A more indolent course, frequently allowing confirmation by echocardiography, may allow transportation of the patient back to the operating room.

Constriction of the heart by pericardium that has been tightly closed may present in an identical manner to that caused by hemopericardium.

Patients on warfarin may develop a large and occasionally symptomatic hemopericardium or pericardial effusion 4 to 7 days after surgery, after removal of chest drains. Our practice has been to evacuate this collection in the operating room by reopening only the lower portion of the incision, thereby allowing evacuation of the collection and placement of a chest tube which is left in place overnight.

Shock or Cardiac Arrest

Hemodynamic collapse may require emergent chest reopening for diagnosis and treatment. Inability to achieve adequate cardiac output by closed cardiac massage is an indication for emergent chest reopening.

Resternotomy for shock or cardiac arrest may allow diagnosis of graft problems, including kinking, spasm or thrombosis, problems with a prosthetic valve, tamponade due to hemorrhage and/or pericardial constriction, or major hemorrhage.

Immediate treatment of a kinked graft, graft spasm, tamponade, or control of hemorrhage may then be effected.

Sternal Osteomyelitis or Mediastinitis

The diagnosis of a deep sternal infection or mediastinitis is clinical, based on pain, fever, sternal instability, and leukocytosis with or without purulent discharge from the wound. Ancillary investigations are usually not required but may include computerized tomographic (CT) scanning to demonstrate bony destruction of the sternum or mediastinal fluid collections, and nuclear imaging to demonstrate localization of leukocytes.

Early reoperation is favored. In many patients, this approach permits debridement of the infected sternum and subcutaneous tissue, confirmation of vascularity of the remaining tissue, and repeat closure of the sternum as per routine. In a few patients, extensive involvement of the sternum mandates sternectomy and placement of muscle flaps. This aggressive approach has decreased the mortality of deep sternal infection to 1.9% at our institution in the last 4 years.

Sternal Dehiscence

Dehiscence usually presents with copious serosanguineous drainage from the sternal incision coupled with varying degrees of sternal instability.

Treatment consists of early resternotomy, intraoperative cultures to rule out infection, sternal rewiring, and routine wound closure.

Redo Surgery

Reoperation for early failure of a graft, valve repair, prosthetic valve, or other indications may be required in rare circumstances. Routine use of intraoperative Doppler or transesophageal echocardiography to assess bypass grafts and valve repair or replacement at initial surgery should limit the need for reopening on this basis.

TECHNIQUE OF EMERGENCY CHEST REOPENING

Equipment

An emergency resternotomy tray should be kept on hand in the CVICU and in every ward. This tray should contain all the instruments necessary for rapid chest reopening and initial interventions, including scalpels, wire cutters, a sternal retractor, internal defibrillator paddles, and temporary epicardial pacing wires.

In addition, a mobile cart with ancillary supplies such as skin preparation solutions, surgical drapes, sterile surgical gloves, gowns, masks, sutures, and suction tubing should also be available.

Portable operating lights and cautery machines may be obtained from the operating suites if necessary.

Personnel

- Besides the operating surgeon, the presence of a surgical assistant is helpful.
- A nurse, respiratory therapist, or anesthetist can ventilate the patient by bagging with 100% oxygen (O_2). If the patient had previously been extubated, emergency reintubation by a physician or trained respiratory therapist is mandatory.
- An anesthetist or intensivist, if available, can attend to anesthetic considerations and supervise pharmacologic circulatory support.
- Notification of the operating suites when an emergency reopening is underway will allow the preparation of an operating room and a cardiopulmonary bypass circuit if one is required, as well as recall of operating room nurses, a perfusionist, and an anesthetist.

Opening

- Rapid skin preparation and draping is performed with the patient in the ICU bed.
- It is important that the sternal incision never be closed at the skin level at the time of the original operation with surgical clips, as subsequent rapid reentry with a scalpel is then impeded.
- The subcutaneous and fascial layers are opened, the sternal wires cut and removed, and a sternal retractor is placed.

Evaluation and Initial Management

Clinically significant tamponade, if present, can be immediately confirmed and be treated by reopening the pericardium. The volume of blood or clot in the mediastinum and pleural spaces indicates whether major hemorrhage has occurred and usually points to its source.

The primary objective is to support and maintain adequate systemic and cardiac perfusion, which may require reopening alone, internal cardiac massage, or further measures. Internal massage must be performed carefully to avoid injury to the right ventricle, bypass grafts, or the left ventricle in patients with a mitral bioprosthesis.

Careful evaluation of all surgical sites allows identification and control of sources of ongoing hemorrhage if present.

Definitive Management

After chest reopening for hemorrhage or tamponade, the hemopericardium is completely evacuated, and any surgical bleeding sites are controlled. The pericardial space is irrigated with warm saline and suctioned dry to ensure that hemostasis is adequate. When a coagulopathy is identified, administration of plasma, cryoprecipitate, or platelets may be required. Fibrin glue or other topical hemostatic agents may be useful for bleeding from needle holes in long suture lines.

Resternotomy for hemodynamic collapse or cardiac arrest necessitates an exhaustive search for the precipitating cause, including careful evaluation of coronary bypass grafts to rule out kinking, thrombosis, or spasm, and/or evaluation of prosthetic or repaired valves. Doppler assessment of grafts and echocardiographic evaluation of repaired valves or prostheses is required. In a few cases, cardiopulmonary bypass may be required for definitive correction of the problem.

When chest reopening is performed for deep sternal infection or mediastinitis, all collections of blood, fluid, or pus are drained, and all necrotic bony and soft tissues are debrided back to healthy, vascular tissue. Care is taken to avoid breaching intact planes below the level of infection, thereby limiting its spread, and samples of bone and any collections are sent for microbiologic analysis to guide further antibiotic therapy. When the remaining sternum is judged to be adequate, sternal reclosure can be performed, but when the sternum is inadequate or completely excised, one-stage closure with pectoralis major or rectus abdominis flaps can be accomplished, leaving drains in the mediastinum and under the flaps to prevent hematoma formation or reaccumulation of fluid collections. Antibiotic coverage is generally continued for several weeks.

Closure

- Temporary epicardial pacing wires should be checked, as these are frequently dislodged during re-exploration.
- Chest drains should be flushed to ensure patency and may be replaced at the discretion of the surgeon.
- Pericardial closure is at the discretion of the surgeon unless reopening was required for tamponade due to or exacerbated by pericardial constriction.
- Sternal closure is performed in the routine manner, but a horizontal mattress arrangement of paired sternal wires permits greater distribution of stresses and promotes stability in large patients or when the sternum has been friable or unstable.

- Skin closure is performed with an absorbable subcuticular suture or a running vertical mattress closure with polypropylene suture. If the subcutaneous infection has been extensive, the wound may be left partially open at the skin level to promote drainage.

OUTCOMES

Mortality

The need for chest reopening is a marker of unfavorable outcomes and was associated in our experience from 2000 to 2003 with a hospital mortality of 9.0%. Mortality in the subset of patients undergoing resternotomy for hemorrhage was 6.4%, for tamponade was 8.9%, and for redo surgery was 12%, but patients undergoing reopening for shock or cardiac arrest had a mortality of 50%.

Deep Sternal Infection

Deep sternal infection, which occurred in 0.3% of patients in 2003, was too rare an event to determine in multivariable analyses whether the requirement for chest reopening, for reasons other than sternal infection, was associated with the subsequent development of sternal osteomyelitis or mediastinitis.

Length of Stay

Patients requiring chest reopening stayed a mean of 5.4 days in the postcardiac surgical unit and 15.6 days in the hospital (versus 2.5 and 8.5 days, respectively, for patients not requiring resternotomy).

SUMMARY

Chest reopening in the early postoperative period may be required for emergency diagnostic or therapeutic purposes. All CVICUs and wards should have an emergency resternotomy tray and appropriate equipment on hand. Restoration of hemodynamic stability in unstable patients is the first priority, followed by careful evaluation of all surgical sites, grafts, and prosthetic or repaired valves to ascertain what further interventions are required. Reopening is associated with increased mortality, morbidity, and length of stay. Meticulous attention to detail at the time of initial operation will minimize the need for resternotomy.

SUGGESTED READING

Vijay V, Gold JP. Late complications of cardiac surgery. In: Cohn LH, Edmunds LH Jr, eds. *Cardiac surgery in the adult*. New York: McGraw-Hill; 2003:521–537.

Chapter 45

Infection, Sternal Debridement, and Septic Shock

Lois K. Champion

MEDIASTINITIS

Introduction

- The overall incidence of postoperative deep sternal wound infections is approximately 1% to 4%.
- The mortality rate is 10% to 20%, and patients who develop deep sternal wound infections have an increased length of stay and associated hospital costs.
- Early recognition and aggressive therapy with antibiotics and surgical drainage/debridement is vital.

Risk Factors

Patient risk factors include diabetes, obesity, renal failure, increased age, chronic obstructive pulmonary disease, cigarette smoking, repeat sternotomy, and prolonged ventilation. Increased blood glucose levels in the postoperative period are associated with an increased risk of surgical site infection.

Operative factors that increase the risk of sternal infection include increased operative time, bilateral internal mammary artery grafts, and re-exploration.

Prevention

- Preoperative:
  - Preoperative chlorhexidine shower (the night before and morning of surgery).
  - Clipping rather than shaving of hair at surgical site (if required).
  - Antimicrobial prophylaxis.

- Intraoperative:
  - Sterile technique.
  - Antimicrobial prophylaxis: The antibiotic administration should be timed so that a bactericidal concentration is present at the time of skin incision, and therapeutic levels must be maintained until the incision is closed. Cefazolin is the antibiotic of choice for prophylaxis; levels will decrease below therapeutic after approximately 3 to 4 hours, necessitating a repeat intraoperative dose if surgery lasts for more than 4 hours. Vancomycin is an alternative antibiotic for patients with allergy to cephalosporin/penicillin. Vancomycin may also be indicated if there is an outbreak of methicillin-resistant *Staphylococcus aureus* (MRSA) wound infections.
  - Intraoperative treatment of hyperglycemia.
- Postoperative:
  - Intensive blood glucose control and insulin therapy decreases the risk of infection and mortality in patients who are critically ill, including cases of postcardiac surgery. Blood glucose should be maintained between 4.4 and 6.1 mmol/L postoperatively.
  - Strict handwashing before and after examination of the patient decreases the risk of nosocomial infections.
  - Surveillance for infection, including daily examination of the incision site, for early recognition and therapy is important.

Diagnosis

Most patients present with symptoms of mediastinitis within the first 2 weeks; however, late presentations may also be seen. In general, infections due to gram-negative organisms appear early in the postoperative course.

Clinical features include fever, increased white blood cell (WBC) count, incisional pain, erythema, and purulent drainage from the sternal wound. Note, however, that patients may *not* have typical features of infection such as fever. Some patients will present with septic shock. The sternum may be unstable clinically with "clicking" on palpation or obvious rocking with respiration.

Radiologically, the chest x-ray may show a midsternal stripe of air (>3 mm), or displacement, or malalignment of the sternal wires with sternal dehiscence. Computerized tomography (CT) findings in mediastinitis include obliteration of the mediastinal fat planes, mediastinal fluid collections, and sternal dehiscence. Because retrosternal fluid collections, pneumomediastinum, and hematomas are seen in many patients postoperatively for up to 3 weeks, CT scan findings tend to be nonspecific with low sensitivity. WBC scanning may show WBC accumulation within the sternum or mediastinum.

Culture of purulent drainage from the wound will help guide antimicrobial therapy; in addition, mediastinal needle aspiration and culture of epicardial pacing wires have also been described.

Therapy

- Medical management of shock if required (see section on Septic Shock).

■ Antimicrobial therapy: Because most deep-sternal infections are caused by *Staphylococcus* (*S. epidermidis* or *S. aureus* including MRSA), initial antibiotic therapy must include a drug such as vancomycin (alternative antibiotics which are effective against MRSA include linezolid and quinupristin-dalfoprisitin). Pending results of the Gram stain and cultures, a broad-spectrum antibiotic effective against gram-negative organisms may also be used. Antibiotic therapy should be continued for 6 weeks in the case of deep infections or osteomyelitis.

■ Debridement and muscle flap:
  ● Debridement of the infected tissue and rewiring of the sternum is indicated in patients with sternal dehiscence without evidence of osteomyelitis; postoperative irrigation with mediastinal drains may also be used.
  ● Patients with necrotic bone, osteomyelitis, or severe infection require debridement of all infected tissues including bone. If the patient is clinically unstable, or the wound is grossly contaminated, then delayed flap closure should be considered. Primary flap closure may be used in select patients.
  ● Flap reconstruction includes the use of a pectoral or latissimus dorsi muscle flap to provide vascular tissue to fill in the defects in the mediastinum, and provide protection to the mediastinum when the sternum has been debrided and rewiring is not possible.

SEPTIC SHOCK

Introduction

Septic shock is defined as sepsis with evidence of sepsis-induced tissue hypoperfusion (hypotension or lactic acidosis). Septic shock is an emergency, and aggressive, early (in the first 6 hours) goal-directed therapy has been shown to improve survival. Overall mortality for patients with septic shock is 30% to 40%.

Initial Resuscitation

Resuscitation goals should include a mean arterial pressure of >65 mm Hg, central venous pressure of 8 to 12 mm Hg, and urine output of >0.5 mL/kg/hour.

Intravenous fluid resuscitation is needed and patients may require over 5 L of fluid in the first 6 hours of resuscitation. There is no evidence that colloids are superior to crystalloids for volume resuscitation in sepsis.

For ongoing hypotension that does not respond to volume resuscitation, inotropic/vasopressor therapy may be required. If there is evidence of inadequate oxygen delivery (central venous or mixed venous oxygen saturation <70%), a dobutamine infusion can be used. For refractory hypotension, an infusion of norepinephrine, dopamine, or a low-dose vasopressin infusion may be used.

Diagnosis

Cultures should be obtained, including two blood cultures and cultures from potentially infected sites. Other diagnostic studies (e.g., CT scans) should be arranged promptly, but resuscitation and stabilization of the patient takes priority.

Therapy

■ Antibiotics: It is recommended that intravenous antibiotic therapy be started within the first hour of recognition of sepsis, after cultures have been taken. Broad-spectrum empiric therapy is needed, and the antibiotics must be reassessed when the results of the cultures become available. Inadequate or delayed antibiotic therapy is associated with an increase in mortality.

■ Source control: Irrigation and drainage of an abscess or debridement of the infected necrotic tissue.

■ Steroids: Patients with septic shock may have relative adrenal insufficiency, with endogenous cortisol levels that are low, given the patient's "high stress" state. Intravenous corticosteroids (e.g., hydrocortisone 50 mg IV q6h, which may be combined with fludrocortisone 50 μg PO OD) should be considered for patients with septic shock and requiring vasopressor therapy. A 250 μg adrenocorticotropic hormone (ACTH) stimulation test should also be considered before beginning steroid therapy to assess the patient for relative adrenal insufficiency. Intravenous steroids have been associated with a decrease in vasopressor requirements in patients with septic shock. In patients with an inadequate cortisol response to a 250 μg bolus of ACTH (a <250 nmol/L increase in cortisol level from baseline), an improved survival was seen with hydrocortisone/fludrocortisone therapy. Steroids should be discontinued after 7 days; alternatively, steroid therapy should be weaned over several days with a goal of discontinuing it within 7 to 10 days.

■ Recombinant human activated protein C (rhAPC) is recommended for patients with severe sepsis: rhAPC has anticoagulant, antifibrinolytic, and anti-inflammatory properties, and has been shown to improve survival in patients with severe sepsis (acute physiology and chronic health evaluation II scores of $\geq$25, or sepsis-induced multiple organ failure). It is contraindicated in patients with active bleeding or in those at high risk of bleeding complications (such as recent hemorrhagic stroke, epidural catheter, etc.). See product labeling for complete indications and contraindications.

■ Attention to detail is vital in the case of a patient who is critically ill.

● Patients on ventilators should be nursed head up (30 to 45 degrees), which has been shown to decrease the risk of ventilator-associated pneumonia.

● Patients should have prophylaxis for deep vein thrombosis (subcutaneous heparin or sequential compression devices if anticoagulants are contraindicated).

● Patients who are ventilated and/or coagulopathic should receive stress ulcer prophylaxis (ranitidine IV or PO).

● Patients should have adequate nutritional support; for intubated patients this will mean enteral feeding. If enteral nutrition is not possible, total parenteral nutrition is indicated.

● For patients with acute lung injury or acute respiratory distress syndrome, a lung protective ventilation strategy should be used. This requires a tidal volume of approximately 6 mL/kg predicted body weight, and limiting end-inspiratory plateau pressures to <30 cm H_2O.

SUGGESTED READINGS

Centers for Disease Control and Prevention (CDC) Hospital Infection Control Practices Advisory Committee. Guideline for prevention of surgical site infection. *Infect Control Hosp Epidemiol.* 1999;20:247–278.

Dellinger RP, Carlet JM, Masur H, et al. Surviving sepsis campaign guidelines for management of severe sepsis and septic shock. *Crit Care Med.* 2004;32:858–873.

Hotchkiss RS, Karl IE. The pathophysiology and treatment of sepsis. *N Engl J Med.* 2003;348:138–150.

Lowy FD, Waldhausen JA, Miller M, et al. NHLBI-NIAID working group on antimicrobial strategies and cardiothoracic surgery. *Am Heart J.* 2004;147:575–581.

Robicsek F. Postoperative sterno-mediastinitis. *Am Surg.* 2000;66:184–192.

van den Berghe G, Wouters PJ, Weekers F, et al. Intensive insulin therapy in critically ill patients. *N Engl J Med.* 2001;345:1359–1367.

Chapter 46

Difficult Weaning from Mechanical Ventilation and Tracheotomy Care

Thomas L. Higgins and Patrick C. Lee

Anesthesia, thoracotomy, surgical manipulation, and cardiopulmonary bypass (CPB) create transient deleterious effects on pulmonary function even with normal lungs. The effects are worse with pre-existing pulmonary pathology. These include:

- Diminished functional residual capacity (FRC)—causes arterial hypoxemia due to ventilation perfusion (V/Q) mismatch.
- Diminished lung compliance—increases the work of breathing (WOB) and oxygen consumption.
- Transient 50% to 75% reduction in the vital capacity (VC) following median sternotomy and intrathoracic manipulation.

- Atelectasis.
- Increased intravascular lung water.

Changes in spirometric measurements and respiratory muscle strength last up to 8 weeks. Common complications include:

- Prolonged mechanical ventilation (≥72 hours following arrival at the intensive care unit [ICU]) in 8%.
- Reintubation of the trachea either shortly after initial extubation or because of delayed respiratory failure in 7%.
- Acute lung injury (ALI) or acute respiratory distress syndrome (ARDS) in up to 12%.
- Tracheostomy in 1.4%.

RISK FACTORS FOR RESPIRATORY INSUFFICIENCY AFTER CARDIOTHORACIC SURGERY

- Respiratory muscle weakness (note that prophylactic inspiratory muscle training reduces the incidence of postoperative ventilation support required for 24 hours or more from 26% to 5%).
- Patients with severe chronic obstructive pulmonary disease (COPD), especially for patients who are 75 years or more or receiving steroids.
- Intraoperative factors, including transfusion of more than 10 units of blood products or a total CPB time in excess of 120 minutes.
- Predictors of mechanical ventilation for more than 72 hours include prolonged CPB time, sepsis, endocarditis, gastrointestinal (GI) bleeding, renal failure, deep sternal wound infection, new stroke, and bleeding requiring reoperation.
- Prognostic implications of an intra-aortic balloon pump (IABP) depend on the reason for insertion. Mortality and ventilation dependency rates increase over baseline if IABP is placed preoperatively for unstable angina, and highest rates if IABP is placed for cardiogenic shock or to assist in separating from bypass. Some patients may be successfully extubated while on IABP, but the need to lie flat after balloon and sheath removal may dictate continued temporary ventilator support.
- Aspiration of mouth flora or gastric contents (therefore, use oral rather than nasal routes for endotracheal and gastric sump tubes and remove devices at the earliest opportunity).
- Hospital-acquired infections: risk of ventilator-associated pneumonia (VAP) is approximately 1% per day of ventilator support when diagnosed using protected specimen brush and quantitative culture techniques.
  - Strategies effective at reducing the incidence of VAP:
    - ▲ Early removal of nasogastric or endotracheal tubes (ETTs).
    - ▲ Formal infection control programs.
    - ▲ Handwashing.
    - ▲ Semirecumbent positioning of the patient.
    - ▲ Avoidance of unnecessary reintubation.
    - ▲ Provision of adequate nutritional support.
    - ▲ Avoidance of gastric overdistention.
    - ▲ Maintenance of adequate ETT cuff pressure.

- Strategies that are *not* considered effective:
  - ▲ Routine changes of the ventilator circuit.
  - ▲ Dedicated use of disposable suction catheters.
  - ▲ Routine changes of in-line suction catheters.
  - ▲ Daily exchanges of heat and moisture changes.
  - ▲ Chest physiotherapy.
- Strategies recommended but not adequately studied:
  - ▲ Postural changes.
  - ▲ Humidification.
  - ▲ Use of protective gowns and gloves.
  - ▲ Continuous aspiration of subglottic secretions.

ACUTE LUNG INJURY AND ACUTE RESPIRATORY DISTRESS SYNDROME

- Acute lung injury (ALI) and acute respiratory distress syndrome (ARDS) may develop as a sequelae of CPB, cardiogenic shock, sepsis, or multisystem organ failure (MSOF).
- Typical clinical presentation:
  - Acute onset.
  - Severe arterial hypoxemia resistant to oxygen therapy.
  - Oxygen pressure (Pao_2) to fraction of inspired oxygen (Fio_2) (P/F ratio) of <200 mm Hg.
  - Absence of left ventricular failure (hard to distinguish postcoronary artery bypass graft [CABG]).
  - Decreased lung compliance (<80 mL/cm of H_2O).
  - Bilateral infiltrates on chest radiograph.
- Pathophysiology: diffuse alveolar damage resulting from endothelial and type I epithelial cell necrosis and noncardiogenic pulmonary edema due to breakdown of the endothelial barrier, with subsequent vascular permeability.
- Exudative phase of ARDS (days 0 to 3 after the precipitating event) mediated by neutrophil activation and sequestration.
  - Release of mediators causing endothelial damage and increased endothelial permeability.
- Proliferative phase of ARDS (days 3 to 7), in which inflammatory cells accumulate because of chemoattractants released by neutrophils.
- Normal repair process should remove debris and then begin repair.
- Disordered repair process results in fibrosis, stiff lungs, and inefficient gas exchange.
- Management:
  - Address precipitating factors (e.g., drain closed-space infections).
  - Compromised lung is no longer homogeneous and ventilation can further damage remaining normal lung:
    - ▲ Over-distention (volutrauma).
    - ▲ High pressures (barotrauma).
    - ▲ Shear injury from repetitive opening and closing.
    - ▲ "Biotrauma" as a result of inflammatory mediator release.
  - Limit inflation pressures with known or suspected lung injury:
    - ▲ Maximal "safe" inflation pressure is not known.

- ▲ Keep peak inspiratory pressures <35 cm H$_2$O.
- ▲ Restrict V$_T$ to 6 mL or less per kg of ideal body weight.
- ▲ ARDS net trial randomized patients to 6 mL/kg V$_T$ versus 12 mL/kg of ideal body weight—decreased interleukin-6 release and significant difference in 28-day survival with the low V$_T$ strategy.
- ▲ Lower tidal volumes with higher amounts of positive end-expiratory pressure (PEEP) may increase alveolar recruitment and thereby improve oxygenation.
- ■ Additional therapies with ALI/ARDS:
  - ● PEEP involves cardiac/pulmonary trade-offs:
    - ▲ PEEP (without volume loading) can decrease cardiac output.
    - ▲ PEEP does not protect against the development of ARDS.
    - ▲ With ALI or ARDS, higher levels of PEEP (often 8 to 15+ cm H$_2$O) are usually necessary to maintain oxygenation levels.
    - ▲ Lung recruitment maneuvers.
    - ▲ Goal is to re-expand collapsed lung so that ventilation occurs on the pressure–volume curve above a critical closing pressure while avoiding overinflation.
    - ▲ Short-term effects of recruitment maneuvers are highly variable and should be performed cautiously because increased airway pressure may decrease venous return and cardiac output.
  - ● Fluid restriction: Effectiveness is unknown. Current National Institutes of Health (NIH) trial is evaluating the effect of liberal versus conservative fluid management, as well as the use of pulmonary artery catheterization in the ARDS population.
  - ● Permissive hypercapnea, if normal Pco$_2$ levels cannot be achieved with low V$_T$.
  - ● Paco$_2$ levels of up to 60 mm Hg acceptable, if pH is >7.30.
  - ● Normal kidneys compensate for Pco$_2$ induced pH change in 12 to 36 hours.
  - ● Hypothesis: Elevated Pco$_2$ levels might be protective, and efforts to lower Pco$_2$ could play a role in organ injury.
  - ● Prone positioning does not improve outcome in ARDS, although one *post hoc* analysis found lower mortality in patients who are critically ill.
  - ● Corticosteroids: therapy involving prolonged lower dose methylprednisolone in cases of unresolving ARDS improves the P/F ratio, ICU survival, and shortens the duration of mechanical ventilation. This is controversial, as emerging ARDS net data argues against the use of steroids.
  - ● Experimental techniques:
    - ▲ Extracorporeal carbon dioxide (CO$_2$) removal (ECCO$_2$R).
    - ▲ Extracorporeal membrane oxygenation (ECMO).
    - ▲ Partial liquid ventilation.
    - ▲ Inhaled nitric oxide.
    - ▲ Inhaled prostacyclin.
    - ▲ None of the above is documented to improve outcome but may temporize worsening of outcome while the underlying process improves.

GENERAL SUPPORT ISSUES

- ■ Common complications in patients with ventilator assistance include:
  - ● Venous thromboembolism (VTE).
  - ● Catheter-related bloodstream infections.

- Surgical site infections:
  - ▲ VAP.
  - ▲ Pressure ulcers.
  - ▲ Nutritional depletion.
  - ▲ Delirium.
  - ▲ GI bleeding.
- Current recommendations:
  - Appropriate VTE prophylaxis (anticoagulants or pneumatic boots).
  - Use of maximum sterile barriers during catheter insertion.
  - Appropriate perioperative prophylaxis with an antistaphylococcal agent.
  - Prophylaxis against GI bleeding with histamine blockers or proton pump inhibitors, especially if not receiving continuous gastric feedings.
  - Head of bed elevation to 30 degrees or more if hemodynamically stable.
  - Brief daily wake up to avoid excessive sedation.
  - Use of in-line suction catheters.
  - Tight glucose control.
- Daily goals forms or computerized systems are helpful.

IMPEDIMENTS TO WEANING AND EXTUBATION

Agitation

- Delirium.
- Transient postoperative delirium occurs in approximately 7% of patients and generally resolves by postoperative day 6.
- Alcohol or benzodiazepine withdrawal should be considered in the differential diagnosis of delirium.
- Pain may precipitate delirium or agitation.
- Use an appropriate drug for an appropriate indication: haloperidol for delirium, benzodiazepines for withdrawal syndromes and sedation, opioids for analgesia.
- Titrate sedatives to effect, monitor using sedation scale, and minimize sedative accumulation in adipose tissue.

Diaphragmatic Paralysis

- More common following reoperation (possible phrenic nerve injury while dissecting fibrotic pericardial tissue).
- Suspect if patient fails to wean from mechanical ventilation.
- Watch for paradoxical movement of diaphragm during inspiration.
- Measure the difference in VC and V_T in the supine and seated positions; differences of >15% are suggestive.

Critical Illness Polyneuropathy

- Seen with systemic inflammatory response syndrome (SIRS).
- Disuse atrophy and steroid administration also contribute.
- Full recovery of diaphragmatic function may take 4 months to more than 2 years; partial recovery is apparent when the patient can lie flat without dyspnea.

Cardiac Failure

- Acute myocardial dysfunction is common; the nadir of cardiac function is typically 2 to 6 hours after termination of CPB.
- Persistent low-output syndrome is associated with multisystem failure (e.g., renal failure, respiratory failure, disseminated intravascular coagulation, and GI bleeding).
- Acute left ventricular dysfunction may occur in patients with COPD during the shift from mechanical to spontaneous ventilation.
- Watch fluid balance; diurese (or ultrafiltrate with continuous venovenous hemofiltration [CVVH]).
- Patients may be "unweanable" until fluid removal reduces body weight to several kilograms below the preoperative weight.

Renal Failure and Fluid Overload

- Incidence of acute renal failure post-CABG: 1% to 4%.
- Lesser degrees of renal dysfunction (elevated levels of serum creatinine) common (up to 30%).

Wound Infections

- Mediastinitis and/or sternal dehiscence: approximately 1% but with a high mortality rate (approximately 13%) and high incidence of ventilator dependency.
- Mediastinal infection: unexplained fever, an unstable sternum, and failure to wean
  - Drainage and debridement.
  - Appropriate antibiotics—often encounter resistant organisms.
  - Additional management may include primary or delayed sternal closure using pectoralis or omental flaps.
- Maintaining perioperative blood glucose <200 mg/dL reduces the sternal wound infection rate from 2.4% to 1.5%.

Ventilator-associated Pneumonia

- Difficult to differentiate from colonization or tracheobronchitis. Protected tip suction catheters, bronchoalveolar lavage (BAL), or protected brush specimens improve diagnostic specificity.
- Continuous lateral rotational therapy reduces the prevalence of pneumonia, but not mortality or ventilator days.

Gastrointestinal Complications

- Upper gastrointestinal (UGI) bleeding requiring transfusion (1% to 3%):
  - Minimize risk in patients with histamine blockers and on ventilator assistance, proton pump inhibitors, or barrier protective agents (sucralfate).
  - Enteral nutritional support may also be protective.
- Postoperative ileus affects diaphragmatic excursion and increases WOB.
- Pancreatitis, mesenteric ischemia, perforation, and bleeding elsewhere in the GI tract are problems of any critically ill patient.

- Diarrhea: differential includes mesenteric ischemia, and *Clostridium difficile* overgrowth in patients treated with antibiotics (especially later generation cephalosporins).
  - Rapid assay for *C. difficile* does not capture all strains.
  - Culture of stool is more reliable but takes longer.
  - Treatment of *C. difficile* colitis:
    - Oral or intravenous metronidazole *or*
    - Oral vancomycin (*not* IV—poor gut penetration).
- Toxic megacolon is a surgical emergency.

Nutritional Support and Weaning

- Institute support early, before serious depletion occurs.
- Use appropriate mix of fat and carbohydrate to maintain a respiratory quotient <1.0 (high carbohydrate loads increase CO_2 production, which increases respiratory workload).
- Weekly transferrin or prealbumin levels monitor change in nutritional status—an increase predicts the eventual ability to wean.
- Weaning success in approximately 93% of those with adequate nutritional repletion.
- Weaning failure occurs in 50% of those with inadequate nutrition.

MODES OF VENTILATOR SUPPORT

Assist-control Mode

- Specified volume delivered for both patient-triggered and machine-triggered breaths. Assist-control (A/C) rate of 12 with V_T of 600 mL, for example, will deliver a minimum of 7.2 L/minute ventilation; more is delivered if the patient is breathing over the set rate.
- As with all volume-cycled modes, peak inspiratory pressure is determined by ventilator settings (i.e., flow rate, inspiratory time, and volume to be delivered), the compliance of the patient's lungs and chest wall, and the patient's degree of synchrony with the ventilator. Primary use of A/C is during full mechanical ventilation support in the critically ill, which is generally not a weaning mode (see section on "On-Off" mode in the following text).
- If patient is sedated or paralyzed and not breathing over the set rate, A/C becomes control-mode ventilation.
- A/C mode can produce respiratory alkalosis in patients with neurologic tachypnea.

Synchronized Intermittent Mandatory Ventilation

- Specified V_T delivered for machine breaths; patient's own inspiratory effort will determine additional minute ventilation.
- Often used as a routine weaning mode, because synchronized intermittent mandatory ventilation (SIMV) rate can be decreased as the patient takes over more of the respiratory work.
- SIMV is most appropriate for short-term mechanical ventilation in patients recovering from opioid anesthesia.

- SIMV mode has been used for weaning complex patients, but the weaning effort may stall at very low IMV rates if patients cannot achieve spontaneous volumes sufficient to activate their pulmonary stretch receptors. Under these circumstances, a patient is likely to become tachypneic, and weaning attempts fail.

Traditional or "On-Off" Weaning

- Traditional weaning can be used with any ventilation mode, although it has been most commonly combined with A/C support.
- Disconnect the patient from the ventilator and allow to breathe through a "T-piece" with supplemental oxygen, with or without continuous positive airway pressure (CPAP).
- Initial weaning attempts may run for less than a minute: the time gradually lengthens as patient strength improves.
- This is a time-consuming method because the active participation of a nurse or respiratory therapist is needed during each weaning trial, often several times per day.
- V_T, apnea, pressure alarms, and capnography are disabled during the T-piece trial.

Pressure Support Ventilation

- Pressure support ventilation (PSV) can be used with CPAP or combined with SIMV.
- PSV assists each spontaneous patient breath by increasing airway pressure during inspiratory phase.
- It is analogous to bilevel positive airway pressure (BiPAP) noninvasive ventilation, with the CPAP level corresponding to expiratory pressure, and the sum of CPAP and PSV level corresponding to the inspiratory pressure.
- PSV level is titrated to keep the patient's spontaneous respiratory rate in the range of 16 to 24 breaths/minute; this is enough to allow the patient to work his or her muscles without overstressing them.
- Tidal volume will vary with the patient's lung compliance; continuous monitoring with pulse oximetry and end-tidal CO_2 is helpful.
- During weaning trials, it is common to "work" the patient during the day with CPAP/PSV and return them to higher levels of ventilation support (A/C, SIMV at high respiratory rates, or higher levels of PSV) at night to allow them to rest and recover.

OVERVIEW OF WEANING (LIBERATION FROM MECHANICAL VENTILATORY SUPPORT)

- Weaning from ventilator support is not synonymous with extubation.
- Conditions where weaning is possible, but extubation is not:
  - Upper airway edema or compression.
  - Glottic dysfunction with aspiration.
  - Neurologic dysfunction or other inability to protect the airway.
- Formal weaning is not necessary in most (healthy) patients.
  - SIMV or PSV weaning may be convenient.
  - Absence of significant cardiopulmonary dysfunction, extubation after short-term support depends more on a stable clinical condition, adequate rewarming, elimination and metabolism of anesthetics, and reversal of neuromuscular blockade.

- Weaning strategies are almost always required after more than 3 days of ventilation support.

READINESS FOR WEANING: TWO ESSENTIAL QUESTIONS

1. Has the original indication for mechanical ventilation resolved?
   - Sepsis or other infection: increases minute ventilation needs.
   - Low cardiac output: cannot impose additional WOB if cardiac output is already marginal or if additional work will precipitate ischemia.
   - Fluid overload—often with renal dysfunction.
   - Open chest, open abdomen, ascites, and pleural effusions—all represent physical impediments to spontaneous respiration.
   - Thick or copious respiratory secretions.
   - Neurologic complications, especially those affecting the respiratory control center or ability to protect the airway.
   - Malnutrition, either pre-existing or developing during the acute illness.
2. Does the patient have sufficient pulmonary and muscle function to support his or her own minute ventilation needs?
   - Adequate oxygenation (typically a $Pao_2 > 60$ mm Hg on 35% inspired oxygen and low levels of PEEP).
   - Adequate ability to respond to CO_2 stimuli.
   - Adequate respiratory mechanics (V_T, maximal inspiratory pressure).
   - Adequate respiratory reserve (minute ventilation at rest of <10 L/minute) and a low frequency to V_T ratio ($f/V_T < 100$) indicating adequate volume at a sustainable respiratory rate.

OBJECTIVE MEASURES OF PATIENT STRENGTH AND ENDURANCE

- A variety of parameters are used; few have been verified.
- VC (volume of gas exhaled after maximal inspiration) is normally >70 mL/kg. A clinical readiness threshold of 10 to 15 mL/kg has been proposed, but that is neither sensitive nor specific.
- Ability to maintain a pH >7.35 while the IMV rate is decreased to CPAP—valid for short-term patients, but not for the difficult population.
- Maximal inspiratory pressure >30 cm H_2O is associated with a moderate false-positive and 100% false-negative rate.
- Resting minute ventilation rate <10 L/minute has a false-positive rate of 11% and a false-negative rate of 75% in predicting successful extubation.
- Frequency to tidal volume ratio (f/V_T):
  - f is measured in breaths per minute; V_T in liters.
  - 20 breaths per minute with 0.4 L V_T would give f/V_T of 50.
  - The greater the f/V_T value, the more rapid and shallow the respirations; and the shorter the expiratory time when diaphragmatic blood flow occurs.
  - $f/V_T > 105$ has a predictive value of 89% for weaning failure.

- Measured respiratory parameters or scoring systems assess pulmonary function but do not include the nonrespiratory parameters affecting weaning (see Table 46-1).

WEANING: THE PROCESS

- Must be individualized for the patient.
- Gradual decrease in SIMV rate in increments of two breaths per minute generally works for short-term ventilatory support.
- Long-term patients often have difficulty making the transition from low SIMV rates to CPAP.
- Pressure support with CPAP or SIMV:
  - It is common to use CPAP with pressure support alone (i.e., no additional IMV rate) because mechanical ventilation introduces one more variable into the evaluation of a patient's progress.
  - Sufficient CPAP is supplied to maintain open alveoli (generally 5 to 8 cm H_2O but often higher when recovering from ALI/ARDS), and then the pressure support level is titrated to provide the patient with sufficient volume and a respiratory rate <24 breaths/minute.
  - As the patient's exercise tolerance improves, the pressure support level can be lowered in increments of 2 to 3 cm H_2O.
  - It is usually necessary to address fluid overload, nutritional support, and other nonpulmonary factors in order to successfully reduce level of PSV.
- End each weaning trial with success rather than failure:
  - Never stress the patient to the point of fatigue.
  - Respiratory rate is the most sensitive clinical marker of fatigue.
  - Other clinical markers are increase in respiratory rate, respiratory alternans, and abdominal paradox.
  - Increased $Paco_2$ levels and acidemia are late findings.

▶ **TABLE 46-1 Nonrespiratory Factors Affecting Weaning**

■ Cardiac function
■ Nutritional status
■ Renal function/fluid overload
■ Sepsis/infection
■ Anemia
■ Metabolic disturbance/thyroid function
■ Excessive sedation/active metabolites
■ Neurologic compromise
■ Neuropsychiatric issues/delirium
■ Sleep deprivation
■ Endotracheal tube size
■ Patient's perception of breathing

MECHANICAL IMPEDIMENTS TO WEANING

- Insufficient inspiratory flow rate may present as "air-hunger."
- Pulmonary effusions and pneumothorax.
- Stacking of breaths or auto-PEEP, especially with obstructive disease.
- Altered chest cage compliance due to increased intercostal muscle tone or increased intra-abdominal pressure.
- Ventilator dys-synchrony: patient actively attempting to impede flow during the inspiratory cycle, a process referred to as "fighting," being "out of phase," or "breathing against" the ventilator. It is commonly due to hypercarbia, acidemia, hypoxia, central nervous system (CNS) dysfunction, pain, anxiety, or agitation.
- Assisting the patient with manual ventilation or switching to assist modes for a short time may allow the patient to settle down and return to synchrony with the ventilator. Evaluate and treat the underlying cause: endotracheal cuff leak, misplaced ETT, inadequate inspiratory flow rates, pneumothorax, abdominal distention, pain, and anxiety should all be considered.

MUSCLE WEAKNESS AND CRITICAL ILLNESS POLYNEUROPATHY

- Long-term administration of neuromuscular blocking agents, particularly with a steroidlike structure, has been associated with persistent paralysis but can be seen with any agent.
- Accumulation of the metabolite 3-desacetylvecuronium is rarely seen in patients with normal renal function, but is quite common in patients with MSOF, especially with renal dysfunction.
- Neurogenic atrophy occurs with prolonged paralysis, resulting in a flaccid quadriplegia or more localized weakness of respiratory muscles.

PSYCHIATRIC ISSUES

- Prolonged ICU stay may precipitate psychosis even in healthy patients.
- These issues are more common in patients with an underlying psychiatric history.
- Continuous light, noise, and sleep deprivation can change the patient's perception of reality: maintain a normal diurnal variation, ensure adequate sleep, create a quiet ICU environment, use pharmacologic agents such as haloperidol as needed, and involve the patient and family as participants in the weaning process.

TRACHEOSTOMY

- Prolonged endotracheal intubation results in injury to the respiratory epithelium and cilia, and may lead to vocal cord damage and airway stenosis.
- Other indications for tracheostomy include copious or tenacious secretions in debilitated patients who are unable to clear them spontaneously.

- Complications include pneumothorax, pneumomediastinum, subcutaneous emphysema, incisional hemorrhage, late tracheal stenosis or tracheomalacia, stomal infections, and, rarely, tracheoinnominate fistula.
- Tracheostomy has been relatively contraindicated with ongoing potential cross-contamination of the sternotomy from colonized tracheal secretions. Percutaneous dilatational tracheostomy may offer a long-term secure airway with less dissection.
- Percutaneous dilatational tracheostomy can be accomplished with commercially available kits using straight dilators (Portex/Smiths Group, Keene, New Hampshire), and angled dilators.
- A swallowing dysfunction may occur following tracheostomy or after prolonged endotracheal intubation, introducing the risk of aspiration pneumonia or respiratory failure.
- Swallowing evaluation is indicated before the first oral feeding after tracheostomy. Dysphagia or aspiration may be noted by nurses during attempted feedings.

INABILITY TO WEAN

- A small percentage of patients will not be able to be weaned from ventilator support despite all efforts. Predictive models, however, are rarely useful for deciding which individuals will not benefit from further intensive care.
- Accumulation of multiple morbidities creates a situation in which the patient may become life-long ventilator dependent. Frank discussions with the patient (if he/she has decisional capacity) or the health care proxy can be helpful in defining the potential benefits and burdens of further therapy and the patient's desires. Consultation from the hospital's ethics team may be very helpful.
- Patients who remain in a low cardiac output state and who have sustained multiple organ failure, rarely, if ever, end their dependence on high-technology support, including ventilation and hemodialysis. Malnutrition and deconditioning, in the absence of ongoing sepsis and organ system failure, sometimes respond to prolonged rehabilitation that may be better handled by a long-term ventilator facility than the acute care hospital.

TAKE-HOME POINTS

- Weaning success requires an individualized and holistic approach to the patient.
- Weaning should be the first priority for the day, and all other demands (e.g., trips to the computed tomographic [CT] scan, wound debridement) should be minimized if possible.
- Avoid disrupting the patient's nighttime sleep so that the patient can be rested and ready to participate in the weaning process.
- Give detailed and full instructions to the patient, and include select family members so that they can serve as adjunct respiratory coaches.
- Avoid pushing the patient to the point of exhaustion or panic. Set conservative and reachable goals so that weaning trials always end with a sense of accomplishment rather than of failure.

SUGGESTED READINGS

The Acute Respiratory Distress Syndrome Network. Ventilation with lower tidal volumes as compared with traditional tidal volumes for acute lung injury and the acute respiratory distress syndrome. *N Engl J Med*. 2000;342:1301–1308.

Canver CC, Chanda J. Intraoperative and postoperative risk factors for respiratory failure after coronary bypass. *Ann Thorac Surg*. 2003;75:853–857.

Chastre J, Fagon J-Y. Ventilator-associated pneumonia. *Am J Respir Crit Care Med*. 2002;165: 867–903.

Freeman BD, Isabella K, Cobb P, et al. A prospective, randomized study comparing percutaneous with surgical tracheostomy in critically ill patients. *Crit Care Med*. 2001;29:926–930.

Kress JP, Pohlman AS, O'Connor MF, et al. Daily interruption of sedative infusions in critically ill patients undergoing mechanical ventilation. *N Engl J Med*. 2000;342:1471–1477.

Laffrey JG, Kavanagh BP. Carbon dioxide and the critically ill—too little of a good thing? *Lancet*. 1999;354:1283–1286.

Rady MY, Ryan T. Perioperative predictors of extubation failure and the effect on clinical outcomes after cardiac surgery. *Crit Care Med*. 1999;27:340–347.

Rady MY, Ryan T, Staff NJ. Early onset of acute pulmonary dysfunction after cardiovascular surgery: risk factors and clinical outcome. *Crit Care Med*. 1997;25:11, 1831.

Richard J-C, Brochard L, Vandelet P, et al. Respective effects of end-expiratory and end-inspiratory pressures on alveolar recruitment in acute lung injury. *Crit Care Med*. 2003;31:89–92.

Samuels LE, Kaufman MS, Rohinton BA, et al. Coronary artery bypass grafting in patients with COPD. *Chest*. 1998;113:878–882.

Chapter 47

Renal Failure and Dialysis

Atilio Barbeito and Mark Stafford-Smith

Acute renal dysfunction is a common serious complication of cardiac surgery. All degrees of renal dysfunction after cardiac surgery are associated with increased short- and long-term morbidity, mortality, and cost. Acute renal failure (ARF) requiring dialysis is independently associated with mortality risk. One study demonstrated a 64% mortality rate for patients requiring dialysis following cardiac surgery after adjusting for other postoperative complications and comorbidities compared to a 4% mortality rate for patients with normal renal function.

The pathophysiology of ARF is only partially understood and, with the exception of developments in replacement therapy, care for this complication has progressed little in the last four decades. With older patients undergoing more radical procedures, and an increased number of patients being supported through multisystem organ failure, the incidence of ARF following cardiac surgery is expected to increase. In the absence of effective treatments, identifying those at risk for perioperative renal dysfunction and implementing strategies aimed at avoiding ARF are essential for the successful management of the patient undergoing cardiac surgery.

This chapter reviews the incidence of ARF in the perioperative period of cardiac surgery patients, the risk factors for ARF, the main pathophysiologic mechanisms leading to renal injury, the approach to the patient with renal dysfunction, and the intraoperative and postoperative management of oliguria and renal failure.

INCIDENCE AND RISK FACTORS

All patients suffer some degree of renal dysfunction following cardiac surgery, and each surgical procedure has its own typical pattern of renal injury and recovery, including incidence of acute renal injury requiring dialysis.

Most cases of mild and moderate postoperative renal dysfunction resolve within days or weeks, unless additional renal insults follow the primary injury (e.g., nephrotoxic drugs) or a perpetuating cause exists (e.g., low cardiac output state).

For coronary bypass surgery with cardiopulmonary bypass (CPB), the average creatinine level rise is 22%, with 8% to 15% of patients sustaining moderate renal impairment (>1 mg/dL peak creatinine rise) and 1% to 5% requiring dialysis. In cases where recovery occurs, typically creatinine peaks on the second postoperative day and returns to baseline by the fourth or fifth day.

Identifying the High-Risk Patient

The primary goal of preoperative assessment and/or initial evaluation upon admission to the intensive care unit (ICU) is to identify the patient at risk for postoperative ARF.

Preoperative Risk Factors

- Pre-existing renal dysfunction: Up to 20% of individuals presenting for coronary bypass surgery have pre-existing renal disease. These patients are no more likely to suffer renal injury than patients with healthy kidneys, but their reduced renal reserve means that they are more likely to reach the threshold where dialysis is required.
- Systemic diseases associated with chronic renal failure: diabetes, hypertension, carotid and peripheral vascular disease, coronary artery disease.
- Increased age: Glomerular filtration rate (GFR) declines progressively with advancing age from about 125 mL/minute in young adults to about 80 mL/minute at age 60 and approximately 60 mL/minute at age 80. Elderly patients have a more limited renal reserve, but also sustain, on average, greater renal insults.
- Increased body weight: Patients who are obese, on average, sustain greater renal insults, possibly owing to an exaggerated inflammatory response to CPB.
- Genetic predisposition: Patients with the E4 phenotype of the apolipoprotein E (Apo E) gene have a lower risk of acute renal injury after coronary bypass surgery when compared to patients with the E2 and E3 phenotypes.
- Exposure to nephrotoxic drugs: Nephrotoxic drugs commonly used in patients undergoing cardiac surgery are presented in Table 47-1.

Risk Factors Related to the Surgical Procedure

- Use of CPB: Extended CPB duration is associated with increased renal injury. Pulsatile CPB flow does not have a protective effect in patients with previously normal renal function. Off-pump surgery and changes in CPB perfusion pressure and temperature management have not demonstrated any major effect on postoperative acute renal injury.
- Intraoperative glucose control: Diabetes and hyperglycemia are associated with increased acute renal injury. Renal reuptake of filtered glucose increases oxygen consumption because of the higher activity of the Na^+/glucose cotransporter.

▶ **TABLE 47-1** Nephrotoxic Drugs Commonly Used in Patients of Cardiac Surgery

Drug	Mechanism
ACE inhibitors	Impair renal autoregulation
Aminoglycosides	Proximal tubular necrosis
Amphotericin B	Glomerulonephritis and acute tubular necrosis
β-lactams	Interstitial nephritis
Cimetidine, ranitidine	Interstitial nephritis
Cyclosporin A	Renal vasoconstriction
Intravenous radiocontrast	Distal tubular necrosis
Metoclopramide	Inhibits renal D_2 receptors
NSAIDs (e.g., ketorolac, indomethacin)	Impair renal autoregulation
Sulfonamides	Interstitial nephritis

ACE, angiotensin converting enzyme; NSAIDs, nonsteroidal anti-inflammatory drugs.

- Aortic manipulation/cross clamping and intra-aortic balloon counterpulsation (IABP): Atheroembolism is a potential complication of these interventions. Suprarenal and infrarenal cross clamping both reduce renal blood flow; the former by a direct mechanism, the latter by an increase in renal vascular resistance caused by activation of the renin-angiotensin system, the sympathetic system, and other mediators.
- Hemodilution: there is an association between CPB hematocrit and renal dysfunction in obese patients, with lower hematocrits corresponding to worsening renal injury.
- Transfusion: A rise in creatinine levels has been independently associated with transfusion of red cells.
- Complex/open chamber procedures: These procedures generally require longer CPB times and add the potential for air and tissue embolism.

Factors That Prevent Recovery of Renal Injury in the Postoperative Period
- Low cardiac output states: The resultant low renal blood flow perpetuates renal injury.
- Sepsis: The associated vasodilatory state decreases effective intravascular volume.
- Use of inotropic agents: α-adrenergic agonist agents cause renal vasoconstriction and renal ischemia.
- Use of nephrotoxins: Many drugs commonly used in the postoperative period are nephrotoxic and may also contribute to renal dysfunction. Notably, aprotinin and lysine-analog antifibrinolytic agents (e.g., tranexamic acid, epsilon aminocaproic acid) have been implicated as nephrotoxic, but current studies have not confirmed that this is the case.

PATHOPHYSIOLOGY

The etiology of acute renal injury postcardiac surgery is thought to be multifactorial. Ischemia-reperfusion, inflammation, and atheroembolism are three common sources of renal injury, whereas other nephropathies may also contribute to renal injury in select patients (e.g., rhabdomyolysis, drug-related, etc.).

■ Renal hypoperfusion: Tubular damage occurs within 25 minutes of critical ischemia. Even when renal blood flow is restored completely after 60 to 120 minutes of ischemia, GFR may be reduced for several weeks. Events or conditions that limit perfusion to the kidneys intraoperatively and postoperatively are outlined in Table 47-2.

As renal blood flow falls, the kidneys maintain GFR by: (a) dilation of the glomerular afferent arteriole by renal prostaglandins and constriction of the efferent arteriole by angiotensin II (tubuloglomerular feedback) and norepinephrine; and (b) secretion of antidiuretic hormone, which promotes reabsorption of water in the collecting ducts, generating smaller amounts of concentrated urine. Nonsteroidal anti-inflammatory drugs (NSAIDs) inhibit prostaglandin production,

▶ **TABLE 47-2 Conditions that can Decrease Renal Perfusion**

A. Decreased preload
1. Decreased intravascular volume
   Hemorrhage
   Gastrointestinal losses (diarrhea, vomiting, nasogastric suctioning)
   Renal losses (diuretics, glycosuria)
2. Decreased effective intravascular volume
   Vasodilation secondary to drugs (nitroglycerin, sodium nitroprusside, anesthetics)
   Sepsis
3. Decreased venous return to the LV
   Positive pressure ventilation
   Pulmonary embolism
   Atrial fibrillation
   Cardiac tamponade
   Tension pneumothorax

B. Decreased contractility/myocardial efficiency
1. Myocardial ischemia
2. Nonischemic cardiomyopathy
3. Valvular dysfunction
4. Negative inotropic drugs

C. Impaired renal perfusion (despite normal preload and cardiac output)
1. Renal artery stenosis or thrombosis
2. Dissecting aortic aneurysm
3. Malpositioned IABP
4. Suprarenal aortic cross clamp
5. Infrarenal aortic cross clamp

D. Impaired renal autoregulation
1. Inhibition of vasodilating renal prostaglandins (NSAIDs)
2. Inhibition of glomerular efferent artery vasoconstriction (ACE inhibitors)
3. Inhibition of dopaminergic receptors (metoclopramide)
4. Blood pressure management below the range of normal renal autoregulation (MAP <80–90 mm Hg)

LV, left ventricle; IABP, intra-aortal balloon pump; NSAIDs, nonsteroidal anti-inflammatory drugs; ACE, angiotensin converting enzyme; MAP, mean arterial pressure.

and angiotensin-conversion enzyme inhibitors (ACEI) hamper the conversion of angiotensin I to angiotensin II, thereby abolishing these compensatory mechanisms and contributing to the development of ARF.

Further declines in renal blood flow overwhelm these compensatory mechanisms, and excessive vasoconstrictive forces cause afferent arteriolar vasoconstriction and a decrease in filtration fraction, evidenced clinically as oliguria. Intense renal vasoconstriction also limits blood flow to the renal tubules, causing tubular cell swelling, sloughing of the "brush border," and even shedding of intact cells into the tubular lumen and formation of obstructive casts, with "backleak" of solute into the circulation, cellular death, and apoptosis.

- Embolism nephropathy: Manipulation of diseased aortic regions during surgery can result in detachment of atheromatous material and downstream embolism. Other contributors to embolic renal injury include thrombus, lipid, air, and other particulate emboli such as tissue fragments.

  Owing to the organization of the renal vasculature, embolic arterial obstruction is poorly compensated for by collateral flow and affects related regions of cortex and medulla, resulting in wedge-shaped infarcts.

- Inflammatory nephropathy: The inflammatory response to surgery, including CPB, generates cytokines (e.g., tumor necrosis factor alpha [TNFα] and interleukin 6 [IL-6]) both systemically and locally in the kidney, which have major effects on the renal microcirculation and may lead to tubular injury.

APPROACH TO THE PATIENT WITH RENAL DYSFUNCTION UNDERGOING CARDIAC SURGERY

Preoperative Assessment of Renal Function

- Conditions associated with postoperative ARF (e.g., hyperglycemia) should be identified (see Section II), and their management optimized to limit renal risk.
- Medications should be reviewed, and potentially nephrotoxic ones should be discontinued whenever possible.
- Preoperative blood urea nitrogen (BUN) and creatinine (Cr) values are usually sufficient to determine any baseline renal dysfunction, although it is important to consider that serum creatinine level does not usually rise until GFR falls below 50 mL/minute, so preoperative BUN and Cr may be normal in patients with some degree of renal dysfunction.
- GFR is a better indicator of renal function than serum creatinine. The Cockroft-Gault equation allows estimation of the GFR on the basis of the patient's age, weight, serum creatinine level, and gender.

$$GFR = (140 - age) \times weight (kg)/(C_r \times 72) \ (\times 0.85 \ for \ women)$$

Note that urine output is generally a very poor indicator of renal function.

- Cardiac catheterization and/or angiography reports should be obtained and any significant renal artery stenosis should be noted. Renal dysfunction related to contrast nephropathy may warrant delay of elective surgery.
- Patients receiving dialysis preoperatively should be evaluated for signs and symptoms of uremia, fluid overload, or electrolyte imbalances. Their treatment schedule

should be reviewed and their dry weight noted. Ideally, dialysis should be carried out the day before surgery to avoid acute fluid and electrolyte shifts.

Monitoring Renal Function in the Operating Room

- A reliable intraoperative monitor for renal function does not currently exist.
- Urine output is a very poor indicator of renal injury, but is readily available and easily measured. It is typically elevated in the presence of high CPB perfusion pressure, diuretics and hyperglycemia, and even in the setting of hypovolemia. Urine color is a very imprecise method of determining urine density; hemolysis related to CPB may make this sign even more unreliable.
- Hemodynamic parameters (invasive arterial pressure monitoring, systolic pressure variation, central venous pressure [CVP], pulmonary capillary wedge pressure [PCWP]) should be considered indirect monitors of renal perfusion in the absence of localized obstruction of blood flow to the kidneys (suprarenal aortic cross clamp, renal artery stenosis, abdominal compartment syndrome). Urine output during CPB is most highly correlated with mean arterial blood pressure.

Determinations of BUN, Cr, urine Na$^+$, and osmolarity are useful in the postoperative period but impractical in the operating room. Intraoperative and immediate postoperative BUN and Cr values may reflect dilutional effects of intraoperative fluids and ultrafiltration during CPB.

Evaluation of Renal Function in the Postoperative Period

Although oliguria (<400 mL urine per day) is a useful marker of hypovolemia and may reflect impending "prerenal" renal failure, most episodes of postoperative ARF develop in the presence of normal urine output.

- A review of vital signs and physical examination to assess volume status may identify treatable causes of renal stress including true hypovolemia and decreased effective arterial volume, as in congestive heart failure.
- Creatinine clearance (C_{Cr}) parallels GFR and is a useful measure of renal filtration in the postoperative period. Two-hour measurements of urine and serum creatinine levels and urine volume are a useful and quick way to assess GFR. It is calculated using the following formula:

$$C_{Cr} \text{ (mL/min)} = U_{Cr} \text{ (mg/dL)} \times V \text{ (mL)}/P_{Cr} \text{ (mg/dL)} \times \text{time (min)}$$

where U_{Cr} = urine creatinine, V = total volume of urine collected, P_{Cr} = plasma creatinine, and time = collection time.

When a reduction in GFR is confirmed (see Table 47-3), reversible causes (e.g., hypovolemia) should be distinguished from irreversible renal injury. Reversible causes are reflected by the continued ability to produce concentrated urine (see Table 47-4). In contrast, the injured kidney will generate urine that more closely resembles the solute content of filtered plasma.

▶ **TABLE 47-3** Creatinine Clearance

Value	Implication
120	Normal (healthy, 20 year old)
80	Normal (healthy, 60 year old)
25–50	Creatinine may become abnormal; adjust drug dosages
15–25	Prerenal ARF, nonoliguric ATN
<10	Oliguric ARF

ARF, acute renal failure; ATN, acute tubular necrosis.
Modified from Lee HT, Sladen RN. Chapter 42 – Perioperative renal protection. In: Murray MJ, Coursin DB, Pearl RG et al., eds. *Critical care medicine, perioperative management.* 2nd ed. Philadelphia, PA: Lippincott Williams & Wilkins; 2002:503–520.

- In the presence of hypovolemia, relative or absolute, the normal kidney generates concentrated urine with a low sodium content (<20 mEq/L). Concentrating ability is lost with established renal injury, and the kidneys eliminate urine with a lower osmolarity and higher sodium content; urine sodium in this case exceeds 80 mEq/L.
- The fractional excretion of sodium (FE_{Na}) compares sodium excretion with creatinine excretion; it is calculated from a spot sample of urine and blood and may be useful in distinguishing hypovolemia from renal injury:

$$FE_{Na} = U_{Na}/P_{Na} \times P_{Cr}/U_{Cr} \times 100$$

where U_{Na} = urine sodium, P_{Na} = plasma sodium, U_{Cr} = urine creatinine, and P_{Cr} = plasma creatinine.

MANAGEMENT

Preoperative Considerations

- Preoperative risk stratification-prevention is preferable.
- High-risk patients may be considered for hydration and prophylactic oral *N*-acetylcysteine therapy before intravenous (IV) contrast administration.

▶ **TABLE 47-4** Laboratory Evaluation of Oliguric Acute Renal Failure

Test	U/P Cr	U_{Na}	FE_{Na} [a] (%)	U osmolarity
Prerenal ARF	>40	<20	<1	>500
ATN	<20	>40	>1	<350

U, urine; P, plasma; Cr, creatinine; U_{Na}, urine sodium; FE_{Na}, fractional excretion of sodium; ARF, acute renal failure; ATN, acute tubular necrosis.
[a]FE_{Na} is invalid within 6 to 8 hours of diuretic use.

- Intravascular volume and cardiac output should be optimal throughout surgery to ensure adequate renal perfusion.
- Procedure planning should include consideration of renal risk (e.g., if epiaortic scanning shows atheromatous plaque, an aortic "no-touch" technique may reduce the possibility of atheroembolism).
- Intraoperative techniques that have not proven to be beneficial include CPB hypothermia, CPB perfusion pressure when normal flow is maintained, surface cooling of the kidneys, selective renal perfusion with Ringer lactate solution and intravenous infusion of inosine, among others.

Management of Intraoperative Oliguria

- The complete absence of urine should prompt the suspicion of a misplaced or obstructed bladder catheter. The catheter should be flushed with 60 mL of sterile water using a Tomey syringe; return of urine confirms correct positioning.
- Oliguria ($<$0.5 mL urine/kg/hr) is always an indicator of reduced GFR, but this often represents an attempt by the kidneys to conserve water during periods of reduced renal blood flow: Renal "success" rather than dysfunction. Hemodynamic parameters should be reviewed, and fluid administered if hypovolemia is suspected. It is easier to treat mild pulmonary edema than established ARF. Although many therapies have been studied and are currently used to prevent or treat postcardiac surgery ARF, none have been proven to be clinically useful (or have U.S. Food and Drug Administration [FDA] approval) in humans, including dopaminergic agonists, loop diuretics, mannitol, atrial natriuretic peptide (ANP, anaritide), calcium channel blockers (CCB), endothelin receptor antagonists, and α2-adrenergic agonists.

Management of Patients with Postoperative Renal Dysfunction

Because recovery of renal function usually takes days or weeks, the goal is to support the patient through this period and prevent any further insults to the kidneys.

Patients with serious renal dysfunction have severe limitations in their ability to regulate volume, electrolyte, or acid-base homeostasis. Guidelines to avoid the complications of ARF by creating an environment that does not exceed the renal homeostatic reserve apply to all patients with renal dysfunction and are outlined in the following text. More severe cases of renal impairment require more rigorous adherence to protocols aimed at limiting complications. When these guidelines are insufficient, dialysis is generally required.

Volume Homeostasis

Normal kidneys adjust for free water excess or deficit by eliminating more or less dilute urine, respectively. Failure to maintain volume homeostasis is most commonly associated with the elimination of a fixed amount of isosmotic urine. When the kidneys fail, they lose the ability to adapt to a changing environment. The goal then is to maintain euvolemia through control of fluid administration that keeps volume status within normal limits without the involvement of the failing kidneys.

- Determine the volume status of the patient by physical examination (peripheral or pulmonary edema, skin turgor, mucous membranes, orthostasis, CVP, PCWP) and review the fluid balance.
- Fluids should be prescribed based on this exam; as a general rule, the euvolemic patient should be provided with a volume of fluid equal to the daily urine output, plus an additional 500 mL/day to replace insensible fluid losses. A sodium intake of 2 g/day or less should also be prescribed. Fluid overloaded patients should be fluid restricted (fluid intake less than total output). Hypovolemia should also be avoided because it may worsen renal injury or delay recovery. In the hypovolemic patient, a positive fluid balance should be sought.
- Disorders of sodium balance are generally linked to volume management and should be corrected.
- Postoperative hyponatremia is often the result of excess free water intake relative to solute from administration of hypotonic parenteral fluids. To correct this, the sodium content of the administered solutions should be increased (e.g., normal saline can be used instead of 5% dextrose as diluent for parenteral antibiotics).
- Hypernatremia is typically the result of insufficient free water intake. The free water deficit can be calculated using the following formula:

$$\text{Water deficit} = \text{TBW} \times (P_{Na} - 140 \text{ mEq/L})/140 \text{ mEq/L}$$

TBW = total body water [weight (kg) $\times$ 0.6 for men, weight (kg) $\times$ 0.5 for women]

The calculated volume should be administered as 5% dextrose in water over 48 hours in addition to the maintenance of fluids. Serial serum osmolarities and plasma sodium values should be obtained during treatment; in general, sodium should be corrected at <0.5 mEq/L/hour to reduce the likelihood of cerebral edema.

Electrolyte Homeostasis

- As a general rule, potassium, magnesium, and phosphorus should not be added to parenteral solutions. They should be repleted only when a specific deficit occurs in order to prevent potentially dangerous accumulations.
- Hyperkalemia is in most cases only the consequence of a reduced excretory capacity of the kidney for this electrolyte and can be prevented by restriction of potassium intake in parenteral solutions and diet. Attention should be paid to surreptitious forms of potassium administered in drugs (e.g., potassium penicillin) or parenteral nutrition solutions.
- If restriction of potassium intake is inadequate to prevent hyperkalemia, potassium binding resins such as sodium polystyrene sulfonate (Kayexalate) can be used. Each gram of resin binds up to 1 mEq of K^+ and releases 1.5 mEq of Na^+; the dose is 15 to 30 g in 100 mL of 20% sorbitol orally or rectally. Oral administration is contraindicated with intestinal ileus or obstruction. Diarrhea is a predictable consequence.
- If a potassium-free parenteral fluid plan or drugs fail to control the hyperkalemia, dialysis is indicated, and should also be a clue for the search of an endogenous source of potassium such as hyperglycemia, severe acidosis, or rhabdomyolysis. Potassium removal with hemodialysis approaches 50 mEq/hour, compared with 10 to 15 mEq/hour for peritoneal dialysis (PD).

- Hyperkalemia that produces cardiac dysrhythmias should be treated emergently (e.g., IV calcium chloride or calcium gluconate). IV calcium partially antagonizes the cardiac effects of hyperkalemia but does not reduce the total potassium content in the body. Inhaled β agonists and an IV infusion of glucose and insulin (50 g of glucose per 10 units or regular insulin) or sodium bicarbonate can also be used to shift potassium intracellularly. Elimination of the excess body potassium in patients with ARF can only be accomplished with resins or dialysis.
- Hypocalcemia is common in ARF but infrequently causes tetany or cardiac dysrhythmias. It is usually accompanied by hypomagnesemia, which inhibits the release of parathyroid hormone. This functional hypoparathyroidism, together with the decreased synthesis of 1,25 dihydroxyvitamin D by the failing kidney, are the factors responsible for the hypocalcemia. Calcium and magnesium should be supplemented orally or intravenously.
- Phosphorus is ingested in the diet and usually accumulates in patients with ARF. Hyperphosphatemia can be prevented by phosphorus restriction and by the administration of calcium salts or aluminum hydroxide gels.

Acid-base Homeostasis
Failing kidneys are unable to eliminate the acid load produced by catabolism of protein and cannot reclaim bicarbonate filtered into tubular fluid, eventually leading to an anion gap metabolic acidosis.

- Acidosis that is severe or appears early in the course of ARF indicates that other causes of acidosis such as lactic or ketoacidosis may be present.
- The acid load is usually reduced by restricting protein intake to 0.6 to 0.8 g/kg of body weight, but this is undesirable in the hypercatabolic state of the postoperative period. In these cases, administration of sodium bicarbonate or acetate can reverse acidosis. Three ampules of hypertonic sodium bicarbonate (50 mEq/50 mL) can be added to 1,000 mL of 5% dextrose in water and administered intravenously, taking into consideration the volume and sodium load.

Uremia
Uremia is a syndrome characterized by fatigue, lethargy, anorexia, nausea, and hiccups; it results from the accumulation of nitrogenous waste products. BUN measurement can be used as a marker of waste accumulation.

- As a general rule, BUN values <70 mg/dL are rarely associated with symptoms, and BUN values >100 mg/dL are almost always associated with symptoms. During the postoperative period, for the reasons mentioned in the earlier text, protein restriction is not advisable.
- Dialysis should be instituted when uremic symptoms develop.

Nutrition
Adequate nutrition is essential for recovery in the postoperative period, and the benefits of avoiding short-term dialysis by protein restriction should be weighed against this.

- Enteral or parenteral nutrition should provide a minimum of 1.0 to 1.2 g/kg of protein per day and 30 to 35 kcal/kg.

■ Sodium acetate or bicarbonate should be added to buffer the acid generated by protein breakdown (60 to 80 mEq/day).

Drug Dosing

■ ARF brings on changes in volume of distribution, plasma protein binding, renal metabolism, and accumulation of drugs and active metabolites.
■ All medications should be reviewed and, for those eliminated by the kidney, dosing should be adjusted on the basis of the estimated GFR. Modified dosing guidelines for renal impairment are generally provided as part of the product monograph for agents that are primarily cleared by the kidney. Drugs that may cause further renal injury must be discontinued.
■ The choice of muscle relaxants drugs should take into consideration their route of elimination. For example, the duration of paralysis from pancuronium is considerably extended in the presence of impaired renal function. Atracurium and cis-atracurium undergo spontaneous hydrolysis at normal pH and temperature (Hoffman elimination); atracurium is also hydrolyzed by nonspecific plasma esterases. This makes them the agents of choice in renal failure.
■ Analgesics with no active metabolites such as fentanyl should be chosen over others with longer half lives and active, renally excreted metabolites (e.g., morphine).
■ Aminoglycoside antibiotics and most vasopressor drugs are removed with dialysis, and dosing should be adjusted to compensate for dialytic losses.
  A summary of the basic guidelines for management of the patient undergoing cardiac surgery who has serious renal dysfunction is provided in Table 47-5.

RENAL REPLACEMENT THERAPY (DIALYSIS)

Criteria for Dialysis

■ Absolute indications for initiating dialysis therapy include fluid overload, refractory hyperkalemia or acidosis, and severe uremic symptoms.
■ The decision to initiate dialysis is otherwise based on the clinical condition of the patient rather than a single laboratory value. The dialysis plan for an oliguric, hypercatabolic, postoperative patient undergoing cardiac surgery in the ICU is different than for patients with chronic renal failure. Although the latter usually receives 3 to 4 hours of hemodialysis treatments three times a week, the former may require daily hemodialysis or continuous venovenous hemodialysis (CVVHD) to control hyperkalemia and limit uremic symptoms, and to remove the fluid administered with parenteral inotropic drugs, antibiotics, and nutrition.
■ Absolute and relative indications for dialysis are outlined in Table 47-6.

Types of Renal Replacement Therapy

Intermittent Renal Replacement Therapy
Hemodialysis:
■ It is the most efficient form of fluid and solute removal.
■ It involves removal of blood from a large vein and its passage across one side of a semipermeable membrane, where solutes diffuse into the dyalisate (a solution with

▶ **TABLE 47-5 Guidelines to Management of Serious Renal Dysfunction or Acute Renal Failure**

1. What is the volume status of the patient?
   - Normal: Fluid intake = urine output + 500 mL/d
               Sodium intake 2 g/d
   - Overloaded: Fluid intake < urine output
               Sodium intake <2 g/d
               Try loop diuretic
               Consider dialysis
   - Depleted: Restore intravascular volume with isotonic saline, then prescribe fluid
               Fluid intake = urine output + 500 mL/d
               Sodium intake 2 g/d
2. Is the patient hyperkalemic?
   - No: Potassium intake = 50 mEq/d
   - Yes: Look for source of potassium
          Eliminate parenteral potassium
          Reduce dietary intake to <50 mEq/d
          Potasium binding resin
          Consider dialysis
3. Is the patient acidemic?
   - No: Protein intake 1.2 g/kg/d
   - Yes: Look for cause of acidosis
          Maintain protein intake 1.0–1.2 g/kg/d if postoperative/catabolic
          Isotonic intravenous bicarbonate
          Consider dialysis
4. Is the patient uremic?
   Check for gastrointestinal bleeding, steroid administration or hyperalimentation
   Consider dialysis
5. Nutrition
   Assess need for enteral or parenteral nutrition
   Provide balanced nutrition with 35 kcal/kg/d and 1.0–1.2 g/kg/d of protein
6. Medications
   Check medication list; replace nephrotoxic agents, adjust dosage for
     drugs eliminated renally

Modified from Hutchison FN. Management of acute renal failure. In: Greenberg A, ed. *Primer on kidney diseases*. San Diego, CA: Academic Press; 2001:275–280.

lower concentrations of the undesired solutes present in the patient's blood). Excess fluid is removed by ultrafiltration. Older cellulose-based membranes caused complement activation and neutrophil deposition into the kidneys, causing further ischemic and inflammatory damage. Newer synthetic "biocompatible" membranes have shown better patient outcomes including improved survival and more rapid renal recovery.

■ It requires temporary vascular access, typically with internal jugular or femoral vein cannulas. The subclavian vein should be avoided for concerns of stenosis that may compromise future arm grafts and the possibility of uncontrolled bleeding.

▌TABLE 47-6 Indications for Dialysis

Relative Indications	Absolute Indications
Dialysis will be required if conservative treatments fail or are unsuccessful Volume overload Hyperkalemia Other electrolyte abnormalities Metabolic acidosis	Dialysis is the only possible treatment Uremic symptoms Uremic pericarditis

Modified from Hutchison FN. Chapter 39 – Management of acute renal failure. In: Greenberg A, ed. *Primer on kidney diseases*, Chap. 39. San Diego, CA: Academic Press; 2001:275–280.

■ Side effects include vascular access complications, hypotension, and cerebral edema (dialysis disequilibrium syndrome) caused by rapid osmolar shifts.

Continuous Renal Replacement Therapy

These forms of renal replacement therapy (RRT) are less efficient than intermittent hemodialysis, but are better tolerated by the patient who is hemodynamically unstable. Despite this, no survival benefit has been demonstrated for continuous versus intermittent forms of dialysis.

Continuous RRT almost always requires some form of anticoagulation:
■ Systemic heparin anticoagulation.
■ Regional heparin anticoagulation: infusion of heparin to blood entering the circuit and neutralization with protamine as it exits.
■ Citrate anticoagulation: Citrate is infused as blood enters the circuit to lower serum calcium, which is necessary for clotting; calcium is reinfused as blood exits the dialysis circuit. Systemic ionized calcium levels must be monitored closely and the infusion adjusted accordingly.

Continuous venovenous hemodialysis:
■ Blood is continuously drawn from a large vein at a low rate. Solute is removed by diffusion into the dialysate, which flows in a countercurrent direction to the blood. Ultrafiltration is used to remove excess volume if desired.
■ CVVHD only requires venous access and therefore uses a blood pump to drive the system.
■ Complications are generally related to the anticoagulation method (bleeding, clotting of the access lines, hypocalcemia).

Continuous arteriovenous hemodialysis:
■ Continuous arteriovenous hemodialysis (CAVHD) utilizes the same principle as CVVHD, but blood is drawn from an arterial site, thereby utilizing the patient's blood pressure as the driving force.

- CAVHD requires arterial catheterization, making hemorrhage and atheroembolism common complications of this type of therapy. For this reason, CAVHD is rarely employed in the ICU.

Peritoneal dialysis:

- Dialysate (1 to 2 L) is introduced into the peritoneal space over 30 to 60 minutes through a catheter placed for this purpose. The solution removes solutes by simple diffusion from the blood perfusing the peritoneum; it is then drained over 30 to 120 minutes.
- Peritoneal dialysis (PD) requires no anticoagulation or extracorporeal circuit, making it less costly and less labor intensive.
- PD is hemodynamically well tolerated; however, for patients with compromised respiratory function, the increased intra-abdominal volume and pressure may not be well tolerated.

SUGGESTED READINGS

Conlon PJ, Stafford-Smith M, White WD, et al. Acute renal failure following cardiac surgery. *Nephrol Dial Transplant*. 1999;14:1158–1162.

Hutchison FN. Chapter 39 – Management of acute renal failure. In: Greenberg A, ed. Primer on kidney diseases, Chap. 39. San Diego, CA: Academic Press; 2001:275–280.

Lassnigg A, Donner E, Grubhofer G, et al. Lack of renoprotective effects of dopamine and furosemide during cardiac surgery. *J Am Soc Nephrol*. 2000;11:97–104.

Lee HT, Sladen RN. Chapter 42 – Perioperative renal protection. In: Murray MJ, Coursin DB, Pearl RG et al., eds. *Critical care medicine, perioperative management*. 2nd ed. Philadelphia, PA: Lippincott Williams & Wilkins; 2002:503–520.

Michelle A, Hladunewich RAL. Chapter 43 – Management of acute renal failure in the critically ill patient. In: Murray MJ, Coursin DB, Pearl RG et al., eds. *Critical care medicine, perioperative management*. 2nd ed. Philadelphia, PA: Lippincott Williams & Wilkins; 2002:521–532.

Stafford-Smith M. Chapter 5 – Perioperative renal dysfunction: implications and strategies for protection. In: Newman MF, ed. *Society of cardiovascular anesthesiologists monograph – perioperative organ protection*. Philadelphia, PA: Lippincott Williams & Wilkins; 2003:124.

Swaminathan M, Phillips-Bute BG, Conlon PJ, et al. The association of lowest hematocrit during cardiopulmonary bypass with acute renal injury after coronary artery bypass surgery. *Ann Thorac Surg*. 2003;76:784–791; discussion 792.

Wilson WC, Aronson S. Oliguria: a sign of renal success or impending renal failure? *Anesthesiol Clin North America*. 2001;19:841–883.

Chapter 48

Neurologic Complications and Management

Ronald J. Butler

Neurologic complications after cardiac surgery include cerebral injuries and peripheral neuropathies. Acute changes in cerebral function after cardiac surgery are relatively common. The brain may be injured owing to an embolism (e.g., atherosclerotic plaque, thrombus, or air), reduced cerebral blood flow, or a local or systemic inflammatory response. The clinical presentation of cerebral problems have been divided into the following:

- Type I problems, including death due to stroke or hypoxic encephalopathy, nonfatal stroke, transient ischemic attack (TIA), or stupor or coma at the time of discharge.
  - Incidence rate: 3.1% following elective bypass procedures.
- Type II problems, including a new deterioration in cerebral function, confusion, agitation, disorientation, memory deficit, or seizure without evidence of focal injury.
  - Incidence rate: 3.0% following elective bypass procedures.
- Type I events were associated with a 10-fold increase in in-hospital mortality, and type II events were associated with a fivefold increase in in-hospital mortality. Both type I and type II events are associated with longer intensive care unit (ICU) and hospital stays compared to patients without an adverse cerebral event.
- The incidence of neurocognitive decline following cardiac surgery as assessed by neuropsychologic testing is much greater, with an incidence that has been reported to be as high as 60% in the first week following surgery; persistent decreases exist in 24% of patients at 6 months.

PREOPERATIVE ASSESSMENT AND PREPARATION

A number of factors have been shown to increase the risk of type I and type II complications (see Table 48-1).

▶ **TABLE 48-1 Risk Factors for Type I and Type II Adverse Cerebral Complications after Cardiac Surgery**

Type I	Type II
Proximal aortic atherosclerosis	History of pulmonary disease
History of neurologic disease	Older age
Use of intraoperative balloon pump	Systolic BP >160 mm Hg on admission
Diabetes mellitus	History of excessive alcohol consumption
History of pulmonary disease	History of CABG
History of unstable angina	Dysrhythmia on day of surgery
Older age	Antihypertensive therapy

BP, blood pressure; CABG, coronary artery bypass graft.
Modified from Roach GW, Kanchuger M, Mangano CM, et al. Adverse cerebral outcomes after coronary bypass surgery. *N Engl J Med.* 1996;335(25):1857–1863.

Approximately 30% of postoperative strokes are associated with carotid artery stenosis of 50% or more. These strokes often occur postoperatively after surgery and after an initial uneventful recovery. Screening patients who have undergone cardiac surgery has shown an incidence of 17% to 22% for moderate stenosis and a 6% to 12% incidence of severe stenosis. Moderate stenosis is associated with a 10% risk of stroke, and severe stenosis is associated with an 11% to 19% incidence of stroke. In experienced hands, prophylactic carotid endarterectomy is superior to conservative therapy for the prevention of stroke and carotid endarterectomy, followed by coronary bypass or concurrent combined procedures, and has been shown to reduce the risk of stroke with a mortality risk of 3% to 4%. Risk factors associated with severe carotid disease include age 65 years or greater, previous TIA or stroke, history of smoking, left main disease, and peripheral vascular disease.

Closed-chamber procedures have a lower risk of stroke than open-chamber procedures.

INTRAOPERATIVE CONSIDERATION AND MANAGEMENT

The intraoperative management of patients with cardiac disorders can considerably reduce the risk of brain injury.

The greatest risk factor for postoperative stroke is the presence of proximal aortic atherosclerosis. This can be detected by manual palpation of the aorta at surgery or can be picked up with greater sensitivity using transesophageal echocardiography, or better still using epiaortic ultrasound scanning. Manipulation of the vessel wall during cannulation/decannulation and clamping/unclamping the aorta, as well as a misdirected cannula jet may result in embolism. Compared to reported rates of stroke, the use of epiaortic scanning to identify and modify cannulation sites resulted in lower rates of stroke. Modifications in technique include cannulating nondiseased segments of the aorta or using subclavian or femoral cannulation sites, modifying the clamping site, and use of both internal thoracic arteries to avoid aortic clamping and off-pump bypass surgery.

Hypothermia has been shown to reduce the risk of neurologic injuries in animal models and has been demonstrated to improve neurologic outcome following anoxic brain injury. The benefit of hypothermia may be attenuated if rapid rewarming is used and there is overshoot in the brain temperature. Slower rewarming and leaving patients mildly hypothermic reduces the incidence of postoperative cognitive decline.

The cerebral perfusion pressure is defined as the difference between mean arterial pressure (MAP) and the intracranial pressure or the central venous pressure (CVP), whichever is higher. Cerebral perfusion is autoregulated within a range of MAP between 60 mm Hg and 160 mm Hg. However, in patients with longstanding hypertension, the autoregulation curve may be shifted to the right, resulting in cerebral hypoperfusion above a MAP of 60 mm Hg. It is possible during the manipulation of the heart to have considerable increases in the CVP, potentially compromising the cerebral perfusion pressure. Major carotid stenosis may also result in cerebral hypoperfusion beyond the stenosis if there is a decrease in MAP.

Alpha-stat acid–base management (pH and Pco_2 uncorrected for body temperature) resulted in less postoperative adverse cerebral events compared to pH-stat (pH and Pco_2 corrected for body temperature) management.

Blood glucose level is often increased in patients with or without diabetes who are undergoing cardiac surgery. The use of glucose-containing solutions, stress response, hypothermia, and the use of exogenous catecholamine infusions contribute to the problem. Hyperglycemia has been demonstrated to worsen outcome following stroke in animal models, as well as in observational studies in humans. Intraoperative monitoring of glucose and treatment of hyperglycemia with insulin to maintain normoglycemia is a goal both intraoperatively and postoperatively.

POSTOPERATIVE ASSESSMENT AND MANAGEMENT
Stroke

Persistent nonawakening following cardiac surgery usually represents the most severe form of neurologic injury. Careful attention to optimizing hemodynamics, and oxygen delivery, and searching for and correcting electrolyte and metabolic factors is the first step. Occasionally, delayed clearance of sedatives and narcotics may delay awakening. Patients who have had reversible metabolic factors excluded should undergo brain imaging with computerized tomography (CT) scanning or magnetic resonance imaging (MRI) of the head and assessment with electroencephalogram (EEG). Serial studies are useful to determine the etiology and to provide accurate prognostication. More commonly, the diagnosis of a new neurologic injury depends upon careful clinical assessment to determine new focal deficits. Up to one third of patients develop their cerebral injury after an initial period of uneventful recovery postoperatively. Focal signs that are identified on clinical examination should be evaluated with a CT scan or MRI of the head. Primary intracranial hemorrhage is extremely uncommon following cardiac surgery, but patients undergoing cardiac surgery for endocarditis are at higher risk for hemorrhage following anticoagulation for surgery. Patients who develop large ischemic strokes are at risk for cerebral edema and hemorrhagic conversion of their stroke.

Initial management of patients with stroke includes maintaining adequate perfusion pressure, normoglycemia, avoidance of dextrose containing intravenous (IV) solutions, and avoidance of hypotonic IV solutions to limit cerebral edema.

Postoperative arrhythmias, particularly atrial fibrillation, can lead to new onset of stroke. Anticoagulation for atrial fibrillation should be considered as soon as it is considered safe in the postoperative period. Patients who have had a small or moderate-sized stroke, and have a persistent source of cardiac emboli, should be anticoagulated with heparin.

Seizures

Seizures occur in 0.4% of patients following cardiac surgery. Seizures may result from metabolic factors, new cerebral injury, or exacerbation of an underlying seizure disorder. The principal goals are to control the seizures and search for and correct reversible factors (see Table 48-2). Initial control of a generalized seizure can be obtained with IV benzodiazepine. IV lorazepam in doses of 0.02 to 0.20 mg/kg have been effective in terminating seizures. IV phenytoin can be used to prevent recurrence of seizures. A loading dose of 20 mg/kg can be given (not to be infused more quickly than 50 mg/minute), followed by a maintenance dosing of 100 mg IV q8h, and then the dose is adjusted to maintain therapeutic levels.

Delirium

Delirium is diagnosed when there is an acute onset of mental status changes (or a fluctuating mental status) *and* evidence of inattention, as well as either disorganized thinking *or* an altered level of consciousness. Delirium is very common in ICU patients. Delirium is associated with an increase in mortality, as well as in increased ICU and hospital length of stay.

Most patients with delirium are agitated, but as many as 30% may present as hypoactive delirium. This form of delirium is easy to overlook and can be misinterpreted as depression by health care providers.

It is important to look for underlying causes and treat them. Supportive treatment is both pharmacologic and nonpharmacologic. Pharmacologic treatment with haloperidol is the therapy of choice in the ICU. Haloperidol has a minimal side effect profile and a low incidence of extrapyramidal effects (IV lower than PO). It can cause prolongation of the QT interval and can lead to torsade de pointes when used in large doses or in conjunction with other drugs that cause QT interval prolongation. Haloperidol can

▶ **TABLE 48-2 Metabolic Causes of Seizures**

Hypoxemia
Hypoglycemia
Hypocalcemia
Hypomagnesemia
Hyponatremia

be combined with lorazepam when agitation is a major component of the delirium and is most effective when used in the ratio 2:1, haloperidol to lorazepam. The drugs should be dosed regularly q6h, with a larger dose at bedtime. The doses should be escalated to gain control and then the drugs should be tapered off 3 to 5 days after symptoms have been controlled.

Nonpharmacologic therapy includes providing reorientation to the environment; attempting to improve the sleep–wake cycle with noise and light reduction at night and minimizing night time interventions.

Delirium tremens is a special case of delirium where the therapy of choice is benzodiazepines instead of Haldol. Delirium can be controlled by repeated dosing of intravenous diazepam until the patient is sedated. The long half-life of diazepam and the multiple active metabolites allows the drug to self-taper. Alternatively, lorazepam can be dosed regularly q6h with prn doses added until the delirium is controlled. The total dose required is then given daily in divided doses and is tapered off in 3 to 5 days.

Peripheral Neuropathy

Peripheral neuropathy can occur following cardiac surgery. Upper extremity peripheral neuropathy occurs in 2% to 15% of patients. This typically presents with numbness, weakness, discoordination of an extremity, and pain. Symptoms improve or resolve in 3 weeks in most patients following cardiac surgery, suggesting a neuropraxic injury rather than an axonal injury. Electromyography and nerve conduction studies can delineate the site and type of injury.

Phrenic nerve injury occurs with cooling the heart with slushed ice. Previously reported to occur in up to 30% of patients, the incidence of this injury has declined considerably with changes in surgical technique.

Intercostal nerve injury can occur with internal thoracic artery dissection, and it can lead to a burning dysesthetic pain over the sternum and left chest wall. These symptoms can be prolonged although most resolve by 4 months postoperatively.

SUGGESTED READINGS

Ahonen J, Salmenpera M. Brain injury after adult cardiac surgery. *Acta Anaesthesiol Scand.* 2004; 48:4–19.
Grigore AM, Grocott HP, Matthew JP, et al. The rewarming rate and increased peak temperature alter neurocognitive outcome after cardiac surgery. *Anesth Analg.* 2002;94:4–10.
Newman MF, Kirchner JL, Phillips-Bute B, et al. Longitudinal assessment of neurocognitive function after coronary-artery bypass surgery. *N Engl J Med.* 2001;344(6):395–402.
Roach GW, Kanchuger M, Mangano CM, et al. Adverse cerebral outcomes after coronary bypass surgery. *N Engl J Med.* 1996;335(25):1857–1863.
Van Dijk D, Jansen WLJ, Hijman R. Cognitive outcome after off-pump and on-pump coronary artery bypass graft surgery. *JAMA.* 2002;287(11):1405–1412.

Surgical Ward Management

Routine Surgical Ward Care

Susan C. M. Lenkei-Kerwin and Stephanie J. Brister

Severity of illness and comorbid conditions are steadily increasing in patients undergoing cardiac surgery. Health care professionals are under intense pressure to minimize hospital stay by discharging patients as early as possible. To do so, increased attention must be focused on specific patient needs. Ward care can no longer be considered as being "routine." Many modalities of care are available. This chapter outlines an approach to postoperative care of the patient undergoing cardiac surgery.

GENERAL CARE

Patients who are hemodynamically stable and who do not need assisted ventilation are transferred out of the intensive care unit (ICU) to the surgical ward within 24 hours. Standardized ICU discharge orders and summaries of the ICU and operative course facilitate care on the ward. All patients should be monitored by telemetry for 24 to 48 hours in the ward. Telemetry is then discontinued, provided the cardiac rhythm has been stable. Vital signs are recorded every 4 hours for the first 24 hours and every 8 hours thereafter. Body weight is recorded daily. Foley catheters should remain in place until ambulation is commenced, usually on the second postoperative day (POD).

All patients should be placed on a fluid restriction of 1,500 mL/day following cardiac surgery. Antidiuretic hormone production is increased in the early postoperative period, predisposing patients to fluid retention.

Pleural, pericardial, and mediastinal chest drains are removed usually in the ICU after 24 hours unless there has been excessive drainage. Drainage in excess of 100 mL in 8 hours is abnormal and requires further observation and/or intervention. An air leak through a chest tube is abnormal; therefore, the chest tube should remain in place until the air leak has stopped.

External pacing wires are usually removed on the third POD unless there is a cardiac dysrhythmia. Pacer wires should be removed completely. If they are cut flush with the skin, problems with late infection can arise. In patients who are taking anticoagulation, wires are removed when the international normalized ratio (INR) is <3.0. If patients are receiving intravenous heparin, the heparin should be discontinued for 2 hours before the removal of the pacer wires and should be resumed 2 hours following removal of the wires. Patients should remain in bed for 2 hours following removal of pacer wires.

Early ambulation is encouraged. Because atelectasis is common following cardiac surgery, patients are instructed preoperatively about respiratory exercises. Postoperatively, they are reminded daily by all health care professionals involved in their care to cough and take deep breaths because they may not be seen routinely by physiotherapists.

Patient and family should attend discharge classes. Instructions about the activities of daily living, exercise, diet, and follow-up care are given. In addition, a comprehensive booklet dealing with concerns during convalescence should be provided. This allows the patient and the family to address issues of concern as they arise.

LABORATORY TESTS

Standard postoperative orders include daily complete blood count, electrolyte concentration, and creatinine level during the first 3 days. The liver function test is evaluated in all patients requiring anticoagulation if the evaluation was abnormal preoperatively or abnormal in the ICU. INR is checked daily in patients who are started on warfarin sodium. Electrocardiograms are taken daily during the first 3 days and on the day before discharge. Chest x-rays are done before and following the removal of chest tubes, as well as before discharge. Echocardiograms should be performed on all patients who have undergone valve surgery. All other tests are ordered as clinically indicated.

WOUND CARE

Surgical wounds are inspected daily and covered with sterile dressings for the first 2 days, after which time they are left exposed to dry. Patients with a sternal click on palpation have a higher risk of dehiscence and/or infection. If a sternal click develops, patients are provided with a chest binder to give added stability when coughing and moving. In cases of instability, rewiring of the sternum should be undertaken.

NAUSEA AND VOMITING

Nausea and vomiting are common following open-heart surgery. The etiology is multifactorial but is most often related to medication intolerance. Discontinuation of the responsible drug and administration of antiemetic agents are the first lines of therapy. If there is evidence of bowel distention, the patient should be placed NPO (nothing by mouth) and a nasogastric tube should be inserted. More serious conditions such as bowel obstruction, cholecystitis, or pancreatitis should be considered.

CONSTIPATION

Constipation is common in all patients because of narcotic administration. A bowel protocol should be in place and should include a daily laxative and enemas if needed. We routinely use Colace, 100 mg PO b.i.d., and lactulose, 15 to 30 mL PO q.i.d., may also be used.

PAIN CONTROL

Management of pain is an important aspect of postoperative care. Initially, morphine sulfate 1 to 4 mg intravenously (IV) q 1–2 h is administered on the first and second POD. When a patient has adequate oral intake, morphine is discontinued and oral oxycodone and Tylenol are administered prn. Nonsteroidal anti-inflammatory drugs (NSAIDs) are effective for pain and can be used in patients who do not tolerate narcotics. NSAID suppositories can be administered to those patients who are unable to take anything by mouth. NSAIDs are contraindicated in patients with elevated creatinine levels, diabetes, or peptic ulcer disease. Gastric protection agents such as a proton pump inhibitor or mucosal protective agents should accompany oral NSAID administration. It is important to note recent literature suggests that selective COX-II inhibitor is contraindicated in cardiac surgical patients. For patients with a history of difficult pain management problems, the Pain Service should be consulted preoperatively and patient-specific protocols should be instituted.

ANTICOAGULATION

Patients who undergo cardiac surgery may develop a hyper-coagulable state postoperatively placing them at risk for thrombotic events. Postoperatively, prophylactic subcutaneous unfractionated heparin or low-molecular-weight heparin should be administered routinely. When the patient is ambulating adequately, prophylactic treatment is discontinued.

All patients with mechanical valves require permanent oral anticoagulation with warfarin sodium to maintain an INR of 2 to 3 for aortic prostheses and 2.5 to 3.5 for mitral valve prostheses. In some institutions, aspirin 81 mg daily is added to warfarin sodium. Patients with mechanical valves should be started on intravenous heparin or low-molecular-weight heparin following removal of chest drains. Therapeutic partial thromboplastin time should be maintained until an INR of 2.0 is reached.

Patients who have had mitral valve replacement with a bioprosthesis or mitral valve repair should be anticoagulated for 3 months if they are in sinus rhythm or permanently if they are in chronic atrial fibrillation (AF). The INR should be maintained between 2 and 3. Patients who had aortic valve replacement with bioprostheses or biologic valves do not need to be anticoagulated with warfarin sodium if they are in sinus rhythm. However, oral anticoagulation during the first 3 months is used in some centers.

Platelet count should be monitored in patients on heparin because of the risk of heparin-induced thrombocytopenia (HIT). If the platelet count drops below 100,000, heparin is discontinued and an HIT assay is ordered. If the patient with HIT requires ongoing anticoagulation, an alternative such as a direct thrombin inhibitor can be used.

All patients with chronic AF or with AF for >48 hours or intermittent AF require oral anticoagulation with warfarin sodium. The target INR is 2.0 to 2.5. The patients should receive concurrent unfractionated or low-molecular-weight heparin until the INR is 2.0.

ATRIAL FIBRILLATION PROPHYLAXIS AND TREATMENT

AF is a common complication following open-heart surgery, occurring in 10% to 40% of patients. Preoperative clinical predictors are age, sex, past history of AF, paroxysmal or new onset of AF, left ventricular dysfunction, congestive heart failure, withdrawal of β-blockers, and preoperative interarterial conduction delay. Operative predictors include the number of coronary artery bypass grafts, as well as concomitant heart valve surgery. Efforts to prevent AF postoperatively have included perioperative administration of β-blockers or amiodarone. Both have proven efficacious, but the incidence of postoperative AF remains at 20% to 40%.

AF postoperatively is usually well tolerated. The aim is first to control the ventricular rate and, when feasible, to revert the patient to sinus rhythm. There is no clinical evidence that the antiarrhythmic conversion strategy is superior to the rate-control strategy. Therefore, in the presence of normal left ventricular function, there is no urgency to achieve sinus rhythm. For postoperative AF in the absence of contraindications, we believe that β-blockers and/or amiodarone are the drugs of choice. If there are contraindications to β-blockers or amiodarone, a calcium channel blocker is used together with digoxin for rate control. Other agents are available but are associated with increased proarrhythmic tendencies. If the patient is hemodynamically compromised, intravenous amiodarone is used and, if necessary, electrical cardioversion is done. However, in our experience, unless the patient is medically pretreated, cardioversion is efficacious only for a limited period of time.

Resumption of sinus rhythm can often be achieved within 48 hours. If sinus rhythm is not restored within 48 hours, anticoagulation is mandatory. In patients who have mitral valve surgery and who develop postoperative AF, only rate control is recommended because these patients will have to remain on anticoagulants. If left ventricular dysfunction is present, rate control is achieved with intravenous amiodarone followed by an oral loading dose.

DIABETES

The Endocrine Service should follow up all patients with type-1 or type-2 diabetes. Tight control of blood sugars is maintained utilizing oral medication or subcutaneous or intravenous insulin.

LEFT VENTRICULAR DYSFUNCTION

For patients with considerable left ventricular dysfunction, angiotensin converting enzyme (ACE) inhibition should be reinstituted before intravascular euvolemia is achieved. Renal function must be carefully monitored because of the concomitant use of diuretics.

PROPHYLAXIS FOR DRESSLER SYNDROME

All patients younger than 50 years who have undergone heart valve or aortic surgery should be placed on high-dose enteric-coated aspirin to prevent Dressler syndrome or postpericardiotomy syndrome. Gastric protection is added.

CORONARY ENDARTERECTOMY

Approximately 30% of coronary arteries that underwent endarterectomy occlude within 1 year. Antiplatelet agents are important to enhance early- and late-patency rates. The combination of aspirin and clopidogrel may be more efficacious than the combination of aspirin and dipyridamole.

DISCHARGE PLANNING

Discharge planning begins before admission. Elderly patients often require additional support in the community and it should be arranged preoperatively. Most patients can be safely discharged on the fifth or sixth POD. Criteria for discharge are listed in Table 49-1. Discharge medications for coronary artery bypass patients should include antiplatelet agents and statins. A hospital pharmacist, a knowledgeable nurse, or a physician should review all medications with the patient and family. Side effects and drug interactions should be outlined. A discharge letter describing the patient's surgery, hospital course, discharge medications, and follow-up care should be given to all patients, with copies to the family physician and the referring cardiologist. A schedule of appointments with the family physician, cardiologist, and surgeon should also be given. This provides seamless transition from in-hospital to community care.

▌ **TABLE 49-1 Criteria for Hospital Discharge**

Afebrile for 24 h
No signs of infection
Weight at or below preoperative level
No drainage from wounds
Absence of heart failure
Blood pressure and rhythm control
Therapeutic anticoagulation
Oxygen saturation satisfactory on room air
Independent ambulation

SUMMARY

The approaches to postoperative care in the patient undergoing cardiac surgery outlined in the preceding pages have proven effective in our institution. A collaborative effort by all health care professionals utilizing the plans outlined has led to a consistent decline in morbidity and mortality and length of stay despite a continued rise in acuity.

SUGGESTED READINGS

Kouthoukos NT, Blackstone EH, Doty DB, et al. Postoperative care. *Kirklin/Barratt-boyes cardiac surgery*. 3rd ed. Salt Lake City, UT: Churchill Livingston/Elesevier Science, 2003.
Martin DO, Saliba W, McCarthy PM, et al. Approaches to restoring and maintaining sinus rhythm. *Cleve Clin J.* 2003;70(3):S12–S30.

Chapter 50

Common Ward Complications and Management

Stephanie J. Brister and Susan C. M. Lenkei-Kerwin

Mortality associated with cardiac surgery has progressively decreased over the last decades. However, with increasing comorbid conditions, the frequency of serious postoperative complications has increased. This chapter outlines common complications, which can be encountered in a postoperative cardiac surgical ward. With early recognition of the complications and prompt institution of therapy, patient disability can be minimized and length of stay in the hospital can be reduced.

POSTOPERATIVE DYSRHYTHMIAS

Cardiac dysrhythmias are common complications after cardiac surgery. Premature atrial and ventricular beats, tachyarrhythmias, and bradyarrhythmias occur in 30% to 50% of patients after coronary artery bypass graft (CABG) and even more frequently after heart valve and combined heart valve/CABG procedures.

Atrial Dysrhythmias

Postoperative sinus tachycardia indicates increased adrenergic tone and is a normal response to stress of surgery. Treatment should be directed at the underlying cause, that is, fever, pain, anxiety, rebound adrenergic tone, or anemia. In the presence of normal left ventricular function, sinus tachycardia has no adverse effect and should not be treated in and of itself. Premature atrial contractions are benign but may herald the onset of atrial tachyarrhythmias.

Atrial flutter and atrial flutter-fibrillation affect 10% to 40% of patients following isolated CABG and up to 50% of patients after heart valve surgery. Peak occurrence is between 1 and 3 days postoperatively. In patients with normal left ventricular function, atrial tachyarrhythmias are well tolerated.

Management of postoperative atrial fibrillation is described in Chapter 49.

Even if the patient resumes sinus rhythm, if there is left atrial enlargement, the patient is at risk for recurrent paroxysmal atrial fibrillation and, therefore, should be discharged on an oral anticoagulant.

Ventricular Dysrhythmias

Premature ventricular contractions can be ignored in the presence of normal left ventricular function and in the absence of any electrolyte imbalance. If ventricular premature beats occur in salvos and are multifocal, or in the presence of impaired left ventricular function, the underlying abnormalities should be investigated and corrected. Ventricular tachycardia and/or fibrillation should be treated aggressively with medication and/or defibrillation. After the patient has been stabilized, the underlying cause should be identified. Electrolytes (K^+, Mg^{2+}) should be optimized. If there is evidence of underlying ischemia, appropriate medical therapy is administered and further investigation is warranted. Ventricular tachycardia in the patient who is hemodynamically stable should be treated immediately with intravenous amiodarone 150 mg bolus up to 450 mg. With the resumption of normal sinus rhythm, a continuous infusion of amiodarone should be initiated. If ventricular tachycardia persists, electrical cardioversion is undertaken. If the patient is hemodynamically unstable, immediate electrical cardioversion should be done, with concomitant administration of a continuous infusion of an antiarrhythmic such as amiodarone. Amiodarone should only be administered through a large-bore intravenous catheter to avoid chemical thrombophlebitis.

Bradyarrhythmias

If a patient develops sick sinus syndrome, Mobitz type II or type III atrioventricular block, permanent pacemaker implantation should be considered. Asymptomatic first-degree heart block should not be treated.

CONGESTIVE HEART FAILURE

Congestive heart failure (CHF) is a common problem in patients with impaired left ventricular function. The patient's weight is obtained daily, and aggressive diuresis is instituted such that weight is lower than or equal to the preoperative weight by discharge.

The management of CHF includes:

- Fluid restriction of 1,000 to 1,200 mL/day.
- Sodium restriction of 1 g/day.

- Diuresis (a combination of furosemide and metolazone has proven effective).
- K^+ and Mg^{2+} levels supplemented as required.
- Angiotensin converting enzyme (ACE) inhibitors can be administered in conjunction with diuresis; doses are titrated to blood pressure and serum creatinine level is carefully monitored.
- β-blockade is instituted before ACE inhibition is maximized.

POSTOPERATIVE CHEST PAIN

The most important aspect of management of postoperative chest pain is to differentiate incisional pain from other types of pain such as pain from myocardial ischemia, pericarditis, acute aortic dissection, pleuritis, pulmonary embolism, esophagitis, and peptic ulcer disease. Most patients who have had ischemic chest pain preoperatively can differentiate ischemic pain from other types of pain. A detailed functional enquiry is fundamental for an accurate diagnosis of pain. All patients with chest pain should have a 12-lead electrocardiogram, which is compared with the previous ones. If ischemic pain is suspected, sublingual nitroglycerin 0.3 to 0.6 mg and/or morphine 1 to 5 mg intravenous should be administered. If there is objective evidence of ischemia, the patient should be transferred to the intensive care unit (ICU). If ischemia is excluded, further investigation of chest pain should be undertaken.

INFECTION

Atelectasis is a frequent cause of low-grade fever, but spiking temperatures imply a more serious cause. Common infections following cardiac surgery include wound infection, pneumonia, urinary tract infection, and septicemia. All patients who develop fever postoperatively should have a thorough functional inquiry and physical examination. Investigation should include complete blood count (CBC), blood cultures (if temperature is $>38.5°C$), sputum culture, urine culture, and chest x-ray. Oral or intravenous antibiotic therapy should be instituted in a timely fashion.

Wound infections most commonly occur between the fifth and tenth postoperative day (POD). All drainage from wounds is cultured, and appropriate antibiotic therapy is instituted. Superficial wound infections are treated with drainage, packing, and antibiotics. Deep sternal wound infections are treated with debridement, drainage and rewiring, or muscle flaps, if necessary. Before surgery, a computed tomographic (CT) scan may provide additional information about the extent of the mediastinal involvement. Duration of antibiotic treatment should be guided by the underlying cardiac operation and the severity of the mediastinal infection.

LEG WOUND

Leg wound problems include numbness along the site of the incisions, fluid collection, edema, and infection. These problems are usually self-limiting and resolve slowly over 6 to 12 months. Collection of fluid or hematoma may be managed with close observation, but if it is large and painful for the patient, it can be treated with drainage. Edema is managed with leg elevation and diuretics. Leg stockings are not routinely used. Areas of necrosis in the leg will usually heal with conservative treatment, but it may, in unusual circumstances, require debridement and possibly a skin graft. Endoscopic techniques of vein harvesting have decreased the rate of leg wound problems.

PLEURAL SPACE COMPLICATIONS

Pneumothorax

The common causes of pneumothorax are unsuspected compromise of the pleural space in the operating room, rupture of a lung bullae, or following the removal of chest tubes. The diagnosis should be confirmed by a chest x-ray. If the patient is symptomatic or the pneumothorax is >20%, a chest tube should be inserted.

Tension pneumothorax is a clinical diagnosis that can be confirmed with a chest x-ray. A chest tube should be inserted immediately if the patient is unstable and if the diagnosis is suspected.

Pleural Effusion

The most common cause of pleural effusion is retained blood or serosanguineous fluid, particularly when the pleural cavities have been entered during surgery. If the collection is large, percutaneous drainage should be done. Heart failure is also a common cause of effusion and is treated with aggressive diuresis.

Empyema

Empyema can develop secondary to nonsterile insertion of chest tubes but is more often related to an underlying pneumonic process. Whenever percutaneous drainage of a pleural effusion is done, fluid is sent for culture. If the culture is positive, a chest tube is inserted and antibiotic treatment is instituted. Surgical drainage and/or pleurectomy may be required.

PERICARDIAL COMPLICATIONS

Pericarditis

Pericarditis is common after cardiac procedures but the patient is generally asymptomatic. If the patient is having pain, high-dose acetylsalicylic acid (ASA) (1,300 to 2,600 mg/day) should be initiated with appropriate gastric protection therapy.

Acute Pericardial Tamponade

Acute pericardial tamponade may occur on a cardiac surgical ward following removal of temporary pacing wires or mediastinal chest tubes. It is a clinical diagnosis requiring emergency surgical intervention.

Delayed Pericardial Tamponade

Delayed pericardial tamponade is uncommon after cardiac surgery but can be fatal if it is not recognized and treated appropriately. Most cases of delayed tamponade are due to accumulation of serosanguineous fluid secondary to pericarditis in patients who are anticoagulated. Patients are usually discharged on the fifth to seventh POD. Therefore, patients at risk should have a transthoracic echocardiogram before discharge. If a small effusion is detected, the patient should be followed closely and the echocardiogram repeated in 3 to 5 days. If there is hemodynamic compromise, appropriate drainage is performed. Surgical insertion of a large drain in the subxiphoid area under local or general anesthesia is all that is required. The drain should be left in for 24 to 48 hours. Delayed tamponade secondary to hemorrhage should be treated with reopening of the chest, evacuation of blood clots, lavage of the pericardial cavity, and achievement of hemostasis.

CONFUSION/AGITATION

Confusion and disorientation are common with the aging patient population and they increase comorbidity. The problem is exacerbated by the administration of narcotics and/or sedatives. Offending medications should be discontinued. Metabolic problems should be ruled out (i.e., check electrolyte levels, glucose levels, renal function, and oxygen saturation levels). In our institution, physical restraints are not used. Constant care attendants are provided.

RENAL FAILURE

Risk factors for postoperative renal failure include older age, diabetes, hypertension, preoperative renal dysfunction, and prolonged cardiopulmonary bypass. Management of postoperative renal dysfunction begins with the identification of etiology. Intravascular volume status should be optimized. If oliguria persists or hyperkalemia develops, the Nephrology Department is contacted and dialysis may be required.

NEUROLOGIC COMPLICATIONS

Neurocognitive deficits can be identified with psychometric testing in up to 50% of patients following cardiac surgery. The incidence of this complication may be less if CABG is done off pump. Most patients are clinically asymptomatic, but those with deficits will improve substantially by 6 to 8 weeks, and deficits will have completely resolved by 6 months in most patients.

Stroke occurs in 1% to 3% of the patients who have undergone cardiac surgery and is usually a perioperative event. Stroke is most often diagnosed in the ICU, however, it can occur on the surgical ward. Cerebrovascular accidents of this type may be embolism secondary to atrial fibrillation or left ventricular thrombus, or hemorrhagic secondary to postoperative antiplatelet or antithrombotic therapy or oral anticoagulation. A CT scan or magnetic resonance imaging (MRI) should be obtained immediately to determine if the stroke is hemorrhagic or ischemic because the mode of treatment is different for each.

DEEP VENOUS THROMBOSIS AND PULMONARY EMBOLISM

Deep venous thrombosis and pulmonary embolism are often unrecognized after cardiac operations. A high index of suspicion is required in any patient with tachycardia, hypoxia, shortness of breath, chest pain, leg edema, and/or low-grade fever. Diagnosis can be made with venous Doppler and/or a spiral CT scan. A ventilation-perfusion scan is often not diagnostic because of postoperative pulmonary changes. Treatment is anticoagulation, initially with heparin and subsequently with Coumadin. In rare circumstances, thrombectomy may be required.

PERIPHERAL NERVE INJURIES

Nerve injuries are often the result of intraoperative trauma. They may not become apparent until the patient is transferred to the ward. Rib compression secondary to the sternal retractor can lead to brachial plexus injury. Caudal placement of the retractor and limited chest opening minimizes the risk. Radial nerve injuries can result from compression of the arm by inappropriate positioning. Ulnar nerve problems develop owing to poor padding at the elbow with excessive rotation of the hand or compression of the elbow. Most patients with nerve injuries will improve within 6 months.

SUMMARY

High-quality health care by all health care professionals is essential for patients with cardiac disorders to minimize the occurrence of complications. However, complications will still arise. Early recognition and immediate institution of appropriate treatment will minimize the sequelae for patients and decrease health care costs.

SUGGESTED READINGS

Kouchokos NT, Blackstone EH, Doty DB, et al. Postoperative care. *Kirklin/Barratt-Boyes cardiac surgery*. 3rd ed.. Salt Lake City, UT: Churchill Livingston, Elsevier Science; 2003:195–253.
Waldhausen JA, Orringer MB. *Complications in cardiothoracic surgery*. St. Louis, MO: Mosby Year Book; 1991.

SECTION VI

Appendices

POSTOPERATIVE TGH/CVICU MEDICAL ADMISSION FORM

UHN TGH - CVICU ADMISSION NOTE
Must be completed and placed in the chart

58502

MRN ☐☐☐☐☐☐

(dd/mm/yyyy)
Date: ☐☐ / ☐☐ / ☐☐☐☐

Allergies: ○ No ○ Yes _____

Addressograph

History:
Sex: ○ M ○ F   **Age** ☐☐

Cardiac:
HTN: ○ No ○ Yes

PVD: ○ No ○ Yes

CHF: ○ No ○ Yes (within 2 weeks)

Angina: ○ No ○ I-III ○ IV ○ UAP (on IV meds)

MI: ○ No ○ <7 d ○ 7-30 d ○ >30 d ○ ?

Vessels: ○ Nr ○ LM >90% ○ LM 50-90%
○ LAD >70% ○ Cx >70% ○ RCA >70%

Valvular: ○ Nr ○ AS ○ AI ○ PS ○ PI
*moderate or severe ○ MS ○ MR ○ TS ○ TR

LV: ○ Nr ○ dilated ○ aneurysmal
○ gr.I ○ gr.II ○ gr.III ○ gr.IV ○ No data

Preop. IABP: ○ No ○ Yes

Pulm. HTN: ○ No ○ Yes (>30 mean or >50 systolic)

Endocarditis: ○ No ○ Yes (within 2 weeks)

Arrhythmia: ○ No ○ Atrial ○ Ventricular (within 2 weeks)

Pacemaker: ○ No ○ Permanent ○ Temp.

Other: ○ No ○ Yes: _____

Resp: ○ NR ○ Smoker (current) ○ Other:
○ COPD/Asthma
○ Sleep Apnea

GI/Renal: ○ NR ○ Peptic Ulcer ○ Other:
○ Liver dysfunction
○ Dialysis dependent

Endo: ○ NR ○ Diabetes, Type I ○ Other:
○ Diabetes, Type II
○ Thyroid

Neuro: ○ NR ○ Stroke ○ Other:
○ TIA
○ Seizures
○ R carotid stenosis >50%
○ L carotid stenosis >50%

Misc: ○ No ○ Coagulopathy ○ Other:
○ Haemoglobinopathy
○ HIT
○ Immunosupressed
○ Malignancy
○ Infection (specify)

Preop. Medications:
○ Beta Blocker
○ Calcium Blocker
○ ACE Inhibitor
○ Diuretic
○ Amiodarone
○ Digoxin

○ Bronchodilators
○ Systemic steroids
○ ASA —— ○ <7 days
○ Coumadin— ○ <5 days
○ IV/LMW Heparin
○ Other:

Preop. Labs:
Creat: ☐☐☐
Hb: ☐☐☐
Plts: ☐☐☐
INR: ☐.☐☐

Surgery:
○ First-time
○ REDO # ☐

Priority (see definitions)
○ Elective
○ Triage/Semi-urgent
○ Urgent
○ Emergent

○ ACB x ☐
Graft Sources
○ SVG ○ Radial
○ LITA ○ Other:
○ RITA
All diseased vessels grafted?
○ Yes: ○ No
Endarterectomy
○ Yes: ○ No

○ Valve
Aortic
○ Repair ○ Replace
○ Tissue ○ Mech.
Mitral
○ Repair ○ Replace
○ Tissue ○ Mech.

Pulmonic
○ Repair ○ Replace
○ Tissue ○ Mech.
Tricuspid
○ Repair ○ Replace
○ Tissue ○ Mech.

Other:
○ LV aneurysmectomy
○ Aortic root repair/replacement
○ ASD repair
○ VSD repair
○ Other Congenital
○ Ross
○ Maze
○ Heart transplant
○ Carotid endarterectomy
○ Other (describe below)

FORM # D-2788 (Rev. 04/99)

58502

MRN ☐☐☐☐☐☐ Date: _____ Name: _____

Intraop:

(duration in minutes)

Pump: ○ No ○ Yes CPB ☐☐☐ x-Clamp ☐☐☐ Circ. arrest ☐☐☐

(units)

Bloods: ○ No ○ Yes PRBC ☐☐ PLT ☐☐ FFP ☐☐ CRYO ☐☐ DDAVP ☐☐

Events: ○ No ○ Yes _____

Last Labs: PaO2: ☐☐☐ Hct: ☐☐.☐ K+: ☐.☐ Fluids: Urine (cc): ☐☐☐☐ Balance (cc): ☐☐☐☐

CVICU:

Intubated: ○ No ○ Yes **A/E Bilateral:** ○ Y ○ N _____

Swan Ganz: ○ No ○ Yes **<50 cm:** ○ Y ○ N _____

Paced: ○ No ○ Yes **Type:** ○ A ○ V ○ A-V _____

IABP: ○ No ○ Yes **Pulse:** ○ Checked **Position:** ○ Checked _____

Bleeding: ○ No ○ Yes _____

Stable: ○ No ○ Yes _____

Inotropes: ○ No ○ Yes ○ Dopamine ○ Epi. ○ Norepi. ○ Dobut. ○ Isopryl ○ Milrinone

Vasodilators: ○ No ○ Yes ○ NTG ○ Nipride ○ Nitric Oxide ──────────

Antiarrhythmics: ○ No ○ Yes ○ Lidocaine ○ Amiodarone ──────────

HR: ☐☐ BP: ☐☐☐ / ☐☐☐ Temp: ☐☐.☐

CVP: ☐☐ PAP: ☐☐ / ☐☐ CO: ☐☐.☐ CI: ☐.☐ SVR: ☐☐☐☐

ECG: ○ ST Elevation ○ Atrial Arrhythmia **CXR:** ○ No ○ Yes
○ ST Depression ○ Ventricular Arrhythmia
○ Other _____

Sig. ECG change from preop: ○ No ○ Yes _____

Plan: _____

_____

_____

_____

Signature: _____

POSTCARDIAC SURGERY MEDICAL ADMISSION ORDERS (TGH/CVICU)

University Health Network

Toronto General Hospital Toronto Western Hospital Princess Margaret Hospital

Doctor's Order Sheet

POSTOPERATIVE ORDERS FOR

CARDIAC SURGERY

Addressograph

PLEASE USE BLACK OR BLUE BALLPOINT PEN, PRESS FIRMLY	**ALLERGIES:** NO KNOWN ALLERGIES ☐ KNOWN ALLERGIES (Specify) ☐

DATE AND TIME ORDERED	PHYSICIAN'S ORDER AND SIGNATURE	SIGNATURE(S) AND POSITION	ACTION TAKEN	PHARMACY

Pre-op orders for CVICU I and II entered in computer

1. Vital signs q 15 min x 1 h, then q 1 h when stable. Post extubation: Vital signs q 2 h when hemodynamically stable.

2. Urine output q 1 h post extubation: Urine output q 2 h when hemodynamically stable.

3. Chest tubes at - 20 cm H_2O suction. Record chest loss q 15 min x 1 h then q 1 h if patient hemodynamically stable

4. Auto-transfuse chest drainage as per CVICU policy   ☐ No ☐ Yes

5. Nasogastric tube to gravity drainage (if present).

6. Cardiac outputs and hemodynamic calculations now and q 6 h and pm (if PA catheter present).

7. IABP frequency _____ : _____

8. Check peripheral pulses q 1 h x 4 then q 4 h.

9. Central line IV, D5W at KVO.

10. K^+ replacement as per guidelines. First hour post-operative give KCI _____ mmol/L.

11. Peripheral IV Normal Saline 0.9% NaCl at KVO

12. 12 Lead ECG now then daily x 3 days then reassess.

13. Ventilation   VT _____ mL   Rate _____ min

       FiO_2 _____   Peep _____ cm/H_2O

14. Titrate FiO2 to

       Keep PO_2 ≥ _____

       OR

       O_2 Saturation ≥ _____

RT to maintain pH between

_____ to _____

OR

maintain $PaCO_2$

between _____ to ____

as per protocol

15. Suction ETT pm and chest care as per assessment.

16. Physiotherapy: Assessment and treatment.

17. Pacemaker connected and checked by M.D.

18. **MEDICATIONS:**

    a) Morphine Sulphate _____ - _____ mg IV q 1 h pm   ☐ No ☐ Yes

    b) Indomethacin Suppository _____ mg pr q h x _____ doses

    c) Acetaminophen Suppository _____ mg pr q 4 h pun if T° > 38.5°C

    d) Gravol Suppository _____ mg IV/tM q 4 h pm x 48 hours.

Form D.2074 (Rev. 11/94)   COPIES: ORIGINAL - RETAIN IN CHART.   YELLOW - PHARMACY

PLEASE USE BLACK OR BLUE BALLPOINT PEN, PRESS FIRMLY	**ALLERGIES:** NO KNOWN ALLERGIES KNOWN ALLERGIES (Specify)				
DATE AND TIME ORDERED	PHYSICIAN'S ORDER AND SIGNATURE		SIGNATURE(S) AND POSITION	ACTION TAKEN	PHARMACY

MEDICATION CONTINUED
Antibiotics:
  e) Cefazofin Suppository _____ g IV q 8 h in _____ mL D5W
     x 6 doses   ☐ No ☐ Yes
     OR
     Vancomycin _____ mg IV q 12 h in _____ mL D5W over
     12 hours x _____ doses   ☐ No ☐ Yes
     Last dose antibiotic in OR at _____ h.
  f) Propofol _____ mg IV in _____ mL D5W at _____ mL/h ☐ No ☐ Yes
     D/C at _____ h.
  g) Sodium Nitroprusside _____ mg IV in _____ mL D5W to keep
     SBP < _____ mmHg ☐ No ☐ Yes
  h) Nitroglycerin _____ mg IV in _____ mL D5W at _____ mL/h ☐ No ☐ Yes
  i) Dopamine _____ mg IV in _____ mL D5W at _____ mcg/kg/h if necessary
     to keep SBP > _____ mmHg.
  j) Nifidepine _____ - _____ mg intranasally/po q 4 h pm for SBP > 130 mmHg.
  k) Protamine _____ mg IV   ☐ No ☐ Yes
  l) Albumin 5% _____ mL IV now   ☐ No ☐ Yes
     OR
     Pendaspan _____ mL IV now   ☐ No ☐ Yes
     Reversed in O.R. ☐ No ☐ Yes

EXTUBATION:
1. Extubation ☐ No ☐ Yes as per CVICU policy.
2. Respirations q 15 min x 1 h then q 1 h when stable.
3. FiO_2 _____ via face mask. Nasal prongs when eating.
4. Oxygen saturation monitor until AM.
5. Incentive spirometer q 1 h.
6. D/C N/G tube   ☐ No ☐ Yes
   D/C chest tube   ☐ No ☐ Yes (to decide in AM rounds) (if yes, Chest X-Ray
   post removal)
8. D/C Pulmonary artery catheter   ☐ No ☐ Yes
9. Total IV/po _____ mL/24 hours.
   Clear fluids   ☐ No ☐ Yes
   Advance to LAF/NAS if tolerated   ☐ No ☐ Yes

MEDICATIONS:
  a) PCA treatment as per portocol   ☐ No ☐ Yes
     OR
     Morphine Sulphate _____ - _____ mg IV q 1 h pm   ☐ No ☐ Yes
  b) Tylenol #3 _____ tabs po q 3 h pm   ☐ No ☐ Yes
  c) ECASA _____ mg po od   ☐ No ☐ Yes
     OR
     ASA suppository _____ mg P/R od   ☐ No ☐ Yes (start day after surgery for
     post-operative ACB).
  d) HS Sedation _____ - _____ mg po q h pm.
  e) Heparin _____ u S/C q 12 h when chest tubes D/C   ☐ No ☐ Yes

Physician's Signature _____   Date _____

POSTCARDIAC SURGERY MEDICAL ADMISSION ORDERS (LHSC/CSRU)

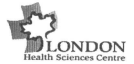

LONDON
Health Sciences Centre

Critical Care

**POSTCARDIAC SURGERY PATIENTS
PREPRINTED ORDER**

KEY: R-REQUISITIONED   P-PROCESSED (KARDEX)   P & T 0000/00

NON-MEDICATION ORDERS	R	P

* **Reason for Exam / Clinical History and Contact # required for all Radiology / Medical Imaging orders.**

ON ARRIVAL IN THE INTENSIVE CARE UNIT/PACU

1. Continuous ECG monitoring (Ld II & V5).
2. SBP target of _____ to _____ mm Hg.
3. Vital Signs q30 min. × 4 then q1h.
4. O_2 to maintain satn. > 93%.
5. Cardiac Outputs (if P.A. catheter) p.r.n. for hemodynamic instability and drug changes.
6. CT to 20 cm H_2O suction.
7. ☐ CXR* _____.
8. ECG (bedside).
9. Labs: STAT: Nova Stat, CBC, INR/PTT, Electrolytes, Mg^{2+}, PO_4, Glucose.
10. Monitor q hourly urine output, if < 30 mL × 2 hrs, call M.D.
11. Repeat ABG's p.r.n.
12. Repeat CBC, INR/PTT if CT drainage > 200 mL/30 min. p.r.n.
13. Oral gastric tube to low interm suction.

4. HOURS POST-OP

1. Cardiac Outputs (if P.A. catheter).
2. Labs: STAT CBC, INR/PTT, Elecrolytes, Urea, Creatinine, Glucose, Mg^{2+}, PO_4.
3. For minithoracotomy CABG patients, dangle/stand at bedside if patient stable.

8 HOURS POST-OP

1. Change to SBP ≤ _____ after 8 hrs if hemodynamically stable and no significant bleeding.
2. Discontinue femoral line if hemodynamically stable & INR/PTT normalized.

POST-OPERATIVE DAY #1

1. 12 Lead ECG.
2. Chest X-ray* _____
3. Labs: ASAP CBC, Electrolytes, Mg^{2+}, PO_4, Glucose, Urea & Creatinine (INR/PTT if prior results elevated)
4. Dangle prior to CT removal.
5. Physiotherapy.

MEDICATION ORDERS	P

1. I.V. 0.9% NaCl @ _____ mL/hr. Change to D5.9 if on insulin protocol.
2. Antibiotic _____
   Until chest tubes discontinued.
3. Heparin infusion to Tycos per protocol.
4. Saline Flush to peripheral lines per protocol.
5. Heparin flush to central line per protocol.
6. P.R.N.: Analgesic: _____
   Sedative: _____
   Antiemetic: _____
7. ☐ ASA (acetylsalicylic acid) 80 mg NG or PR 6 hours post-op CABG (SVG). (Hold if platelet count < 60000 or chest tube drainage > 600 mL or > 100 mL / hour).
☐ _____
☐ _____

VASODILATORS

Aim to keep SBP between _____ and _____ mmHg.

☐ Nitroglycerin 50 mg in 250 D5W.
   Start at _____ ug/min to maximum 150 ug/min.

   When maximum of NTG

☐ Nitroprusside 50mg in 250 mL D5W.
   Start at _____ ug/kg/min to maximum 3 ug/kg/min.

INOTROPES/VASOPRESSORS

☐ Epinephrine 4 mg/250 D5W.
   Start @ _____ ug/min to maximum _____ ug/min.
   Aim to keep SBP > _____ and CI > _____.

☐ Milrinone 20 mg/100 mL D5W @ _____ ug/kg/min.
☐ _____
☐ _____

CRITERIA FOR WEANING OF INOTROPES/VASOPRESSORS

At 8 hours if hemodynamically stable and no significant bleeding wean to maintain: SBP>_____mmHg; CI _____; PA< _____ Titrate the following:

☐ Epinephrine to off or _____ ug/min
☐ Milrinone to off or _____ ug/kg/min
☐ _____
☐ _____

PRESCRIBER'S PRINTED NAME / SIGNATURE / CONTACT			DATE (YYYY/MM/DD):		TIME:
PROCESSOR'S INITIALS:	DATE (YYYY/MM/DD):	TIME:	R/N INITIALS:	DATE (YYYY/MM/DD):	TIME:

NS1134 (Rev 2005/02/24)

TGH/CVICU MEDICAL DISCHARGE FORMS

UHN TGH - CVICU DISCHARGE NOTE
Must be completed and placed in the chart

53440

MRN ☐☐☐☐☐☐☐

(dd/mm/yyyy)
Date: ☐☐ / ☐☐ / 2 0 0 ☐

Addressograph

Allergies: ○ No   ○ Yes:

(dd/mm/yyyy)
OR Date: ☐☐ / ☐☐ / 2 0 0 ☐   **Procedure:**

Was patient re-admitted to CVICU?
○ No   ○ Yes, reason & date:

Other Procedures?   ### Details (date, reason, etc.):

○ No   ○ Yes   ○ Re-opening without CPB   Reason for re-opening: ○ Bleeding   ○ Tamponade   ○ Arrest   ○ Other
              ○ Re-opening with CPB
              ○ Pacemaker insertion
              ○ Sternal rewiring
              ○ Sternal debridement
              ○ Muscle flap
              ○ Tracheostomy
              ○ Laparotomy
              ○ Other:_____

PERIOPERATIVE COURSE (See CVICU admission note for Past History)

EVENTS   **Description / Current Status / Follow up**
(see definitions)

○ **Mortality**   Give date and complete all applicable sections below

Cardiovascular   ○ NIL   IABP postop.: ○ No   ○ Yes   **Preop. LV grade:** ○ I   ○ II   ○ III   ○ IV
○ Perioperative MI   **Postop. LV grade:** ○ I   ○ II   ○ III   ○ IV
○ Heart failure
○ Atrial arrhythmia
○ Ventricular arrhythmia
○ Bradycardia/heart block
○ Cardiac arrest
○ Tamponade
○ Pericardial effusion   **Plan:**
○ Other:_____
                                  Telemetry: ○ No   ○ Yes   **Needs 2D-echo/TEE:** ○ No   ○ Yes

Respiratory   ○ NIL
○ Difficult Intubation
○ Re-intubated
○ Respiratory insufficiency
○ Pulmonary embolism
○ Pneumothorax
○ Pleural effusion
○ Pulmonary aspiration
○ Other:_____   **Plan:**

FORM # D-2789 (Rev, 04/99)

53440

MRN ☐☐☐☐☐☐ Date: _____ Name: _____

EVENTS (see definitions)	Description / Current Status / Follow up

Neurologic ○ NIL
○ Seizures
○ Stroke
○ Delirium
○ Peripheral nerve injury
○ Other:_____   **Plan:**

Infectious ○ NIL
○ Wound infection
○ Sternum-deep
○ Endocarditis
○ Pneumonia
○ Urinary tract infection
○ Sepsis
○ Other:_____   **Plan:**

Renal ○ NIL
○ Acute renal failure
○ Acute renal insufficiency
○ Dialysis dependent
○ Other:_____   **Plan:**

GI ○ NIL
○ Liver dysfunction
○ GI bleed
○ Ischemic bowel
○ Other:_____   **Plan:**

Miscellaneous ○ NIL
○ HIT
○ Coagulopathy
○ Skin burns/ulcers
○ Other:_____   **Plan:**

Discharge Medications:

○ Beta-blocker _____   ○ Heparin   Target INR: ☐.☐☐
○ Calcium CB _____   ○ Coumadin
○ ACE-I _____   ○ ASA   _____
○ Diuretic _____   ○ Insulin   _____
○ Amiodarone _____   ○ Oxygen   _____
○ Digoxin _____   ○ Other

Discharge Labs: Creat ☐☐ Hb ☐☐☐ Platelets ☐☐☐ INR ☐.☐☐ PaO2 ☐☐☐

Transfer: Weight (kg) ☐☐ Balance (cc) ☐☐☐☐ ○ Positive
                                                  ○ Negative

Signature:

TGH/CVICU MEDICAL DISCHARGE ORDERS

	THE TORONTO HOSPITAL A University of Toronto Teaching Hospital Doctor's Order Sheet ROUTINE STANDING ORDERS FOR CARDIAC PATIENTS LEAVING ICU	

ALLERGIES NO KNOWN ALLERGIES ☐	Surgery <u>Fill in type of surgery</u> LV Grade

DATE AND TIME	PHYSICIAN'S ORDERS	ACTION TAKEN	SIGNATURE AND POSITION
	1. Cancel all previous orders		
	2. Transfer orders (24 hours or 48 hrs post-op) entered on computers.		
	3. Daily PT, PTT entered on computer No ☐ Yes ☑ ─────▶ only if indicated		
	4. Daily Glucose entered on com puter No ☑ Yes ☐ ─────▶ not done, accucheck on floor		
	5. Clear fluids, LAF, NAS DAT or Diabetic diet 1800 kJ look on admission orders		
	6. Vital Signs q 4 hrs, then qid PRN.		
	7. Intake and output as per unit guidelines.		
	8. Peripheral IV 2/3 - 1/3 or D5W plus _0_ mmol/L KCL at _TKVO_ ml/hr. or saline lock if no infusions		
	9. D/C central line ☐ No ☑ Yes (if no, D5W _____ ml/hr) cordis always removed, unless IV amiodarone		
	10. Total daily fluid allowance (IV & PO) 1500-2000 ml/24 less if need fluid restriction		
	11. Weight as per unit guidelines.		
	12. AAT ☐ No ☑ Yes Other		
	13. Wound care as per unit guidelines		
	14. ECG tomorrow ☐ No ☑ Yes and on 4th & 6th post op days		
	15. D/C pacemaker ☐ No ☑ Yes (if yes, cover pacer wires) unless pacer on standby		
	16. Telemetry ☐ No ☑ Yes yes, if POD #1 or dysrhythmia		
	17. Remove pacer wires prior to discharge.		
	18. Inspirometer q 1 -2 hrs		
	19. Physiotherapy assessment and treatment.		
	20. FiO₂ _____ via face mask / nasal prongs individualize		
	Tandem flow ☑ No ☐ Yes if needed, unusual to send patients on FiO₂ > 60% to floor		
	21. D/C arterial line.		
	22. D/C Foley catheter ☐ No ☑ Yes (Leave in situ if 24 hrs transfer)		
	23. D/C Chest tubes ☐ No ☑ Yes (if yes, CXR post removal)		
	Medications:		
Order either Morphine or demerol	a) PCA Treatment as per protocol ☑ No ☐ Yes OR Most patients don't use PCA		
	Morphine sulphate 1-4 mg IV/IM q 1 hrs x 24 hrs		
	☐ No ☑ Yes OR		
	Demerol 10-30 mg IV/IM q 1 hrs x 24 hrs		
	☐ No ☑ Yes		
Order both tylenol #3 and percocet	b) Tylenol #3 1-2 tabs po q 3 hrs prn x 14 days OR unless codeine allergy		
	Percocet 1-2 Tab po q 4 hrs prn x 14 days		
	c) Gravol 25-50 mg IV/IM q 4 hrs PRN 7 days		
	☐ No ☑ Yes		
	d) HS sedation _____ mg po q hs prn x 14 days Imovane 3.75 mg may repeat x 1		
	e) Colace 100 mg po bid order on all patients		
	f) MOM 30 ml po qhs PRN order on all patients		
	g) Lasix _____ mg po daily x _____ days start on _____ Do not order as both Lasix and Slow K		
	h) Slow K _____ tabs po q _____ hrs x _____ days start on _____ are assessed daily on floor		
	i) Antibiotics _____ as per routine postop schedule or continue SBE treatment		
	j) Anticoagulation		
	1. Heparin 5000 u s/c q 12 hrs. Reassess if platelets < 100,000 Routine ACB patients receive		
	D/C Heparin when fully ambulatory SQ Heparin q 12h and ECASA		
	2. ECASA 325 mg po daily ☐ No ☐ Yes		
	3. Coumadin _____ mg po daily (Target INR _____) ☐ No ☐ Yes		
	4. Heparin _____ u IV in _____ cc D5W at _____ u/hrs		
	☐ No ☐ Yes		
	Reorder non cardiac preop drugs (thyroid, eye drops etc.)		
	Physician's Signature _____ Date _____		

LHSC VENTILATION WEANING AND EXTUBATION PROTOCOL

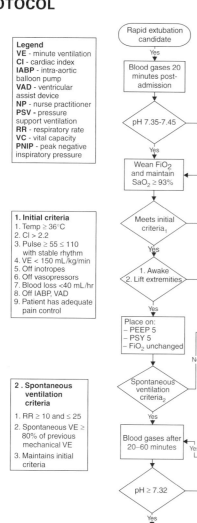

Legend
VE - minute ventilation
CI - cardiac index
IABP - intra-aortic balloon pump
VAD - ventricular assist device
NP - nurse practitioner
PSV - pressure support ventilation
RR - respiratory rate
VC - vital capacity
PNIP - peak negative inspiratory pressure

1. Initial criteria
1. Temp ≥ 36°C
2. CI > 2.2
3. Pulse ≥ 55 ≤ 110 with stable rhythm
4. VE < 150 mL/kg/min
5. Off inotropes
6. Off vasopressors
7. Blood loss <40 mL/hr
8. Off IABP, VAD
9. Patient has adequate pain control

2 . Spontaneous ventilation criteria
1. RR ≥ 10 and ≤ 25
2. Spontaneous VE ≥ 80% of previous mechanical VE
3. Maintains initial criteria

3. Extubation criteria
1. SaO_2 ≥ 93% on FiO_2 ≤ 0.5 PEEP ≤ 5
2. Adequate gag
3. Effective cough
4. Capable of maintaining airway
5. Minimal secretions
6. Perform VC and PNIP (at RTs discretion)

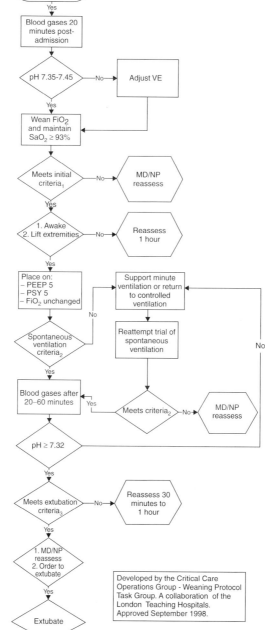

Developed by the Critical Care Operations Group - Weaning Protocol Task Group. A collaboration of the London Teaching Hospitals. Approved September 1998.

Appendix G

PATIENT CONTROL ANALGESIA ORDER

University Health Network

Toronto General Hospital Toronto Western Hospital Princess Margaret Hospital

DOCTOR'S ORDER SHEET
ANAESTHESIA/ACUTE PAIN SERVICE
PATIENT CONTROLLED ANALGESIA
(PCA ORDERS)

Addressograph

ALLERGIES
NO KNOWN ALLERGIES ☐

DATE AND TIME ORDERED	PHYSICIAN'S ORDER	ACTION TAKEN	SIGNATURE AND POSITION
	1. While on PCA device, patient is to receive NO further supplemental Narcotics unless approved by the Anesthesia/Acute Pain Service		

	2. PCA DRUG:
	      Morphine ___ mg/mL
	      Meperidine ___ mg/mL
	      Other: _____ mg/ML		

	3. PUMP SETTINGS:
	      Dose ___ mg to ___ mg
	      Initial Lockout Interval ___ min
	      Four hour limit ___ mg		

	4. MONITORING: Respiratory Rate, Sedation Score q 2 h × 24hr, then q 4 h. record on PCA Flow Sheet		

	5. TREATMENT OF SIDE EFFECTS:
	      Have Naloxone (Narcan) 0.4 mg/mL vial readily available at Nursing Station
	
	      NAUSEA/VOMITING:
	      Dimenhydrinate (Gravol) _____ mg IV/IM q 3 - 4 h prn
	      IV dose to be infused in 15 - 30 min
	
	      ITCHINESS:
	      Diphenhydramine (Benadryl) _____ mg IV/IM q 3 - q4 h prn
	      IV dose to be infused in 15 - 30 min
	      Discontinue Dimenhydrinate (Gravol) and Diphenhydramine (Benadryl) when PCA Stopped		

	6. If patient confused - Hold PCA and Treat Pain with ___ mg IV / SC q ___ h prn		

	7. Call Acute Pain Service if:
	      a) Respiratory Rate less than 10/min
	      b) Blood Pressure less than 90 mmHg systolic
	      c) Pulse less than 50/min
	      d) Sedation Score of 3 (somnolent, difficult to rouse)
	      e) Unsatisfactory analgesia
	      f) If four hour limit of drug dose is reached before 4 hours has elapsed		

	8. In an emergency, if NO response after calling the above Beeper #, call Anaesthesia Resident through locating		
	9. If side effects of slow respiratory rate, hypotension or somnolence occur, STOP PCA Pump immediately and inform attending service as well as Acute Pain Service		
	10. RN will check and verify PCA setting once per shift.		
	11. When tolerating fluids well, D/C PCA then start analgesics with: _____ _____		
	Physician's Signature Date		

449

ANTICOAGULATION GUIDELINE POSTCARDIAC SURGERY

Anticoagulation for Postoperative Cardiac Patients

Division of Cardiovascular Surgery, TGH (1994)

Anticoagulation Guidelines Postcardiac Surgery

1. Valves
mechanical
St. Jude, CarboMedics, Sorin, Medtronic Hall, Bjork-Shiley
- All Positions: Coumadin permanently INR 2.5-3.5
- Closer to 3.5 for mitral and tricuspid
- Closer to 2.5 for aortic
- Heparin until INR therapeutic:
  - Mitral position 8,000 units SQ tid
  - Aortic position 5,000 units SQ tid

bioprosthetic
Hancock Porcine, Carpentier Edwards Pericardial, Medtronic Mosaic Porcine, Toronto Stentless Porcine Valve (SPV), Homograft, Autograft
- Aortic position: ASA 325 mg OD permanently
- Mitral (A. fib): Coumadin permanently INR 2.0-3.0
- Mitral (sinus): Coumadin for 3 months INR 2.0-3.0 then ASA 325 mg OD permanently
- Heparin 5,000 units SQ bid until fully ambulatory

2. Annuloplasty Rings
Types: Duran, Carpentier Edwards
All positions: Coumadin x 3 months, INR 2.0-3.0
After 3 months Coumadin only if indicated for other reasons

3. Aortocoronary Bypass
Heparin 5,000 units SQ bid until ambulatory
ASA 325 mg PO OD
Consider Plavix in cases of coronary endarterectomy or arteries with poor run-off

4. Atrial Fibrillation

Age	Risk Factors	Antithrombotic
<65	no risk factors	ASA or nothing
	risk factors	Warfarin INR 2-3
65–75	no risk factors	Warfarin or ASA
	risk factors	Warfarin INR 2-3
>75	with or without	Warfarin INR 2-3

Risk Factors: previous TIA or stroke, HBP, heart failure, diabetes, clinical coronary disease, mitral stenosis, prosthetic heart valves or thyrotoxicosis

---

Additional comments:

1. Coumadin should be started when the patient can swallow. If the patient cannot swallow by 24 hours after surgery then heparinization is recommended, but the therapeutic level and duration of therapy should be determined by the specific circumstances. Monitor platelets count and think of heparin induced thrombocytopenia (HIT).

2. Patients on Heparin and Coumadin should not receive ASA.
3. Start Coumadin according to the accompanying guidelines, with the newly approved Pharmacy Assisted Warfarin Dosing Program available in CVICU. Starting dose for Coumadin should be 5.0 mg or 7.5 mg if any of the following variables exist:
   - high live r function tests (LFTs) of known liver disease or congestion
   - patients over 70 years of age
   - general condition of patient is frail, undernourished and underweight
   - patients of Chinese descent where dietary habits include dry mushrooms
   - pre-op or postop Amiodarone or medications affecting coagulation
   - fluid retention status is still significantly over pre-op weight, or other signs of heart failure
   - documented coagulopathy of known or unknown origin
4. On discharge letter to the family doctor, write the valve type and anticoagulation required; e.g., Aortic Valve Replacement with St. Jude Mechanical Valve Permanent Coumadin INR to be 2.5–3.5.

Pharmacy Assisted Warfarin Dosing (PAWD)

1. An order written by the ICU Physician is necessary to enroll a patient in the PAWD program. The indication for Coumadin and the target INR must be stated.
2. Coumadin may be started if the chest tubes are removed or they are likely to be removed within 24 hours after the initial dose.
3. Coumadin will not be given to a patient who is pacemaker dependent and may require a permanent pacemaker.
4. A baseline AST will be sent when the order for Coumadin is written. (Postcardiopulmonary bypass patients frequently have an unpredictable rise in AST).
5. Heparin 8000 Units s.c tid will be given to patients with mechanical valves until INR >2.5.
6. Special attention to the rate of increase of INR will be given to patients on Amiodarone, Cipro, Septra, and those with an elevated AST.
7. If INR increased by >1 after any single dose, the ICU Physician will be notified before any further Coumadin is administered.
8. If INR is not >2 after 3 doses of Coumadin, in the patient with a mechanical valve, an ICU Physician will be consulted as to the need for IV Heparin pending therapeutic INR.
9. When patient is on Coumadin treatment, *NO* ASA should be given concomitantly unless approved by cardiologist/cardiovascular surgeon.

INSULIN PROTOCOL FOR GLUCOSE CONTROL

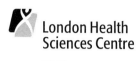

London Health Sciences Centre

CSRU

INSULIN INFUSION PREPRINTED ORDER

KEY: R - REQUISITIONED P - PROCESSED (KARDEX) P & T _____

NON-MEDICATION ORDERS	R	P
1. Target range for glucose for all patients is 4.5 - 6.5 mmol/L. • If any glucose measurement is > 7.5 mmol/L, repeat in 2 hours. If still > 7.5 mmol/L, initiate protocol with above target goal. • This protocol is NOT to be used for patients with diabetic ketoacidosis during the first 48 hours post admission or acute hepatic failure. • Send blood glucose to lab OD with am bloodwork and prn to verify glucometer readings of glucose < 2.5 or > 20 mmol/L.		
2. Draw all glucose measurements from arterial catheter. Obtain capillary sample only when no indwelling access.		
3. Administer insulin by dedicated line. Do not piggyback with other infusions or use line for intermittent medication administration.		
4. Maintenance I.V. must contain dextrose when insulin is administered in the absence of enteral or parenteral feeding (e.g. D5W and 0.9 normal saline).		
5. GLUCOSE MONITORING AND ADJUSTMENT: • Measure glucose and adjust insulin per protocol q 2h until 3 glucose levels within range, then q 4h. • If glucose decreases by 50%, is < 4.5 or decreases by > 2 ranges, measure and adjust insulin per protocol q 1h until 3 glucose levels within range.		
6. If neurological status decreases, suspect hypoglycemia and perform STAT glucose check.		
7. Increase glucose monitoring frequency when sympathomimetic drug infusions are being titrated or intermittent steroid doses are administered.		
8. If TPN is abruptly discontinued (without enteral feeding being established), administer dextrose 10% I.V. at the same rate as the TPN, repeat blood glucose in 1 hour and review orders with physician.		
9. If enteral feeding is stopped or decreased, recheck blood glucose in 1 hour. If feeding is withheld during patient transport for test or procedure, stop insulin infusion. Recheck glucose upon return to unit and restart insulin according to protocol.		
10. Review insulin therapy with anaesthesia prior to transfer to OR.		
11. Continue insulin infusion protocol until patient is discharged. • Continuous insulin therapy may be discontinued when patient has transfer orders and is no longer receiving continuous feeding. • For patients without a previous history of diabetes mellitus who have been stable for at least 48h on an infusion of < 2 u/h, attempt to wean insulin off. Restart if glucose increases above target range.		

MEDICATION ORDERS

MEDICATION ORDERS	P
1. Regular Insulin infusion 2 u/mL concentration in 0.9% NaCl.	
2. Start infusion at 2 u/h (1 u/h). Start at 4 u/h (2 mL/h) if glucose > 13.	
3. Nurses may use discretion when adjusting insulin infusions +/-3 u/h, based on observed trends.	

Glucose Level	
< 2.5	• HOLD insulin infusion • GIVE 25 mL D50W • NOTIFY MD • If patient is an insulin dependent diabetic, leave insulin infusion at 0.5 u/h after giving dextrose bolus
2.5 - 3	• HOLD insulin infusion • RECHECK blood sugar q 1h • GIVE 10 mL D50W • NOTIFY MD if patient is symptomatic • RESTART insulin infusion at 2/3 the previous infusion rate when glucose > * • If patient is an insulin dependent diabetic, leave insulin infusion at 0.5 u/h after giving dextrose bolus
If > 3 and decreased > 50%, or glucose decreases by ≥ 2 ranges	• Decrease infusion rate by 50% and recheck in 1 hour

	Change in glucose since the last check:		
	Increased from a lower range	Is within same range	Decreased from a higher range
3.1 - 4.4	No change	Decrease infusion (Rate Change "A")*	Decrease infusion (Rate Change "B")*
4.5 - 7.0	No change	No change	Decrease infusion (Rate Change "A")*

	Change in glucose since the last check:		
	Decreased by < 2 or increased	Decreased by 2 - 4	Decreased by > 4
7.1 - 8.5	Increase by 1 u/h	No change	Decrease infusion (Rate Change "A")*
8.6 - 18	Increase by 2 u/h	Increase by 1 u/h	No Change
18.1 - 24	Increase by 3 u/h	Increase by 2 u/h	No Change
> 24	Call MD		

* RATE CHANGE CHART IS ON BACK OF THIS PAGE.

NOTE: Changes of glucose readings < 1 may be within glucometer measurement error and should not be considered a significant change.

PRESCRIBER'S PRINTED NAME / SIGNATURE / CONTACT #:		DATE (YYYY/MM/DD):		TIME:
PROCESSOR'S INITIALS:	DATE (YYYY/MM/DD):	TIME:	RN INITIALS:	DATE (YYYY/MM/DD):	TIME:

Distribution: WHITE - Chart   CANARY - Pharmacist   PINK - Nurse

DECREASING INSULIN INFUSION		
CURRENT RATE OF INFUSION	**RATE CHANGE "A"**	**RATE CHANGE "B"**
< 5 units per hour	Reduce by 0.5 units per hour	Reduce by 1 unit per hour
5.5 - 8 units per hour	Reduce by 1 unit per hour	Reduce by 2 units per hour
> 8 units per hour	Reduce by 2 units per hour	Reduce by 3 units per hour

PHARMACOLOGY IN CARDIOVASCULAR ANESTHESIA AND SURGERY

Janet Martin, BScPhm, RPh, PharmD

TABLE (a) Dose, Administration and Mechanism of Action

Drug	Bolus	Infusion Rate	Preparation Concentration	Onset	T$^{1}/_{2}$ β	Metabolism/ Excretion	MOA
Adrenergic Agents							
Clonidine (Catapres)	3–5 μg/kg IV	NA	—	<15 min	6–20 h	Hepatic/urine	Centrally acting α_2-adrenergic agonist/antagonist
	150 μg IT	Epidural infusion: 30 μ/h (titrate carefully, not to exceed 40 μg/h)					
Dexmedetomidine (Precedex)	0.25–1.0 μg/kg IV over 10 min	0.2–0.7 μg/kg/h (infuse for <24 h)	Must be diluted prior to use	<5 min	2 h	Hepatic/urine	Centrally acting α_2-agonist/ antagonist
Dobutamine (Dobutrex)	N/R	1–20 μg/kg/min	250 mg/250 mL 1,000 μg/mL	1–2 min	3 min	Liver/urine	β_1-agonist
Dopamine (Intropin)	N/R	0.5–2 μg/kg/min (low-dose, renal) 2–10 μg/kg/min (intermediate dose, cardiac) 10–20 μg/kg/min (high dose, vascular)	200 mg/250 mL 800 μg/mL	<5 min	2 min	Kidney and plasma (by MAO and COMT)/urine	Endogenous catecholamine
Dopexamine	N/R	0.5–6 μg/kg/min	—	<5 min	7–11 min	Liver/urine	Structural similarity to dopamine
Ephedrine	5–20 mg IV q5 10 min	Not recommended for infusion because of development of tachyphylaxis	—	<5–10 min	3–6 h	Liver (oxidative deamination)/ urine	Noncatecholamine sympathomimetic with direct and indirect α and β adrenergic stimulation

Drug	Dose	Infusion dose	Concentration	Onset	Half-life	Metabolism	Mechanism
Epinephrine (Adrenaline)	1 mg IV push q3–5 min for resuscitation/arrest	0.01–0.30 µg/kg/min 1–10 µg/min	1 mg/250 mL 4 µg/mL	<15 min	2 min	Hepatic/urine	Endogenous catecholamine, activates α and β receptors
Isoproterenol	0.01–0.06 mg IV for heart block	0.01 µg/kg/min titrate to desired effect, up to 0.15 µg/kg/min	1 mg/250 mL 4 µg/mL	<1 min	2–5 min	Liver/urine	Sympathomimetic amine, β_1 and β_2 receptor stimulation
Mephentermine (Wyamine)	20–60 mg IV	1–5 µg/kg/min	—	<2 min (IV) <15 min (IM)	—	Liver/urine	Sympathomimetic α- and β-receptor stimulation
Metaraminol (Aramine)	0.5–5 mg IV or 2–10 mg IM/SC q10min	1 mg/kg SC/IM q10min	—	<2 min (IV) <10 min (IM) <20 min (SC)	5–10 min	—	Sympathomimetic α- and β-receptor stimulation
Methoxamine (Vasoxyl)	2–5 mg IV q15min for shock 10 mg IV over 3–5 min for PSVT	—	—	<2 min (IV) <20 min (IM)	—	Liver/urine	Selective α_1-receptor agonist
Norepinephrine (Levophed)	N/F	Initial: 0.5–1 µg/min, and titrate to response (usually 8–30 µg/min)	4 mg/250 mL 16 µg/mL	<1 min	2 min	Hepatic (via COMT, MAO)/urine	Catecholamine, direct-acting adrenergic agonist
Phenylephrine (Neo-Synephrine)	0.5–1 mg IV, then increase by 0.1–0.2 mg increments	0.15–0.75 µg/kg/min	10 mg/250 mL 40 µg/mL	<2 min (IV)	—	Intestines and liver	Sympathomimetic with direct α-adrenergic stimulation

(continued)

457

◗ **TABLE (a) Dose, Administration and Mechanism of Action** (Continued)

Drug	Bolus	Infusion Rate	Preparation Concentration	Onset	$T^{1}/_{2}\beta$	Metabolism/ Excretion	MOA
Hormones							
Desmopressin DDAVP	2–4 µg/d IV over 15 min	—	—	<30 min	75 min	—	Antidiuretic: ↑ water permeability at renal tubules and collecting ducts Antihemorrhagic: ↑ release endogenous factor VIII
Glucagon (GlucaGen)	1 mg IV, repeat after 15 min	—	—	5–20 min	3–6 min	Liver/urine	↑ Plasma glucose levels, causes smooth muscle relaxation; positive inotrope on myocardium
Prostacyclin (Epoprostenol, PGI₂)	15–20 µg nebulized	2–70 ng/kg/min nebulized or 2–20 ng/kg/min IV	Powder to be mixed with saline for inhalation	Immediate	3–5 min	Plasma hydrolysis/ urine	A naturally occurring prostaglandin with potent vasodilation and inhibitor of PLT aggregation
Triiodothyronine, T₃	0.4 µg/kg	0.4 µg/h for 6 h	—	<1 h	1–2 d	Liver, kidney, intestine/feces	Promotes gluconeogenesis; ↑ metabolic rate of tissue; stimulates protein synthesis; ↑ mobilization of glycogen

Drug	IV push	Infusion	Concentration	Onset	Duration	Metabolism/Excretion	Comments
Vasopressin (Pitressin)	40 U IV push for VF resuscitation/arrest	0.03 U/min to preserve renal function; 0.1 U/min or 1–6 U/h as a vasopressor	40 U/100 mL 0.4 U/mL	<30 min	10–20 min	Liver and kidney/urine	ADH effect at renal tubules, ↑ GI peristalsis, vasoconstriction of capillaries and small arterioles

Vasodilators

Drug	IV push	Infusion	Concentration	Onset	Duration	Metabolism/Excretion	Comments
Amrinone	0.75 mg/kg over 2–3 min	2–10 μg/kg/min (not to exceed total daily dose of 10 mg/kg)	1–3 mg/mL	<5 min	3.6 h	Liver/urine	Inhibitors phosphodiesterase, ↑ myocardial cAMP, arrhythmogenic properties
Hydralazine (Apresoline)	5–20 mg IV	—	—	10–15 min	3–7 h	Liver/urine	Direct vasodilator effect on vascular smooth muscle
Milrinone	25–50 μg/kg	0.25–0.75 μg/kg/min	20 mg/100 mL 200 μg/mL	5–15 min	2–3 h	None/excreted unchanged in urine	Selective inhibitor of cAMP phosphodiesterase (peak III inhibitor); vasodilation
Nitroglycerin	10–200 μg	0.1–5.0 μg/kg/min, titrate to effect, max 200 μg/min (tolerance develops after 24-h infusion)	100 mg/250 mL 400 μg/mL	Immediate	2 min	Plasma, liver/urine	Peripheral vasodilator relaxes vascular smooth muscle
Nitroprusside	1–2 μg/kg	0.2–10 μg/kg/min, titrate to effect (when prolonged infusion >2 μg/kg/min, cyanide accumulates)	50 mg/250 mL 200 μg/mL Unstable in light (protect)	0.5–1 min	<10 min	Plasma, liver/urine	Peripheral vasodilation via direct vascular smooth muscle relaxation

(continued)

TABLE (a) Dose, Administration and Mechanism of Action (Continued)

Drug	Bolus	Infusion Rate	Preparation Concentration	Onset	T½ β	Metabolism/ Excretion	MOA
Fenoldopam (Corlopam)	N/R	0.05–0.1 μg/kg/min renal dose; 0.1–0.3 μg/kg/min dose as a venodilator	10 mg/250 mL 40 μg/mg/mL	<1 min	5–10 min	Liver/urine	Rapid-acting vasodilator; agonist at D1-like dopaminergic receptors and α_2-adrenergic receptors

Antiarrhythmics

Class I (Sodium channel blockers; Class IA—APD prolonged; Class IB—APD shortened; Class IC—APD unchanged)

Drug	Bolus	Infusion Rate	Preparation Concentration	Onset	T½ β	Metabolism/ Excretion	MOA
Lidocaine (Xylocaine) (IB)	1–1.5 mg/kg over 2 min; may repeat 0.5–0.75 mg/kg q5 min up to total of 3 mg/kg	1–4 mg/min	2 g/250 mL 8 mg/mL	<2 min	1–2 h	Liver/urine	Inhibits re-entry, ↓ automaticity, ↓ ERP, ↓ APD
Phenytoin (Dilantin) (IB)	100 mg q5min p.r.n. (max 700 mg/d)	—	—	0.5–1 h	7–30 h	Liver/urine	↓ Sodium ion influx, stabilizes neural membranes, ↓ APD, ↓ ERP, ↓ AT interval, ↑ AV nodal conduction
Procainamide (Pronestyl) (IA)	100 mg given over 5 min, may repeat q5min, upto a maximum total dose of 1 g	2–6 mg/min	2 g/250 mL 8 mg/mL	<30 min	2–5 h	Liver/urine	↓ Myocardial excitability, ↓ automaticity, ↓ CV, ↑ ERP, ↑ APD, anticholinergic activity, ↑ AV nodal conduction

Drug	Dose	Maintenance/infusion	Concentration	Onset	Half-life	Metabolism/excretion	Receptor/effects
Quinidine (Quinora, Quinalan) (IA)	6–10 mg/kg, given slowly (i.e., 10 mg/min)	Up to 20–30 mg/min if tolerated	—	<10 min	6–8 h	Liver/urine	↓Automaticity, ↑ERP, ↑APD, ↓AV nodal refractoriness; anti-ACh effects
Class II (β-blockers)							
Atenolol (Tenormin)	1–5 mg IV over 5 min; repeat once after 10 min	—	—	<5 min	6–7 h	No metabolism/ urine	Selective β₁-antagonist
Esmolol (Brevibloc)	0.5–1 mg/kg IV over 1 min; repeat twice	50–300 μg/kg/min	2.5 g/250 mL 10 mg/mL	<5 min	8–12 min	RBC esterases/ urine	Selective β₁-antagonist
Labetolol (Trandate, Normodyne)	20–80 mg IV over 2 min, repeat q10min intervals, to a maximum of 300 mg (or continuous infusion)	2 mg/min (up to 300 mg maximum total dose)	500 mg/250 mL 2 mg/mL; infusion pump	2–5 min	2.5–8 h	Liver/urine	α₁-antagonist β₁-antagonist β₂-antagonist
Metoprolol (Lopressor)	2.5–5 mg IV q5min	2.5 mg/h, titrate	—	5 min	3–7 h	Liver/urine	β₁-antagonist
Propranolol (Inderal)	1–3 mg IV slow push; repeat q2min p.r.n.	—	—	<2 min	3–5 h	Liver/urine	β₁-antagonist β₂-antagonist
Class III (K⁺ channel blockers; APD and ERP prolonged)							
Amiodarone (Cordarone, Pacerone)	Pulseless VT/VF: 300 mg IV push (diluted in 20 mL NS);	1 mg/min over 6 h; then 0.5 mg/min (maximum daily dose: 2.2 g)	150 mg/100 mL 1.5 mg/mL	5–15 min	7–20 h	Liver/urine, feces	Inhibits adrenergic stimulation, prolongs the action potential and refractory

(continued)

▶ TABLE (a) Dose, Administration and Mechanism of Action (Continued)

Drug	Bolus	Infusion Rate	Preparation Concentration	Onset	T½β	Metabolism/ Excretion	MOA
	then 150 mg IV push (diluted in 20 mL NS) if necessary Breakthrough VT/VF: 150 mg supplemental dose given over 10 min						period in myocardial tissue; decreases AV conduction and sinus node function
Bretylium (Bretylol)	5–10 mg/kg given over 10–30 min. Repeat after 1 h p.r.n. (to a maximum of 30 mg/kg)	1–2 mg/min	—	3–30 min	5–10 h	None/urine	Inhibits repolarization, ↑APD, ↑ERP, transient catecholamine release
Ibutilide (Corvert)	Weight <60 kg: 0.01 mg/kg over 10 min Weight ≥60 kg: 1 mg over 10 min Repeat if necessary after 10 min	—	—	10–90 min	2–12 h	Liver/urine, feces	Unknown MOA; prolongs action potential in cardiac tissues

Class IV (Calcium Channel Blockers)

Drug	IV Dose	Infusion	Preparation	Onset	Duration	Elimination	Mechanism of Action
Diltiazem (Cardizem)	20 mg IV loading over 2 min for SVT (i.e., 0.25 mg/kg); may repeat 20–25 mg IV after 15 min if needed	5–15 mg/h depending on HR and BP (infusions >24 h not recommended, because of reduced clearance, prolonged action)	250 mg/250 mL 1 mg/mL; infusion pump required	<2 min	3–6 h	Liver/urine	Inhibits calcium ion from entering "slow channels" of selected voltage-sensitive areas of vascular smooth muscle and myocardium during depolarization; relaxes coronary vascular smooth muscle and produces coronary vasodilation; slows automaticity and conduction of AV node
Nicardipine (Cardene)	0.625–2.5 mg IV	2.5–15 mg/h (start low, and titrate by 2.5 mg/h q15min p.r.n.)	Dilute to 0.1 mg/mL	2–10 min	2–4 h	Liver/urine	See above
Verapamil (Isoptin)	2.5–10 mg IV over 2 min; repeat in 15–30 min (to maximum 20 mg total dose)	N/R	—	1–2 min	6–12 h	Liver/urine	See above

(continued)

▶ **TABLE (a)** Dose, Administration and Mechanism of Action (Continued)

Drug	Bolus	Infusion Rate	Preparation Concentration	Onset	T½ β	Metabolism/ Excretion	MOA
Miscellaneous Antiarrhythmics							
Adenosine (Adenocard)	6 mg over 1–2 s, via peripheral line; if not effective with in 1–2 min, give 12 mg; repeat 12-mg dose if needed; follow each bolus with NS flush	—	—	Immediate	10 s	Immediate bio-transformation/ cellular uptake	Slows conduction through AV node; inhibits reentry pathways
Atropine	Bradyarrhythmia: 0.5–1 mg q5min (max 3 mg)	—	—	<2 min	2–3 h	Liver/urine	Competitive ACh antagonist at central and peripheral muscarinic receptors
Digoxin (Lanoxin)	0.5–1 mg initially; then 0.1–0.3 mg q8h (up to max 1 mg dose)	—	—	5–30 min	39 h	Liver/urine	Inhibits membrane bound Na^+/K^+-activated ATPase, $\downarrow Ca^{2+}$ current during AP, $\uparrow$ vagal and sympatholytic effects at SA node, $\uparrow$ AV node refractory period, $\downarrow$ AV node conduction, $\downarrow$ SA

Magnesium	1–6 g IV (dilute first, and give over several minutes at a rate not to exceed 150 mg/min)	3–20 mg/min	1–2 g/100 mL (8–16 mEq/100 mL)	Immediate	1 h	None/urine	nodal automaticity, ↑ PVR, ↑ sympathetic outflow, (+) inotrope Decreases ACh in motor nerve terminals and acts on myocardium by slowing rate of AV node impulse formation and prolonging conduction time
Antiplatelets							
ASA (aspirin, acetylsalicylic acid)	—	81–325 mg PO daily for cardiovascular/ cerebrovascular protection Up to 4 g PO daily for analgesia/anti-inflammatory indications	81 mg tabs 325 mg tabs 650 mg tabs	5–15 min	15–30 min	Liver/urine	Inhibits Pg synthesis (↓ cyclooxygenase activity), ↓ thromboxane A_2, ↓ platelet aggregation, peripheral vasodilation
Clopidogrel (Plavix)	300 mg PO loading dose for ACS or for post-PCI	75–300 mg PO daily (no IV availability)	75 mg tabs	2 h	8 h	Liver/urine, feces	Blocks binding of fibrinogen to glycoprotein receptors; ↓ PLT aggregation

(*continued*)

▶ **TABLE (a) Dose, Administration and Mechanism of Action** (Continued)

Drug	Bolus	Infusion Rate	Preparation Concentration	Onset	Metabolism/ T½β	Excretion	MOA
Dipyridamole/ ASA (Aggrenox)	—	200 mg PO b.i.d. of dipyridamole	Combination tabs: 200 mg dipyridamole/25 mg ASA	<30 min	1–2 h	Liver/feces	Inhibits PLT adhesion, serum adenosine deaminase, phosphodiesterase, thromboxane A₂; coronary vasodilator
Dipyridamole (Persantine)	0.14 mg/kg/min IV for 4 min (max: 60 mg) for evaluation of CAD		5 mg/2 mL	<2 min	1–2 h	Liver/feces	*See above*
Ticlopidine (Ticlid)	—	250 mg PO b.i.d. (no IV availability)	250 mg tabs	<1 h	0–15 h (↑ with chronic use)	Liver/urine	Blocks ADP-induced PLT aggregation; prolongs bleeding time
Abciximab (ReoPro)	0.25 mg/kg over 30 min	0.125 μg/kg/min for 12 h (max 10 μg/min)	9 mg/250 mL 35 μg/mL filter	<5 min	30 min (PLT effects, 15 d)	Liver	GP IIb/IIIa inhibiting agents: blocks binding of fibrinogen and von Willebrand factor to platelet glycoprotein IIb/IIIa inhibitor; → PLT aggregation and thrombosis
Eptifibatide (Integrilin)	180 μg/kg over 1–2 min	2 μg/kg/min	Premixed solution does not require dilution	<1 h	2.5 h	Liver/urine	*See above*
Tirofiban (Aggrastat)	0.4 μg/kg/min for 30 min	0.1 μg/kg/min	Premixed solution does not require dilution	<1 h	2 h	None/urine, feces	*See above*

MOA, mechanism of action; NA, not applicable; IT, intrathecal; N/R, not recommended; MAO, monoamine oxidase; ADH, antidiuretic hormone; COMT, catechol-*O*-methyl transferase; PSVT, paroxysmal supraventricular tachycardia; DDAVP, desamino-D-arginine-vasopressin; PGI₂, prostacyclin; PLT, platelet; ADH, antidiuretic hormone; GI, gastrointestinal; cAMP, cyclic adenosine monophosphate; APD, action potential duration; ERP, effective refractory period; AT, antithrombin; AV, atrioventricular; CV, cardiovascular; ACh, acetylcholine; RBC, red blood cell; VT/VF, ventricular tachycardia/ventricular fibrillation; NS, normal saline; SVT, supraventricular tachycardia; HR, heart rate; BP, blood pressure; ATPase, adenosine triphosphatase; AP, action potential; SA, sinoatrial; PVR, pulmonary vascular resistance; ASA, aspirin; tabs, tablets; ACS, acute coronary syndrome; PCI, percutaneous coronary intervention; EtOH, ethanol; CAD, coronary artery disease; ADP, adenosine diphosphate; GP, glycoprotein.

▶ **TABLE (b)** Indications and Effects

Drug	Indications	Contrain-dications	CV	CNS	Pulmo-nary	GI	Other	Drug Interactions	Anesthetic Interactions
Adrenergic Agents									
Clonidine (Catapres)	Hypertension Anesthetic/analgesic adjuvant Opioid withdrawal Postoperative shivering	Porphyria, Raynaud phenomenon Breastfeeding	↓BP ↓SVR ↓HR ↓Renin activity ↑Pedal edema	Drowsiness Dizziness Depression	—	Dry mouth Constipation	Diaphoresis Fluid retention Pruritus ↓Libido	Antagonized by MAOIs and TCAs; cimetidine ↑CNS toxicity; β-blockers enhance bradycardia	↓Anesthetic and analgesic requirements; produces sedation during perioperative period; TTS patch should be applied 1 d prior to surgery; remove patch 2–3 d prior to elective cardioversion
Dexmedeto-midine (Precedex)	Anesthetic/analgesic adjuvant Sedative/analgesic in ICU	Sick sinus syndrome First and second degree AV Hypovolemia	Sympath-olysis ↓HR ↓BP Sinus arrest Oliguria Anemia	Sedation Dizziness Headache Confusion Neuralgias	Hypoxemia Pleural effusion Edema	Dry mouth Nausea Vomiting Thirst Diarrhea	↓ACTH ↓ADH ↓Insulin ↑Growth hormone ↓Shivering ↓Wound healing Leukocytosis	↑Sedation with other CNS depressants	↑Bradycardia with opioids or β-blockers; useful for perioperative hypertension; useful for ↓anesthetic and analgesic requirements
Epinephrine	Anaphylaxis Broncho-spasm Cardiac arrest	β-blocker therapy Hyperthyroidism	↑CO MVO₂	Restless-ness Tremor Headache Confusion Dizziness Weakness	—	Nausea Vomiting ↑Splanchnic blood flow	Hypokalemia Hyperglyc-emia Lipolysis ↑Tempera-ture	α- and β-blockers ↓effects;↑risk of hypertensive crisis with MAOIs, TCAs, antihista-mines, oxytocics, thyroid hormone; ↑insulin require-ments in diabetics	Limit dose to <5 μg/kg with volatile anesthetics to ↓risk arrhythmias Potential for CV tox-icity when com-bined with other sympathomimetics

(*continued*)

TABLE (b) Indications and Effects (Continued)

Drug	Indications	Contraindications	CV	CNS	Pulmonary	GI	Other	Drug Interactions	Anesthetic Interactions
			↑MVO2 ↑SV ↑HR ↑Contractility ↑BP ↑Arrhythmias ↑CBF Vasoconstriction Angina ↓RBF	Cerebral hemorrhage					
Ephedrine	Hypotension Bronchospasm	Hypertension Diabetes Hyperthyroidism Angle-closure glaucoma	↑CO ↑BP ↑HR Arrhythmias Angina ↓RBF	Restlessness Tremor Confusion Dizziness	Bronchodilator Pulmonary edema (rare)	Nausea Vomiting Anorexia	Dysuria Urinary retention	↑Effects of sympathomimetics; MAOIs and TCAs ↑pressor effects Anticholinergics and theophylline decrease HR and BP effects	Volatile anesthetics may ↑arrhythmias
Mephentermine (Wyamine)	Hypotension during spinal anesthesia Ganglionic blockade	Hypertension Hyperthyroidism Hemorrhagic shock	↑BP ↑Contractility	Restlessness ↑CBF	—	—	—	↑Arrhythmias with digoxin; ↑CV toxicity with MAOIs; ↓hypertensive response with phenothiazine, reserpine, guanethidine	↑Volatile anesthetic requirements; increased risk of arrhythmias with volatile anesthetics

Control of Rate and Rhythm (Continued From Tachycardia Overview)

Atrial fibrillation/ atrial flutter with • *Normal heart* • *Impaired heart* • *WPW*	1. Control Rate		2. Convert Rhythm	
	Heart Function Preserved	**Impaired Heart EF <40% or CHF**	**Duration <48 Hours**	**Duration >48 Hours or Unknown**
Normal cardiac function	**Note:** *If AF >48 hours duration, use agents to convert rhythm with extreme caution in patients not receiving adequate anticoagulation because of possible embolic complications.* *Use only one of the following agents (see note below):* • Calcium channel blockers (Class I) • β-Blockers (Class I) • For additional drugs that are Class IIb recommendations, see Guidelines or ACLS text	*(Does not apply)*	**Consider** • DC cardioversion *Use only one of the following agents (see note below):* • Amiodarone (Class IIa) • Ibutilide (Class IIa) • Flecainide (Class IIa) • Propafenone (Class IIa) • Procainamide (Class IIa) • For additional drugs that are Class IIb recommendations, see Guidelines or ACLS text	• **No DC cardioversion!** • **Note:** *Coversion of AF to NSR with drugs or shock may cause embolization of atrial thrombi unless patient has adequate anticoagulation.* • Use antiarrhythmic agents with extreme caution if AF >48 hours duration *(see note above).* *or* ***Delayed cardioversion*** **Anticoagulation** × **3 weeks at proper levels** • Cardioversion, *then* • Anticoagulation × 4 weeks more *or* ***Early cardioversion*** • Begin i.v. heparin at once • TEE to exclude atrial clot *then* • Cardioversion within 24 hours *then* • Anticoagulation × 4 more weeks
Impaired heart (EF <40% or CHF)	*(Does not apply)*	**Note:** *If AF >48 hours duration, use agents to convert rhythm with extreme caution in patients not receiving adequate anticoagulation because of possible embolic complications.* *Use only one of the following agents (see note below):* • Digoxin (Class IIb) • Diltiazem (Class IIb) • Amiodarone (Class IIb)	**Consider** • DC cardioversion *or* • Amiodarone (Class IIb)	• **Anticoagulation** as described above, followed by • **DC cardioversion**

Control of Rate and Rhythm (Continued From Tachycardia Overview)

Atrial fibrillation/ atrial flutter with • *Normal heart* • *Impaired heart* • *WPW*	1. Control Rate		2. Convert Rhythm	
	Heart Function Preserved	**Impaired Heart EF <40% or CHF**	**Duration <48 Hours**	**Duration >48 Hours or Unknown**
WPW	**Note:** *If AF >48 hours duration, use agents to convert rhythm with extreme caution in patients not receiving adequate anticoagulation because of possible embolic complications.* • DC cardioversion *or* • **Primary anti- arrhythmic agents** *Use only one of the following agents (see note below):* • Amiodarone (Class IIb) • Flecainide (Class IIb) • Procainamide (Class IIb) • Propafenone (Class IIb) • Sotalol (Class IIb) ---- ***Class III (can be harmful)*** • Adenosine • β-Blockers • Calcium blockers • Digoxin	**Note:** *If AF >48 hours duration, use agents to convert rhythm with extreme caution in patients not receiving adequate anticoagulation because of possible embolic complications.* • DC cardioversion *or* • Amiodarone (Class IIb)	• DC cardioversion *or* • **Primary anti- arrhythmic agents** *Use only one of the following agents (see note below):* • Amiodarone (Class IIb) • Flecainide (Class IIb) • Procainamide (Class IIb) • Propafenone (Class IIb) • Sotalol (Class IIb) ---- ***Class III (can be harmful)*** • Adenosine • β-Blockers • Calcium blockers • Digoxin	• **Anticoagulation** as described above, followed by • DC cardioversion

WPW indicates Wolff-Parkinson-White syndrome; AF, atrial fibrillation; NSR, normal sinus rhythm; TEE, transesophageal echocardiogram; and EF, ejection fraction.

Note: Occasionally two of the named antiarrhythmic agents may be used, but use of these agents in combination may have proarrhythmic potential. The classes listed represent the Class of Recommendation rather than the Vaughn-Williams classification of antiarrhythmics.

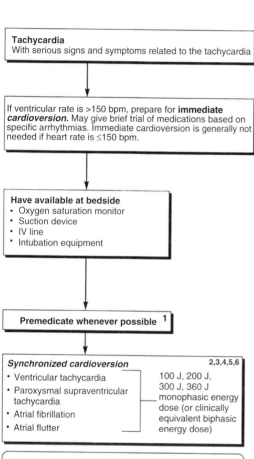

Tachycardia
With serious signs and symptoms related to the tachycardia

If ventricular rate is >150 bpm, prepare for **immediate cardioversion.** May give brief trial of medications based on specific arrhythmias. Immediate cardioversion is generally not needed if heart rate is ≤150 bpm.

Have available at bedside
• Oxygen saturation monitor
• Suction device
• IV line
• Intubation equipment

Premedicate whenever possible ¹

Synchronized cardioversion	2,3,4,5,6
• Ventricular tachycardia • Paroxysmal supraventricular tachycardia • Atrial fibrillation • Atrial flutter	100 J, 200 J, 300 J, 360 J monophasic energy dose (or clinically equivalent biphasic energy dose)

Notes:
1. Effective regimens have included a sedative (e.g., *diazepam, midazolam, barbiturates, etomidate, ketamine, methohexital*) with or without and analgesic agent (e.g., *fentanyl, morphine, meperidine*). Many experts recommend anesthesia if service is readily available.
2. Both monophasic and biphasic waveforms are acceptable if documented as clinically equivalent to reports of monophasic shock success.
3. Note possible need to resynchronize after each cardioversion.
4. If delays in synchronization occur and clinical condition is critical, go immediately to unsynchronized shocks.
5. Treat polymorphic ventricular tachycardia (irregular form and rate) like ventricular fibrillation: see ventricular fibrillation/pulseless ventricular tachycardia algorithm.
6. Paroxysmal supraventricular tachycardia and atrial flutter often respond to lower energy levels (start with 50 J).

Steps for synchronized cardioversion

1. Consider sedation.
2. Turn on defibrillator (monophasic or biphasic).
3. Attach monitor leads to the patient ("white to right, red to ribs, what's left over to the left shoulder") and ensure proper display of the patient's rhythm.
4. Engage the synchronization mode by pressing the "sync" control button.
5. Look for markers on R waves indicating sync mode.
6. If necessary, adjust monitor gain until sync markers occur with each R wave.
7. Select appropriate energy level.
8. Position conductor pads on patient (or apply gel to paddles).
9. Position paddle on patient (sternum-apex).
10. Announce to team members: *"Charging defibrillator—stand clear!"*
11. Press "charge" button on apex paddle (right hand).
12. When the defibrillator is charged, begin the final clearing chant. State firmly in a forceful voice the following chant before each shock:
    • *"I am going to shock on three. One, I'm clear."* (Check to make sure you are clear of contact with the patient, the stretcher, and the equipment.)
    • *"Two, you are clear."* (Make a visual check to ensure that no one continues to touch the patient or stretcher. In particular, do not forget about the person providing ventilations. That person's hands should not be touching the ventilatory adjuncts, including the tracheal tube!)
    • *"Three, everybody's clear."* (Check yourself one more time before pressing the "shock" buttons.)
13. Apply 25 lb pressure on both paddles.
14. Press the "discharge" buttons simultaneously.
15. Check the monitor. If tachycardia persists, increase the joules according to the electrical cardioversion algorithm.
16. **Reset the sync mode after each synchronized cardioversion because most defibrillators default back to unsynchronized mode.** This default allows an immediate defibrillation if the cardioversion produces VF.

PREOPERATIVE CARDIAC TRANSPLANT MEDICAL ORDER

University Health Network

Toronto General Hospital Toronto Western Hospital Princess Margaret Hospital

Doctor's Order Sheet

Multi Organ Transplant Program

Preoperative Cardiac Transplant

Addressograph

PLEASE USE BLACK OR BLUE BALLPOINT PEN, PRESS FIRMLY	ALLERGIES: NO KNOWN ALLERGIES ☐ KNOWN ALLERGIES (Specify) ☐

PHYSICIAN'S ORDER AND SIGNATURE	SIGNATURE(S) AND POSITION	ACTION TAKEN	PHARMACY
(Check ☑ appropriate box(es) and complete orders as required)			
1. ADMISSION:			
a) Admit to CCU under Dr. _____			
b) Admitting Diagnosis: _____			
c) Call medical records for old chart STAT.			
d) Vital Signs.			
e) Pre operative weight.			
f) Activity as tolerated.			
2. OXYGEN THERAPY:			
☐ Administer oxygen via nasal prongs or mask to maintain oxygen saturation greater than _____%			
☐ Other: _____			
3. DIET:			
☐ NPO.			
4. IV THERAPY:			
☐ Start peripheral IV of (specify solution) _____ infuse at _____ mL/h.			
5. LABORATORY TESTS:			
i) **STAT Bloodwork:**			
☐ Sodium, Potassium, Chloride, Magnesium, Glucose, Creatinine, Arterial blood gases, CBC with differential, Platelet Count, Reticulocyte Count, PT/INR, aPTT and AST. Cross and Type for 5 units of PRBC.			
ii) ☐ **Tissue Typing:**			
2 yellow top (7 mL tubes), 1 red top (10 mL tube).			
Send as Routine for all heart transplants.			
iii) **OTHER:**			
☐ CMV - IgG antibody.			

Form D-2120 (Rev. 30/03/2004)

COPIES: ORIGINAL - RETAIN IN CHART,   YELLOW-PHARMACY

	PHYSICIAN'S ORDER AND SIGNATURE	SIGNATURE(S) AND POSITION	ACTION TAKEN	PHARMACY

PLEASE USE BLACK OR BLUE BALLPOINT PEN, PRESS FIRMLY

ALLERGIES:
NO KNOWN ALLERGIES ☐
KNOWN ALLERGIES (Specify) ☐

(Check ☑ appropriate box(es) and complete orders as required)

6. **DIAGNOSTIC TESTS:**
   a) Chest X-Ray STAT
      - ☐ PA and Lateral
      - ☐ Portable
   b) ☐ Right heart catheterization STAT: notify transplant attending physician and surgeon with the Pulmonary Artery Pressure and Trans Pulmonary Gradient (TPG).

7. **MEDICATIONS:**
   - ☐ Stop Warfarin (Coumadin®).
   - ☐ Stop Heparin
   - ☐ Other: _____

   On call to O.R.
   - ☐ Methylprednisolone Sodium Succinate (Solu-Medrol®) _____ g IV in 50 mL D5W infused over 30 – 60 minutes. (Usual dose 1 g).

   - ☐ Cefazolin (Ancef®) _____ g IV in 50 mL D5W infused over 15 – 30 minutes. (Usual dose 1 g).
     OR
   - ☐ If patient is allergic to Cephalosporins/Penicillins, give:
     Vancomycin 1 g IV in 250 mL D5W infused over 1 hour.

   - ☐ Mycophenolate Mofetil (Cellcept®) _____ g IV in 50 mL of D5W infused over 30 minutes. (Usual dose 1gm).

8. **MISCELLANEOUS:**
   - ☐ Surgical skin prep as per coronary artery bypass.

9. **INTRA-OPERATIVE ORDERS:**
   Send with patient to O.R.
   (TO BE GIVEN AFTER THE CROSSCLAMP) by anesthetist.
   - ☐ Methylprednisolone Sodium Succinate (Solu-Medrol®) _____ mg IV in 50 mL D5W
     infused over 30 – 60 minutes. (Usual dose is 500 mg).

   - ☐ Basiliximab (Simulect®) _____ mg IV in 100 mL D5W infused over 15 minutes after cardio pulmonary bypass. (Usual dose is 20 mg).

Physician's Signature: _____ Date: ___/___/___ Time: _____
                                                        dd   mm   yy

MDWF

MEDICAL TRANSFER ORDERS POST HEART TRANSPLANT

University Health Network

Toronto General Hospital Toronto Western Hospital Princess Margaret Hospital

Doctor's Order Sheet

**TRANSFER STANDING ORDERS FROM
CARDIOVASCULAR INTENSIVE CARE TO
MULTI ORGAN TRANSPLANT**

Addressograph

PLEASE USE BLACK OR BLUE BALLPOINT PEN, PRESS FIRMLY	**ALLERGIES:** NO KNOWN ALLERGIES KNOWN ALLERGIES (Specify)		

DATE AND TIME ORDERED	PHYSICIAN'S ORDER AND SIGNATURE	SIGNATURE(S) AND POSITION	ACTION TAKEN	PHARMACY
	I. NURSING ORDERS			
	1. Transfer to Multi Organ Transplant Unit.			
	2. Vital Signs q _____ h.			
	3. diet: _____			
	4. Notify Dietition.			
	5. Fluid restriction _____ mL/day.			
	6. Intake and output q1h.			
	7. Weight q AM.			
	8. Cardiac monitor.			
	9. Notify Physiotherapy.			
	II. STUDIES			
	1. Serum CMV buffy coat AST, ALP, CK, Calcium, Phosphate, Protein, Albumin q Monday.			
	2. CBC and Differential, Serum Creatinine, Sodium, Potassium, Chloride daily.			
	3. Cyclosporine level daily (once started on Cyclosporine).			
	4. Urine and Sputum for C and S and Fungus Monday and Friday.			
	5. PA and Lateral Chest film in department.			
	6. ECG and Echocardiogram once weekly.			
	7. 24 h Holter BP monitoring before discharge.			
	8. Absolute Lymphocyte Count daily while on Rabbit Antithymocyte Serum (RATS).			
	III. DRUGS			
	1. Cyclosporine dose to be ordered daily.			
	2. Prednisone dose to be ordered daily.			
	3. Azathioprine (Imuran) _____ mg daily p.o.			
	4. RATS dose to be ordered daily. Muromonab-CD_3 (Orthoclone OKT_3) dose to be ordered daily.			
	5. Co-Trimoxazole (Bactrim, Septra) _____ tabs _____ daily p.o.			
	6. Nystatin (Mycostatin) mouthwash, swish and swallow _____ units q6h while awake.			
	7. Docusate (Colace) _____ mg p.o. pm.			
	8. Pravastatin (Pravachol) _____ mg p.o. daily.			
	9. Calcium Carbonate _____ mg p.o _____ daily.			
	10. Vitamin D _____ units p.o. daily.			
	11 Ganciclovir _____ mg I.V. q 12 h.			
	12. I.V. _____ to run at _____ mL/h.			
	13. Mycophenolate Mofetil _____ mg daily p.o.			
	14. Other: _____			
	Physician's Signature: _____ Date: __/__/__ Time: _____ dd mm yy			

FORM D-2119 (Rev. 05/98)   COPIES: ORIGINAL-RETAIN IN CHART   YELLOW - PHARMACY

MEDICAL ORDERS FOR CARE OF SPINAL DRAINS

University Health Network

Toronto General Hospital Toronto Western Hospital Princess Margaret Hospital

Doctor's Order Sheet

Cardiovascular Intensive Care Unit

Care of Spinal Drains

Addressograph

PLEASE USE BLACK OR BLUE BALLPOINT PEN, PRESS FIRMLY	**ALLERGIES:** NO KNOWN ALLERGIES KNOWN ALLERGIES (Specify)	☐ ☐

PHYSICIAN'S ORDER AND SIGNATURE	SIGNATURES AND POSITION	ACTION TAKEN	PHARMACY
1. ON ADMISSION TO UNIT:			
a) Spinal Drain to 10 cm H_2O drainage.			
b) Keep system open to drain except during transport and repositioning.			
c) Patient must remain flat with 1 pillow only, may be turned from side to side only.			
2. MONITORING:			
a) Measure CSF drainage and document q 1 h. Notify physician if no CSF drainage in an hour, volume greater than 20 mL/h, or if CSF becomes cloudy or bloody.			
b) Measure Spinal Pressure (ICP) and document pressure reading q 1 h. Notify physician if ICP is less than 5 mm Hg or greater than 15 mm Hg.			
c) Document Mean Arterial Pressure (MAP) q 1 h. Target MAP between 30 and 90 mm Hg.			
d) Calculate the Cerebral Perfusion Pressure (CPP = MAP - ICP) and document the value q 1 h. Notify physician if less than 70 mm Hg.			
e) Assess patient's level of consciousness (LOC) by Glasgow Coma Scale and document findings q 1 h, for 24 hours. Notify physician to reassess need for hourly assessment of LOC after 24 hours.			
3. TESTS:			
a) Culture cerebral spinal fluid q 24 hours for C & S.			
b) Portable Chest X-ray immediately post op.			

Physician's Signature: _____ Date: _____ / _____ / _____ Time: _____
dd   mm   yy

Form D-3273(19/05/2003)   **COPIES:**   ORIGINAL - RETAIN IN CHART,   YELLOW-PHARMACY   YELLOW-PHARMACY

HOSPITAL DISCHARGE INSTRUCTIONS POSTCARDIAC SURGERY

HOSPITAL DISCHARGE INSTRUCTIONS POST CARDIAC SURGERY

Cardiovascular Surgery Services - Toronto General Hospital, University Health Network

Discharge Instructions	Patient: XXX,XXXX
Date of Birth: XX/XX/XX	TTH No. 000000

Admission Date: XX/XX/XX	Date of Procedure: XX/XX/XX
Discharge Date: XX/XX/XX	Left Ventricular Function:

Reason for Hospitalization (Admission Diagnosis):

Procedure(s) Performed:

Postoperative Course:

Activity:
SLOWLY increase your daily activities to return to normal within 2-3 months. Try to walk daily. Rest when you need to. Do not lift objects weighing greater than 5 kg (10 lbs). Do not work with your arms above shoulder height. Return to work 2-3 months after you have been seen by your Cardiologist.
Diet:
Health Diet (low fat, no added salt)

Anticoagulation:
COUMADIN daily order if indicated
Dosage adjusted to maintain Target INR:
Length of Therapy:

Leg Staple Removal:
Removal to be performed by family physician. Recommended Removal Date: XX/XX/XX

Medications Upon Discharge

Additional Instructions:
Patient will be followed by home care nursing.
Please Call your Family Doctor if any of the following should occur:
- You develop a FEVER
- You experience RAPID HEART RATE
- You experience WEIGHT GAIN OF GREATER THAN TWO POUNDS IN 24 HOURS
- You experience SHORTNESS OF BREATH
- There is ABNORMAL DRAINAGE from your incision(s)

BE SURE TO ARRANGE FOLLOW UP APPOINTMENT WITH:
- FAMILY DOCTOR.   Within 7 days of discharge
- CARDIOLOGIST   Within 4 weeks of discharge
- SURGEON   APPROXIMATELY 8 WEEKS AFTER DISCHARGE
YOUR CARDIOVASCULAR SURGEON IS: Dr.

Toronto General Hospital, Division of Cardiovascular Surgery
200 Elizabeth Street
Toronto, ON M5G 2C4   Tel: _____

Completed by: _____ (signature)   Date completed: XX/XX/XX

511

Hypotension
  preoperative, 189
  problems in CSRU, 349, 350t, 351t
  treatment of, 19, 22, 27
Hypothermia
  categories of, 119t
  and circulatory arrest. *See* Hypothermic
    circulatory arrest (HCA)
  deep hypothermia and circulatory arrest, 79
  due to HCA, 38
Hypothermic circulatory arrest (HCA), 37–41
  bleeding and coagulation, 41
  clinical presentation, 37–38
  CPB and, 38
  DHCA, 79, 268–269
  glucose management, 40
  hypothermic cerebral protection, 38–39
  pH management, 40
  with RCP, 37, 39
  renal protection, 40
  with SACP, 37, 39, 40
Hypothermic fibrillation, 196, 197t
Hypovolemia, 19f, 54, 113, 116
Hypoxemia, 47, 59
Hypoxia, 352

I

IMH. *See* Intramural Hematoma (IMH)
Immunosuppression and organ
    transplantation, 299
Implantable cardioverter defibrillators (ICDs).
    See Pacemakers/ICDs
Induction, coma, 77–78
Infection prophylaxis and organ
    transplantation, 299
Infections, postoperative, 380, 381–385, 392, 431
Infectious diseases, 355–356
Informed consent, 8
Inhalational agents and FTCA, 17
Inotropes
  for RV dysfunction and pulmonary
    hypertension, 148, 149t
  for weaning from CPB, 137–143
Insulin, 40, 51t, 126, 143, 453
Integrilin. *See* Eptifibatide (Integrilin)
International normalized ratio (INR), 170,
    240, 247, 256, 360
Intra-aortic balloon pump (IABP)
  augmentation adjustments, 130
  balloon deflation effects, 131, 133f
  balloon inflation effects, 130–131, 133f
  complications and side effects of, 132
  controls found on console, 129–130
  indications/contraindications for use, 129
  mechanical support for weaning from
    CPB, 143
  mechanism of action and role, 128–129
  monitoring, 131–132
  removal techniques, 133–134
  RV dysfunction and, 149t, 150
  timing, conventional vs. real, 130
  timing adjustments, 130

  trigger modes, 130
  weaning from, 132
Intramural Hematoma (IMH), 274, 277
Intrathecal technique, 94, 95t
Ischemia
  acute ischemic MR, 192
  revascularization and, 186–189
  treatment of, 19

K

Kallikrein inhibitor units (KIU), 41, 167
Konno surgical procedure

L

Left internal thoracic artery (LITA), 202
Left ventricle (LV) monitoring, 110–112
Left ventricular assist device (LVAD)
  anesthesia for redo or noncardiac surgery, 68
  contraindications to, 66
  implantation complications, 68
  indications for use of, 65–66
  perioperative considerations, 67–68
  types of, 66–67
Left ventricular reconstruction. *See*
    Ventricular reconstruction
Leg wound complications, 431–432
Length of stay (LOS)
  FTCA management and, 14, 15t
  mean/median in STS database, 3, 208
  predictors of, 4–5
Lepirudin, 176t, 179–180. *See also* Hirudin
    (Lepirudin and Desirudin)
Lesions, CHD, 71–74
Lorazepam (Ativan), 9, 76
LOS. *See* Length of stay (LOS)
Low molecular weight heparin (LMWH), 175
Lung cancer, 45
Lung injury, acute, 389–390
Lung transplantation, 56–61, 295–300
  anesthetic technique, 57–58
  antibiotics and, 60–61
  anticoagulation and, 299
  CPB and, 58, 297t
  donor procedure for, 295
  heart-lung transplant procedure, 297–298
  hematology and fluid management, 60
  hemodynamic management, 59–60
  immunosuppression, 299
  infection prophylaxis, 299
  lung preservation technique for, 296t
  monitors/lines for, 57
  physiologic events, 59
  postoperative care, 61, 298–299
  preoperative recipient management, 57
  recipient characteristics, 56
  ventilation, 59, 299

M

Magnesium management in CSRU, 355
Magnetic resonance imaging (MRI)
  assessment for CPB, 75
  neuraxial block testing, 92